THE PREVENTION OF
Stroke

THE PREVENTION OF
Stroke

Edited by

Philip B. Gorelick, MD, MPH, FACP

Center for Stroke Research, Department of Neurological Sciences,
Rush Medical Center, Chicago, IL

and

Milton Alter, MD, PhD

Department of Neurology, MCP/Hahnemann University,
Philadelphia, PA

The Parthenon Publishing Group
International Publishers in Medicine, Science & Technology

A CRC PRESS COMPANY
BOCA RATON   LONDON   NEW YORK   WASHINGTON, D.C.

Library of Congress Cataloging-in-Publication Data

The prevention of stroke/edited by Philip B. Gorelick and Milton Alter.
    p. ; cm.
  Includes bibliographical references and index.
  ISBN 1-84214-115-5 (alk. paper)
    I. Cerebrovascular disease--Prevention.
    2. Cerebrovascular disease--Risk factors.
    I. Gorelick, Philip B. II. Alter, Milton, 1929-
    [DNLM: 1. Cerebrovascular Disorders–prevention & control. WL 355 59213436 2002]
  RC388.5 .S85292 2002

                          2002017055

British Library Cataloguing in Publication Data

The prevention of stroke
  1. Cerebrovascular disease - Prevention
  I. Gorelick, Philip B. II. Alter, Milton
  616.8′1′05

  ISBN 1842141155

Published in the USA by
The Parthenon Publishing Group
345 Park Avenue South, 10th Floor
New York, NY 10010, USA

Published in the UK and Europe by
The Parthenon Publishing Group
23–25 Blades Court
Deodar Road
London SW15 2NU, UK

Copyright © 2002 The Parthenon Publishing Group

Typeset by Siva Math Setters, Chennai, India
Printed and bound by Bookcraft (Bath) Ltd., Midsomer Norton, UK

Contents

Chapter 17

Chapter 18

Chapter 19

Chapter 20

Chapter 21

Chapter 22

Chapter 23

List of contributors

Robert J. Adams, MS, MD
Department of Neurology
Medical College of Georgia
1467 Harper Street, HB 2060
Augusta, GA 30912
USA

Milton Alter, MD, PhD
Department of Neurology
MCP/Hahnemann University
Broad and Vine Street
Philadelphia, PA 19102
USA

Ambika Babu, MD
Department of Medicine
Rush-Presbyterian-St. Luke's
   Medical Center
1735 West Harrison Street
Chicago, IL 60612
USA

José Biller, MD
Department of Neurology
Indiana University School
   of Medicine
545 Clinical Drive, EH 125
Indianapolis, IN 46202
USA

Bernadette Boden-Albala, MD
Neurological Institute
710 West 168th Street
New York, NY 10032
USA

Monique M.B. Breteler, MD, PhD
Department of Epidemiology and Biostatistics
Erasmus Medical Center Rotterdam
PO Box 1738
3000 DR Rotterdam
The Netherlands

Robin L. Brey, MD
Department of Neurology
University of Texas
7703 Floyd Curl Drive
San Antonio, TX 78229
USA

Stanley N. Cohen, MD
Department of Neurology
Cedars-Sinai Medical Center
8631 W. Third Street, Suite 1145E
Los Angeles, CA 90048
USA

John W. Cole, MD
Department of Neurology
Maryland Stroke Center
22 South Greene Street
Baltimore, MD 21201
USA

Thomas J. DeGraba, MD
Stroke Branch
National Institute of Neurological Disorders
   and Stroke
36 Convent Drive, MSC 4128
Building 36, 4A-03
Bethesda, MD 20892
USA

William J. Elliott, MD, PhD
Department of Preventive Medicine
Rush-Presbyterian-St. Luke's Medical Center
1700 West Van Buren, Suite 470
Chicago, IL 60612
USA

Miriam M. Fay, MPH
Division of Adult and Community Health
National Center for Chronic Disease
    Prevention and Health Promotion
Centers for Disease Control and Prevention
4770 Buford Highway NE, Mailstop K-45
Atlanta, GA 30341
USA

James D. Fleck, MD
Department of Neurology
Indiana University School of Medicine
541 Clinical Drive, CL 365
Indianapolis, IN 46202
USA

Michael Fleming, MA, MS
Health Care Quality Improvement
Anthem Blue Cross and Blue Shield
2 Gannett Drive
South Portland, ME 04106
USA

Jay Garg, MD
Department of Preventative Medicine
Rush-Presbyterian-St. Luke's Medical Center
1700 West Van Buren, Suite 470
Chicago, IL 60612
USA

Glen Geremia, MD
Department of Diagnostic Radiology
Rush-Presbyterian-St. Luke's Medical Center
1653 West Congress Parkway
Chicago, IL 60612
USA

Richard F. Gillum, MD
Department of Health and Human Services
Centers for Disease Control and
    Prevention
National Center for Health Statistics
6525 Belcrest Road, Rm 730
Hyattsville, MD 20782
USA

Larry B. Goldstein, MD
Duke Center for Cerebrovascular Disease
Stroke Policy Program
Center for Clinical Health Policy
    Research
Duke University Medical Center, Box 3651
Durham, NC 27710
USA

Philip B. Gorelick, MD, MPH, FACP
Center for Stroke Research
Department of Neurological Sciences
Rush Medical Center
1645 West Jackson, Suite 400
Chicago, IL 60612
USA

Vladimir Hachinski, MD, FRCPC, DSc
Department of Neurological Sciences
London Health Sciences Center
339 Windemere Road
London, Ontario N6A 5A5
Canada

Dan Heffez, MD, FRCS
Cerebrovascular Surgery
Chicago Institute of Neurosurgery and
    Neuroresearch
Rush University and Rush-Presbyterian-
    St. Luke's Medical Center
Chicago, IL 60612
USA

Monika Hollander, MD
Department of Epidemiology and
  Biostatistics
Erasmus Medical Center Rotterdam
PO Box 1738
3000 DR Rotterdam
The Netherlands

Robert G. Holloway, MD, MPH
Departments of Neurology and Preventive
  and Community Medicine
University of Rochester School of
  Medicine
1351 Mt. Hope Avenue, Suite 220
Rochester, NY 14620
USA

George Howard, PhD
Department of Biostatistics
University of Alabama at Birmingham
327 Ryals Public Health Building
1665 University Boulevard
Birmingham, AL 35294
USA

Virginia J. Howard, PhD
Department of Biostatistics
University of Alabama at Birmingham
327 Ryals Public Health Building
1665 University Boulevard
Birmingham, AL 35294
USA

Munavvar Izhar, MD
Department of Preventative Medicine
Rush-Presbyterian-St. Luke's
  Medical Center
1700 West Van Buren, Suite 470
Chicago, IL 60612
USA

Chakravarthy Kannan, MD
Department of Medicine
Rush-Presbyterian-St. Luke's Medical Center
1735 West Harrison Street
Chicago, IL 60612
USA

Steven J. Kittner, MD, MPH
Department of Neurology
Maryland Stroke Center
22 South Greene Street
Baltimore, MD 21201
USA

Darwin R. Labarthe, MD, MPH, PhD
Division of Adult and Community Health
National Center for Chronic Disease
  Prevention and Health Promotion
Centers for Disease Control and Prevention
4770 Buford Highway NE, Mailstop K-45
Atlanta, GA 30341
USA

Sung B. Lee, MD
Department of Neurology
Medical College of Georgia
1467 Harper Street, HB 2060
Augusta, GA 30912
USA

Theodore Mazzone, MD
Department of Medicine
Rush-Presbyterian-St. Luke's Medical Center
1735 West Harrison Street
Chicago, IL 60612
USA

Nilay Patel, MD
Rush-Presbyterian-St. Luke's Medical Center
1653 West Congress Parkway
Chicago, IL 60612
USA

Sean Ruland, DO
Section of Cerebrovascular Disease and
  Neurologic Critical Care
Rush-Presbyterian-St. Luke's
  Medical Center
1725 West Harrison Street
Chicago, IL 60612
USA

Steven R. Rush, MA
American Academy of Neurology
1080 Montreal Avenue
St. Paul, MN 55116
USA

Ralph L. Sacco, MD
Neurological Institute
710 West 168ᵗʰ Street
New York, NY 10032
USA

Michael J. Schneck, MD
Department of Neurological
  Sciences
Rush Medical Center
1725 West Harrison, Suite 1106
Chicago, IL 60612
USA

Patti Shwayder, MPA
National Stroke Association
9707 East Easter Lane
Englewood, CO 80112
USA

Bradley Strimling, MD
Rush-Presbyterian-St. Luke's
  Medical Center
1653 West Congress Parkway
Chicago, IL 60612
USA

Meredith L. Tipton, PhD, MPH
College of Osteopathic Medicine
University of New England
11 Hills Beach Road
Biddeford, ME 04005
USA

Gretchen E. Tietjen, MD
Department of Neurology
Medical College of Ohio
3120 Glendale Avenue
Toledo, OH 43614
USA

Edward H. Wong, MBChB, FRACP
Department of Neurological Sciences
London Health Sciences Center
339 Windermere Road, Rm 7GE5
London, Ontario N6A 5A5
Canada

Foreword

A substantial gap exists between scientific knowledge about cerebrovascular disease and implementation of this knowledge for the maximal benefit of the general public. The enormous burden that stroke imposes upon affected individuals, their families and, indeed, upon society as a whole demands that more attention be paid to strategies that can reduce this burden. As the third leading cause of death in the United States and the major cause of disability in older individuals, prevention of stroke deserves greater and more dedicated efforts of medical practitioners and health policy planners. Stroke, often descending upon an individual without warning, is the most frequent event that deprives older adults of their independence to manage their own lives. The economic cost of stroke for society is staggering with direct costs estimated at $30 billion in the United States alone. As infections, cardiac disease and cancer are better controlled, individuals can expect to live longer and the population, as a whole, will continue to age. Older individuals are at increased risk of stroke compared with younger individuals. Therefore, in absolute terms, the number of strokes will increase, giving stroke prevention measures an increased imperative and making successful implementation of these measures even more important in the future. Successful implementation of stroke prevention strategies should produce very tangible benefits for large segments of society.

This book emphasizes the stroke risk factors that are amenable to modification and describes ongoing strategies for their amelioration. Primary prevention of risk factors is stressed because intervention before a stroke risk factor appears is clinically likely to yield the highest benefits. But, secondary prevention measures are also recognized as important in reducing the chance of a stroke. A strength of this book is its reliance on well-founded, scientifically derived evidence interpreted by clinically experienced stroke experts. The authors assess the state of our current knowledge of successful stroke prevention measures while pointing out areas where there is a need to develop new and better prevention techniques. The text provides a road map to guide physicians and other health professionals in ways to overcome barriers to stroke prevention practices. For these goals, the book can be highly recommended.

Martha N. Hill, RN, PhD, FAAN
Interim Dean and Professor, Johns Hopkins
University
and
Daniel F. Hanley, MD
Jeffrey and Harriet Legum Professor
Director, Division of Brain Injury Outcomes
Johns Hopkins University Institutions

Dedication

This book is dedicated to the National Stroke Association, American Stroke Association, and the American Academy of Neurology, organizations in the United States that promote stroke prevention, diagnosis, treatment, rehabilitation, and patient advocacy.

Philip B. Gorelick, MD, MPH, FACP
Milton Alter, MD, PhD

Chapter 1

Stroke incidence, mortality, and prevalence

George Howard, PhD, and Virginia J. Howard, PhD

INTRODUCTION

The Centers for Disease Control and Prevention (CDC) list the 'decline in deaths from coronary heart disease and stroke' as one of the ten great public health achievements of the 20th century in the USA (Table 1)[1]. This list acknowledges the remarkable accomplishments in primary prevention and secondary treatment of these diseases, and heart disease and stroke are the only specific diseases explicitly mentioned. In combining coronary heart disease and stroke, however, the list masks the remarkably greater achievement in the reduction of stroke mortality alone. Mortality from heart disease in the USA reached a peak in 1950 with an age-adjusted rate of 307.4 deaths per 100 000, and had decreased by a remarkable 56% by 1996 to a rate of 134.6 per 100 000 (Figure 1)[2]. In comparison, the decline in mortality from stroke has persisted since 1900, a period of decline at least twice as long as the decline in mortality from heart disease. Moreover, from 1950 to 1996, during which heart disease declined 56%, stroke mortality declined an even greater 70%, from 88.8 deaths per 100 000 to 26.5 deaths per 100 000[2]. Thus, the decline in stroke mortality exceeds the decline in coronary disease mortality not only in duration but also in magnitude. Despite this dramatic reduction in mortality, stroke remains the third leading cause of death in the US, accounting for 158 448 of the 2 337 256 total deaths (7%) in 1998[3].

The causes that underlie this dramatic decline in heart disease and stroke mortality are not well understood. While there is evidence of a trend in a reduction in blood pressure since the early 1900s[4], other risk factors such as cigarette smoking showed a general increasing prevalence until the late 1960s and a declining prevalence only after that time[5]. The pattern of smoking prevalence more closely reflects the increase and subsequent

Table 1 Ten great public health achievements – United States, 1900–1999

Vaccination
Motor-vehicle safety
Safer workplaces
Control of infectious diseases
Decline in deaths from coronary heart disease and stroke
Safer foods
Healthier mothers and babies
Family planning
Fluoridation of drinking water
Recognition of tobacco use as a health hazard

Reproduced with permission from Centers for Disease Control, *Morbidity and Mortality Weekly Report* 1999;48: 241–3

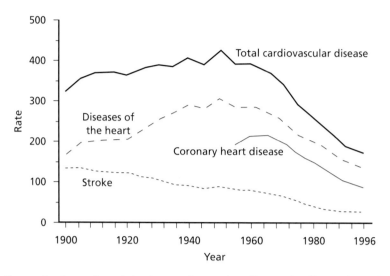

Figure 1 Age-adjusted death rates for total cardiovascular disease (——),
diseases of the heart (– – –), coronary heart disease (——), and stroke (- - - -),
by year for the United States, 1900–1996. Data are given per 100 000 population, standardized to the 1940 US population; diseases are classified according to the *International Classification of Diseases* codes in use when the
deaths were reported. Data from *Morbidity and Mortality Weekly Report*
1999;48:241–3

decrease of heart disease mortality than the
steady decline of stroke mortality since the
1900s. Since a majority of the risk factors for
stroke are shared with heart disease, it is
particularly puzzling why stroke mortality
and heart disease mortality did not change
in a similar manner during the first half of the
last century.

Besides the burden of stroke deaths, the
large number of stroke survivors constitutes
an additional public health burden. The prevalence rate for stroke in the United States
is approximately 11.3 per 1000[6] (or about
4 000 000 individuals[7]). Stroke is the leading
cause of disability among adults in the US[7].
The prevalence of stroke and transient ischemic
attack (TIA) is substantial even among relatively young cohorts, with 5.5% of white and
6.3% of African-Americans having a stroke
between the ages of 45 and 65[8].

INTERNATIONAL PERSPECTIVE

Compared with other countries, the US has a
relatively low stroke mortality rate. Sarti *et al.*
recently reported stroke mortality rates for
men and women aged 35 to 74 and for those
75 and over for the most recent five-year
period available (periods are slightly different
between countries, but generally from the late
1980s through the early 1990s) (Figure 2)[9].
The stroke mortality rate for North American
males between the ages of 35 and 74 is approximately 42 per 100 000, while for women of
the same age it is 33 per 100 000, the fifth
lowest internationally. This is much lower
than in most other countries; e.g. in Kyrgyzs-
tan, the country with the highest mortality
rate, the rate of 314 per 100 000 for men is
7.5 times higher than in the US, while the rate

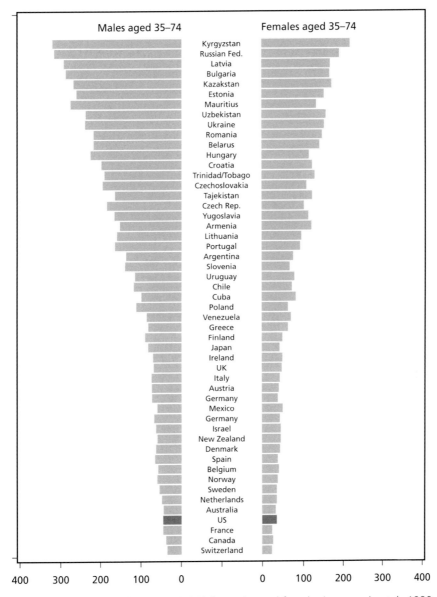

Figure 2 Stroke mortality per 100 000 for males and females in approximately 1990. Data from Sarti *et al.*, *Stroke* 2000,31:1588–601

of 222 per 100 000 women is 6.7 times that in the US. In general, the highest stroke mortality rates tend to be in Eastern Europe. For 29 of the 51 countries (57%), including developed countries such as Finland where over-diagnosis is less likely, the stroke mortality rate for men was at least twice that of the US. Similarly, for women, 28 of the 51 countries (55%) listed have a stroke mortality rate twice that of the US. Among the countries with a lower rate, Canada's rate of 37 per 100 000 was 12% lower than the US rate for men, and Switzerland's rate of 34 per 100 000 was 19% lower than that of the US. In Australia the rate for women of 31 per 100 000 was 6% lower than that in the US, in Canada the rate of 25 per 100 000 was 24% lower than that of the US, in France the rate of 23 per 100 000 was 30% lower than that of the US, and in Switzerland – with the lowest rate, 20 per 100 000 – the rate was 39% lower than that in the US.

Sarti and colleagues also reported the change in stroke mortality rates by country for men and women aged 35–74 for the entire period from 1968 through 1994, and for three other time intervals, the latest being from 1985 to 1994[9]. From these, the change in mortality rates over time could be calculated for 36 countries. The US had the 33rd greatest decline for men and the 28th for women, with an annual decrease of greater than 4% per year (averaged over the entire period from 1968 to 1994) for each sex. Even in the most recent period (from 1985 to 1994), there were above average declines for both US men (an annual decrease of 2.5% for this most recent period) and women (an annual decrease of 2.9% for the most recent period).

Thus, although stroke represents the third leading cause of death in the United States, the US stroke mortality rates are actually among the lowest internationally. Additionally, the US stroke mortality rates have been falling faster than those in most other nations, with the most recent periods still displaying substantial declines in the US.

TEMPORAL PATTERN

Although the long-term decline in stroke mortality over the previous century is evident from the pattern in Figure 1, in more recent decades the rate of decline has substantially fluctuated. As noted by Soltero and colleagues[10], prior to 1972 stroke mortality was declining; however, starting in 1972 the rate of the decline became more rapid. Between 1960 and 1967, stroke mortality for white men had been decreasing at an average rate of 2.6% per year, but between

1968 and 1975 the rate of decrease became more rapid, with average annual estimated declines of 4.8%. Likewise for white women, the rate of decrease changed from 2.8% to 3.8%, for black women from 4.9% to 18.7%, and for black men from an increase of 1.3% to a decrease of 19.7%. Soltero *et al.* calculated that this acceleration in the rate of decline of stroke mortality was responsible for a reduction of 87 600 deaths during this period.

This period of rapid decline in stroke mortality beginning in 1972 requires an explanation, but the reasons remain a matter of debate. Some have suggested that the long-term decline in stroke mortality (as well as the more rapid decline after 1972) reflects a decline in the incidence of stroke attributable to improved hypertension control[11]. While hypertension control was probably not a substantial contributor to the decline prior to 1950, it is likely that it contributed to the rapid decline over the past 40 years.

Because there is no national surveillance system for stroke incidence, the data on temporal changes in incidence are sparse. Perhaps the best data on the temporal trend of stroke incidence is from Olmstead County, Minnesota, where incidence rates have been stable (or slightly increasing) since 1970–5 for men, and since 1965–9 for women (Figure 3)[12,13]. Similar data have been reported from the Oakland Kaiser Permanente population[14] and from Framingham[15], where, despite substantial reductions in cardiovascular mortality over the post-1972 period, there were no improvements in the incidence of stroke. Data from the National Hospital Discharge Survey (NHDS) suggest that the number of hospital admissions for stroke was stable or slightly increasing over the period from 1970 to 1987[16]. Although the interpretation of the NHDS is difficult because the data are not adjusted for recurrent stroke, increasing stroke recurrence would not produce a state hospitalization rate with a 70%

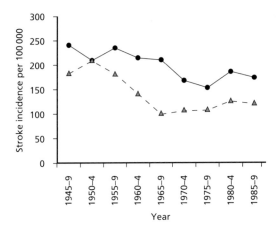

Figure 3 Temporal pattern of annual incidence rates of stroke per 100 000 population during five-year periods in Rochester, MN. Data from Broderick[12] and Brown *et al.*[13]; —●—, male; – ▲ – , female

overall decline in stroke mortality. Therefore, declining incidence does not seem able to account for the rapidly declining stroke mortality after 1972.

It is difficult to reconcile steady or increasing incidence rates with rapid declines in stroke mortality. This observation suggests a possible role for decreasing stroke case fatality. Although data are sparse regarding temporal patterns in survival after stroke, the available data suggest that there have been substantial reductions in fatalities following stroke. In Minnesota between 1980 and 1990, increases in two-year survival following stroke were observed from 64 to 72% for men, and from 57 to 71% for women[17]. Likewise, between 1970 and 1980 in North Carolina, increases were observed in one-year survival following stroke (for men and women combined) from 49 to 63%[18]. For the time period from 1950 to 1970, the Framingham study reported increases in one-year survival following stroke from 67 to 87% for men, and from 79 to 82% for women[15]. Substantial improvements in post-stroke survival were also reported in the

Oakland Kaiser Permanente population, with an approximately 25% lower risk of death (hazard) when comparing the 1980 to 1971 study cohort[14]. With problems due to the inability to identify recurrent versus initial stroke admissions, the data from the NHDS show that in-hospital deaths associated with stroke admissions steadily decreased from 1970 to 1987 from 19 to 10%[16]. Hence, available data describing the post-1972 period of rapidly declining stroke mortality suggest that at least part of the decline in mortality can be attributed to a decreasing case fatality following stroke.

After 1972 there were substantial advances in diagnostic technology, for example CT and MRI, that could have contributed to the identification of milder stroke patients where lower mortality would be expected. The identification of milder cases that in previous years had gone undiagnosed would have the effect of increasing the estimated incidence, and decreasing the estimated case fatality. The identification of milder new cases could bias interpretations to assume that reductions in case fatality from stroke are relatively more important than reductions in stroke incidence in explaining a decline in mortality. However, to attribute observed changes in incidence simply to improved diagnostic technology would require that 40% of strokes diagnosed in 1990 were undiagnosed in 1972. It is, perhaps, more reasonable to expect that improved diagnostic technology mainly affected the ability to provide stroke subtype rather than identifying new and milder stroke cases. For example, between 1980 and 1991 the Pawtucket Heart Study identified a total of 2269 discharges as definite or probable stroke[19]. Over this time period the proportion of stroke cases with a CT rose from approximately 40% to nearly 90%, and the proportion with neurology consults rose from slightly less than 50% to nearly 80%. These changes were associated

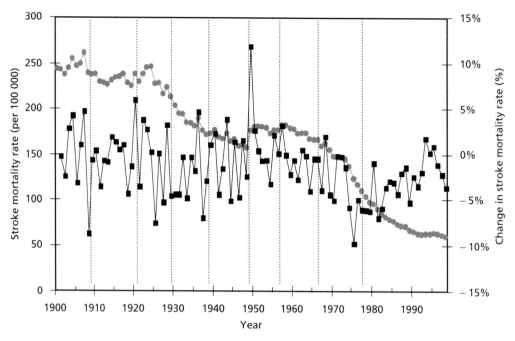

Figure 4 Temporal pattern of stroke mortality rates (per 100 000 population) since 1900 (left vertical axis) and the percent change between subsequent years in stroke mortality (right vertical axis). ●—, Stroke mortality rate; ■—, change in stroke mortality rate

with an improvement in the ability to provide subtype stroke classification with the percent of 'ill-defined' strokes (ICD code 436 or 437) falling from approximately 50% to less than 10%. Moreover, a recent population-based study showed approximately equal survival of stroke patients diagnosed with and without neuro-imaging, suggesting that those with a CT- or MRI-supported diagnosis are not milder cases[20]. Therefore, while the advent of neuroimaging has had a major impact on the accuracy of differential diagnoses, it is not so clear that it has contributed substantially to the number of new and milder cases of stroke that are identified.

The rate of decline in stroke mortality began to slow by 1980 and reached a plateau in the early 1990s for reasons that are poorly understood (Figure 1). After the long history of steadily declining stroke mortality, and particularly after the period of dramatic

declines in stroke mortality starting in 1972, this plateauing of the stroke mortality rates raised concerns that the period of declining stroke mortality may have ended[21,22]. Cooper *et al.* were among the first to note that the rapid rate of decline observed between 1972 and 1978 was not present between the period from 1979 to 1986. Specifically, the rate of decline had slowed by 57% for white men, 58% for white women, 44% for black men and 62% for black women[21]. This 'early warning' was confirmed by subsequent observations. The rate of decline in stroke mortality nearly stopped or may actually have increased after 1990[22].

Figure 4 provides an alternative display of the long-term decline in stroke mortality that adds the year-to-year percent decline of stroke mortality displayed on the right vertical axis with stroke deaths per 100 000 population shown on the left vertical axis. Focusing on the pattern of the annual percent decline offers several insights. While the dramatic declines during the 1970s are striking (six consecutive years of almost 5% decline), a reasonably similar dramatic decline had occurred previously in the early 1930s (four of five consecutive years with approximately 5% decline). Perhaps more importantly, periods with little or no reduction in stroke mortality have previously been observed. For example, starting in approximately 1915, for four consecutive years there was little decline in stroke mortality, and likewise little decline was shown for three consecutive years in the early 1920s, five consecutive years starting in approximately 1955, and three consecutive years starting in 1969. While the overall long-term trend in stroke mortality has been consistently decreasing, Figure 4 shows that short-term periods have shown both bursts and plateaus. The decrease over the century has averaged 1.7%; however, there is considerable year-to-year variation in the decrease. Thus, while the rapid decline in stroke mortality starting in 1972 is gratifying and while the plateauing of stroke mortality rates in the early 1990s may cause concern, short-term trends in similar periods have previously occurred. Only time will tell whether the decline in stroke mortality will continue into the future. New declines in stroke mortality from 1996 to 1998 suggest that additional declines in stroke mortality are possible, but continued and varying changes in the rate of change in stroke mortality can be expected. Therefore, over-interpretation of trends that may simply be short-term fluctuations should be avoided.

STROKE RATES VERSUS THE ABSOLUTE NUMBER OF STROKE EVENTS: THE PUBLIC HEALTH BURDEN

Because age distribution may be different between populations, epidemiologic descriptions of a disease tend to focus on age-adjusted rates per population (normally, per 100 000). For example, if the goal is to compare the stroke risk of men and women, age adjustment is necessary to adjust for proportionately more older women than older men. Likewise, changes in stroke risk over time could be confounded by the temporal shifts toward there being more older people over time. Without the adjustment, stroke risk may appear to have increased since 1900 simply because of the increase in the proportion of elderly individuals who are at higher risk for stroke. Therefore, age-adjustment is necessary to describe the difference in stroke risk between groups or across time; age-adjusted stroke risk has been used in this chapter up to this point. However, age-adjusted rates obscure aspects of the public health burden of a disease. For example, focusing on the rates may lead to the false conclusion that stroke is becoming less of a public health problem as rates continue to decline, or to falsely conclude that more men than women are affected by stroke.

To address this type of public health issue it may be more appropriate to focus on the absolute number of stroke events. Because of the 'graying of America', the number of older people is growing. For example, the US census bureau estimates that in the year 2000, there were 4.3 million people above the age of 85 in the US. This number is anticipated to increase to 5.8 million by the year 2010, and to 19.4 million by 2050[23]. In addition, because life-expectancy is greater for women than men, there are more older women than older men. Under the assumption that the age-specific stroke mortality rates remain constant, the total number of strokes for future years can be estimated by applying the 1998 age-specific rates[24] to the Census Bureau estimates of a future population (Figure 5)[23]. Accordingly, in the year 2000 more stroke deaths are anticipated for women (98 852) than for men (60 243). Figure 5 also shows the striking impact of the 'graying of America'. The number

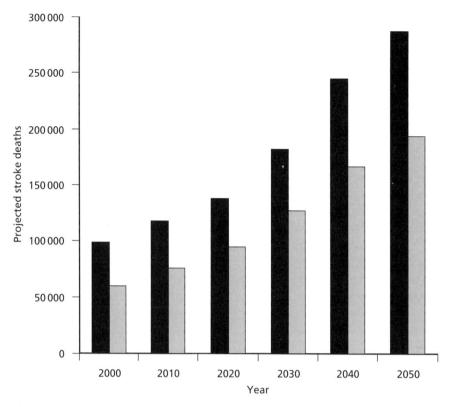

Figure 5 Anticipated number of stroke deaths for future years for men and women. Calculated under the assumption that the observed 1998 age-specific stroke mortality rates[24] continue, and that the population size described by middle series estimates of the US Census Bureau are achieved[23]. ■, female; ▢, male

of anticipated stroke deaths is approximately three times greater in the year 2050 than it was in 2000, with an anticipated 287 879 stroke deaths for women and 193 588 stroke deaths for men. It could easily be argued that the public health burden of stroke may be more closely tied to the absolute number of stroke events than to age-adjusted mortality rates. That is, the need for hospital beds, physicians and nurses, pharmaceutical agents, demands on rehabilitation services, and nursing home beds are all more tied to the absolute number of stroke events than to the stroke incidence rates.

Although it is hoped that stroke mortality rates will continue to decline, it is difficult to conceive the magnitude of the reduction necessary to offset the substantial increase in the absolute size of the older US population. While reductions in stroke mortality rates would lead to lower numbers of estimated deaths from stroke, other demographic changes in the population may increase the frequency of strokes. For example, as the proportion of African-Americans in the population increases (as it is anticipated to do), the higher stroke mortality rates observed among African-Americans would tend to increase the average stroke risk as well as the absolute number of stroke events. While these forecasts could be in error, it does seem likely that the public health burden for stroke will increase substantially in the next half century.

CONCLUSIONS

The decline in stroke mortality since 1900 has been one of the great public health advances of the previous century. This decline has been one of the contributing factors that has led the US to have stroke mortality rates among the lowest in the world. Even at this low mortality rate, stroke remains the third leading cause of mortality in the US, the single largest contributor to adult disability and a relatively common condition, with over 4 000 000 prevalent cases. The causes for the decline in stroke mortality are not well understood. However, the available data suggest a substantial role for decreases in the case fatality rates (that also increases the number of individuals with disability from

stroke). Whether stroke mortality will decline following a recent period of stable rates is unknown; however, it is encouraging to note that the recent stable period is similar to other periods in the past century of several years duration during which stable stroke mortality rates were observed. Thus, the recent stable period may be followed by a continued decline in stroke mortality. However, this declining stroke mortality rate is not likely to offset an anticipated rapidly growing public health burden for stroke attributable to the rapidly increasing number of older people in the population at increased risk of stroke. Only reductions in the incidence of the treatable stroke risk factors can ameliorate this dire prediction.

References

1. Centers for Disease Control. Ten great public health achievements — United States, 1900–1999. *Morbid Mortal Weekly Rep* 1999; 48:241–3
2. Centers for Disease Control. Achievements in public health, 1900–1999: decline in deaths from heart disease and stroke — United States, 1900–1999. *Morbid Mortal Weekly Rep* 1999; 48:649–56
3. National Center for Health Statistics. Deaths and death rates for the 10 leading causes of death in specified age groups, by race and sex: United States, 1998. *Nat Vital Stat Rep* 2000;48: 26–36
4. Goff DC, Howard G, Russell GB, Labarthe DR. Birth cohort evidence of population influences on blood pressure in the United States, 1887–1994. *Ann Epidemiol* 2001;11:271–9
5. US Department of Health and Human Services. *The Health Consequences of Smoking: Nicotine Addiction.* A report of the Surgeon General. Rockville (MD): US Department of Health and Human Services, Public Health Service, Office on Smoking and Health, 1988
6. Adams PF, Hendershot GE, Marano MA. Current estimates from the National Health Interview Survey, 1996. National Center for Health Statistics. *Vital Health Stat* 1999;10:200

7. American Heart Association. *2001 Heart and Stroke Statistical Update.* Dallas, Texas: American Heart Association, 2000
8. Toole JF, Chambless LE, Heiss G, et al. Prevalence of stroke and transient ischemic attacks in the Atherosclerosis Risk in Communities (ARIC) study. *Ann Epidemiol* 1993;3:500–3
9. Sarti C, Rastenyte D, Cepaitis Z, Tuomilehto J. International trends in mortality from stroke, 1968 to 1994. *Stroke* 2000;31:1588–601
10. Soltero I, Liu K, Cooper R, et al. Trends in mortality from cerebrovascular diseases in the United States, 1960 to 1974. *Stroke* 1978;9: 549–58
11. Whisnant JP. The decline of stroke. *Stroke* 1984;15:160–8
12. Broderick JP. Stroke trends in Rochester, Minnesota, during 1945 to 1984. *Ann Epidemiol* 1993;3:476–9
13. Brown RD Jr, Whisnant JP, Sicks J, et al. Stroke incidence, prevalence, and survival: secular trends in Rochester, Minnesota, through 1989. *Stroke* 1996;27:373–80
14. Hann MN, Selby JV, Rice DP, et al. Trends in cardiovascular disease incidence and survival in the elderly. *Ann Epidemiol* 1996;6:348–56
15. Wolf PA, D'Agostino RB, O'Neal MA, et al. Secular trends in stroke incidence and mortality.

The Framingham Study. *Stroke* 1992;23: 1551–5

16. Howard G, Craven TE, Sanders L, Evans GW. Relationship of hospitalized stroke rate and in-hospital mortality to the decline in US stroke mortality. *Neuroepidemiology* 1991;10:251–9

17. Shahar E, McGovern PG, Sprafka JM, *et al.* Improved survival of stroke patients during the 1980s. The Minnesota Stroke Survey. *Stroke* 1995;26:1–6

18. Howard G, Toole JF, Becker C, *et al.* Changes in survival following stroke in five North Carolina counties observed during two different periods. *Stroke* 1989;20:345–50

19. Derby CA, Lapane KL, Feldman HA, Carleton RA. Trends in validated cases of fatal and nonfatal stroke, stroke classification, and risk factors in southeastern New England, 1980 to 1991: data from the Pawtucket Heart Health Program. *Stroke* 2000;31:875–81

20. Barker WH, Mullooly JP. Stroke in a defined elderly population, 1967–1985: a less lethal and disabling but no less common disease. *Stroke* 1997;28:284–90

21. Cooper R, Sempos C, Hsieh SC, Kovar MG. Slowdown in the decline of stroke mortality in the United States, 1978–1986. *Stroke* 1990;21: 1274–9

22. Gillum RF, Sempos CT. The end of the long-term decline in stroke mortality in the United States? *Stroke* 1997;28:1527–9

23. US Census Bureau. Population Projections Program, Population Division, US Census Bureau, Washington, DC: 20233, 2001

24. Centers for Disease Control. National Center for Health Statistics. Death rates for 72 selected causes by 5-year age groups, race, and sex: United States, 1979–1998. Http://www.cdc.gov/nchs/datawh/statab/unpubd/mortabs/gmwk291.htm. Date accessed October 24, 2001

Chapter 2

'Nonmodifiable' risk factors for stroke: age, race, sex, and geography

Virginia J. Howard, PhD, and George Howard, PhD

INTRODUCTION

As the third leading cause of death and the leading cause of adult disability[1], stroke is a major public health burden in the US. This burden is not shared equally among Americans; rather, there are groups defined by 'nonmodifiable' risk factors with substantial disparities in stroke risk. This chapter describes these differences with an emphasis on the risk of stroke by age, race, sex and geographic region of residence.

DIFFERENTIAL STROKE RISK BY AGE

The dramatic increase in stroke mortality rates with increasing age is shown for the 1998 US population (all races, both sexes) in Figure 1. At age 40 to 45 the stroke death rates were 7.6 per 100 000, and these rates increased steadily to a death rate of 1500 per 100 000 for those over 85[1]. Shown on the same graph is the estimated annual percent increase in the risk of dying of a stroke deduced from the death rates in adjacent age strata. For age strata below 69, the risk of death from stroke is increasing at approximately 11% per year, a rate that would double the risk of a stroke death each

6.6 years. Above age 69 there is an increase in the rate at which the stroke mortality rate is increasing, and above age 85 the stroke mortality rate is increasing at approximately 18% per year (a difference that would double the risk of a stroke death each 4.2 years). Hence, not only is stroke mortality increasing with age, but the rate is accelerating at ages above 69 years.

The increase in mortality rates at older ages could, potentially, be due either to increases in incidence rates or to higher case fatality. The prevalence of cerebrovascular risk factors, most notably hypertension and diabetes, is known to increase dramatically with age[2]. Thus, estimating the increase in risk for stroke that is attributable specifically to age requires statistical adjustment for the risk factors that also increase with age. In the Framingham Study, after adjustment for stroke risk factors (specifically, systolic blood pressure, diabetes mellitus, cigarette smoking, cardiovascular disease, atrial fibrillation and left ventricular hypertrophy), a ten-year increase in age was associated with a 1.66 times increase in the risk of a stroke for men, and a 1.93 times increase for women[3]. Similar increases were

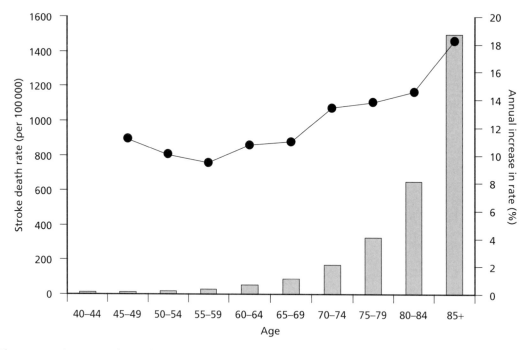

Figure 1 Histogram of overall (all races, both sexes) death rate per 100 000 from cerebrovascular diseases (ICD 430 to 438) during 1998 in the US (bars and scale on left vertical axis) and annual percent increase in stroke death rate estimated from adjacent age strata (line and scale on right vertical axis); data from Centers for Disease Control[1], Death rates for 72 selected causes by 5-year age groups, race and sex: USA, 1979–98

observed in the Cardiovascular Health Study, where after adjustment for a similar array of risk factors – and compared to individuals aged 65 to 69 – the risk of an incident stroke was 1.81 times greater for those aged 70 to 74, 2.96 times greater for those aged 75 to 79, 3.55 times greater for those aged 80 to 84 and 2.86 times greater for individuals over the age of 85[4]. These dramatic increases in risk, coupled with the opportunity to compare individuals who differ in age by 20 or more years, place increasing age among the largest of the risk factors for stroke.

Not surprisingly, with increases in stroke incidence there is also an associated increase in the prevalence rate of stroke. It is estimated that there are 2.0 individuals per 1000 population aged 18–44 who are stroke survivors[5].

This increases to 12.8 per 1000 between the ages of 45 and 64, to 40.2 per 1000 between the ages of 65 and 74, and to 99.4 per 1000 over the age of 75[5]. There is, therefore, a clear pattern of increasing stroke mortality, incidence and prevalence with increasing age.

SEX DIFFERENCES IN THE RISK OF STROKE

For both African-Americans and whites, the age-adjusted stroke mortality is greater for men than women across the time period 1979–97 (Figure 2)[6]. Despite the observed substantial declines in stroke mortality over this time period for all four race–sex groups, the mortality ratio for sex (men relative to women)

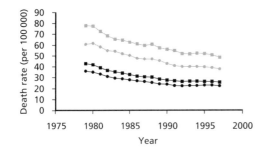

Figure 2 Stroke mortality rate for US African-Americans and whites by year (deaths per 100 000); data from Adams et al.[5] Vital Health Stat 1999: 10(200). ■, white males; •, white females; ▪, black males; ▪, black females

Table 1 Stroke mortality for white men and women by age strata, and age-specific mortality ratio in the USA, 1998

| | Mortality rate (per 100 000 population) | | Mortality ratio |
Age range	Men	Women	
45–49	11.0	8.1	1.36
50–54	18.0	14.9	1.21
55–59	30.4	23.8	1.28
60–64	53.6	40.1	1.34
65–69	93.2	72.6	1.28
70–74	181.5	145.5	1.25
75–79	345.8	297.7	1.16
80–84	665.2	625.5	1.06
85+	1365.9	1598.6	0.85

has fluctuated over a very narrow range of 1.14 to 1.20 for whites and 1.21 to 1.34 for African-Americans. It is apparent that the increased risk of death due to stroke in men is of moderate size and has been relatively stable over time. However, the difference between the sexes is not consistent across the age spectrum but is somewhat larger at younger ages and absent for older ages. Figure 3 shows the mortality ratio (male to female) by race and age strata for 1998[1], and Table 1 shows the mortality due to stroke for white men and women by age. Beginning with the 60 to 64 year age stratum, the excess mortality for men declines until, at ages over 85, women are at greater risk of death due to stroke than their male counterparts[1]. A pattern similar to the male/female mortality ratio has been reported for stroke incidence in several studies, where the majority of the excess events for men occurs at younger ages. For example, in the Cardiovascular Health Study the incidence rate ratio for sex was 1.80 (M, 7.9 : F, 4.4) for study participants aged 65 to 69[4]. This decreased to an incidence rate ratio of 1.52 (M, 12.8 : F, 8.4) between the ages of 70 and 74, to 1.09 (M, 17.7 : F, 16.3) and to 1.00 (M, 22.4 : F, 22.3) for ages above 80[4].

RACE AND ETHNIC DIFFERENCES IN STROKE RISK

The dramatic differences in stroke mortality between African-Americans and whites is shown in Figure 2 where, over the period from 1979 to 1997, the African-American to white mortality ratio ranged between 1.8 and 2.0 for men, and between 1.7 and 1.9 for women[6]. However, as is the case with differences by sex, there are dramatic differences by age in the mortality ratio associated with race. The age-specific stroke death rates for both African-Americans and whites, as well as other racial/ethnic groups, are shown in Figure 4[7]. While clearly the most striking feature of Figure 4 is the dramatic increase in stroke risk with increasing age, these data can also be used to provide a description of ethnic differences in the risk of stroke death. The high death rate due to stroke among African-Americans below the age of 54 is apparent in Figure 4, for example, with mortality rates of 18.2 per 100 000 for African-Americans aged 35 to 44 compared to rates of 4.5 for whites, 8.4 for American Indian/Alaska natives, 5.7 for Asian/Pacific islanders, and 5.8 for Hispanics.

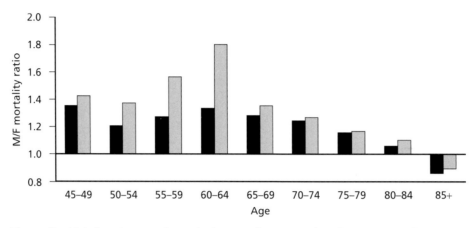

Figure 3 Male/female mortality ratio by race for 1998; data from Centers for Disease Control[1]. ■, whites; ▨, African-Americans

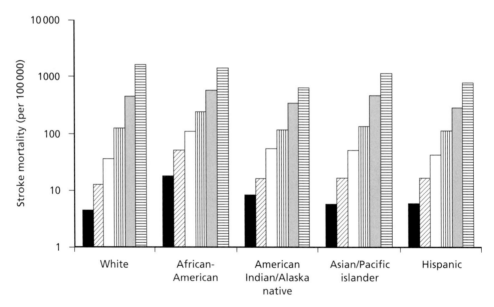

Figure 4 Age and race/ethnic specific stroke mortality rates per 100 000 – United States, 1997. ■, 35–44; ▨, 45–54; □, 55–64; ▥, 65–74; ▨, 75–84; ▤, 85+. Data from Cooper *et al.*, *J Nat Med Assoc* 1993;85:97–100

Using whites as the reference group, racial differences in the risk of stroke death can be seen by expressing the mortality ratio of the ethnic groups compared to whites (Figure 5). The striking feature of Figure 5 is the substantially increased risk for African-Americans in the younger age strata, with African-Americans below the age of 54 having a risk of stroke death that is approximately 4 times that of their white counterparts. This increased risk decreases to 'only' 3 times greater when comparing African-Americans and whites aged 55 to 64. With increasing age, the magnitude of excess risk continues to decline, and for

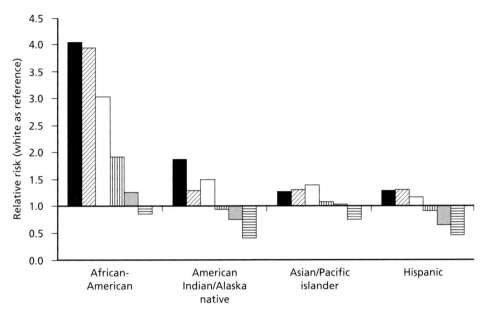

Figure 5 Age and race/ethnic specific relative risk of stroke mortality, white as reference group – United States, 1997. ■, 35–44; ▨, 45–54; □, 55–64; ▥, 65–74; ▨, 75–84; ▤, 85+. Data from Cooper *et al.*, *J Nat Med Assoc* 1993;85:97–100

the oldest age strata (85+), African-Americans are relatively protected compared to their white counterparts. This substantial changing pattern of the African-American to white risk has been previously reported[8-10], and reports have recently begun to focus not on the 'average' risk difference across age strata, but rather on describing the striking difference between African-Americans and whites at ages under 65[2].

It is also apparent from Figure 5 that the differences between white and other race/ethnic groups (American Indian/Alaska native, Asian/Pacific islanders, or Hispanic) are relatively small. The differences that do exist between whites and other race/ethnic groups show a trend for the stroke mortality risk of the other race/ethnic groups to be slightly greater than for whites at ages less than 65 years (Figure 5), and the risk to be slightly below the risk for whites at ages above 75 years. Thus, the largest differences in stroke mortality exist because of the exceptionally high stroke

mortality at young ages for African-Americans. The number of 'excess deaths' can be calculated for African-Americans by first calculating the expected number of deaths that would occur within each age stratum if African-Americans had a death rate similar to whites (or some other group). The excess deaths represent the difference between the actual number of deaths observed and this expected number of deaths. The number of extra deaths in each age stratum for African-Americans (as compared to whites) was calculated for 1997[7], and is presented in Figure 6. In 1997 there was a total of 17 738 stroke deaths among African-Americans in the US. Of these, 5700 (32%) were 'extra stroke deaths' that would not have occurred had African-Americans experienced the stroke death rates of their white counterparts. Of these 5700 extra deaths, 709 (12%) occurred between the ages of 35 and 44. An additional 1283 extra deaths occurred between the ages of 45 and 54, for a total of 1992 extra deaths between the ages of 35 and

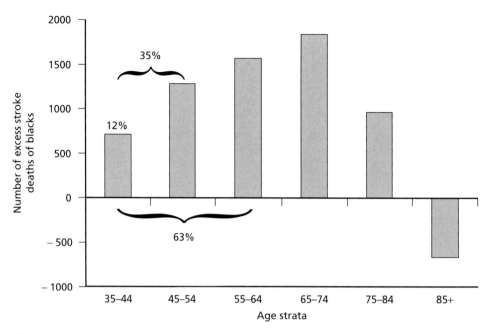

Figure 6   Number of excess deaths among African-Americans by age strata – United States, 1997. Data from Cooper *et al.*, *J Nat Med Assoc* 1993;85:97–100

54 – representing 35% of all of the extra deaths. An additional 1572 extra deaths occurred between the ages of 55 and 64, for a total of 3564 extra deaths between the ages of 35 and 64. Hence, 63% of all of the extra deaths due to stroke among African-Americans occur below the age of 65.

Until recently, most stroke mortality data were available only from predominantly white communities. It has not been clear whether the higher stroke mortality among African-Americans was attributable to a higher incidence rate among African-Americans or to a higher case fatality subsequent to the stroke event. Recently, data on racial differences in stroke mortality have become available from the Greater Cincinnati/Northern Kentucky Stroke Study, showing a pattern for racial difference in stroke incidence that reflects the racial differences in mortality discussed above[2]. This pivotal study gives insights into the importance of efforts to reduce stroke incidence among African-Americans.

GEOGRAPHIC VARIATIONS IN STROKE

The 'stroke belt' was first identified in 1965 as a region of high stroke mortality in the southeast of the USA[11], and it is frequently defined as eight southern states: North Carolina, South Carolina, Georgia, Tennessee, Mississippi, Alabama, Louisiana and Arkansas. This region of excess mortality due to stroke has been shown to exist since at least 1940[12]. Some areas within the stroke belt have an even higher stroke mortality, defining a 'buckle' region along the coastal plain of North Carolina, South Carolina, and Georgia[13].

The geographic variation in stroke mortality rates has been affected by a decline in the stroke mortality rates in the US. Stroke mortality has been declining since the early 1900s, with a period of more rapid decline during the 1970s[2], but the rate of decline slowed during the 1990s to a near plateau[14–16]. Over the 29-year period from 1968 to 1996 there was a

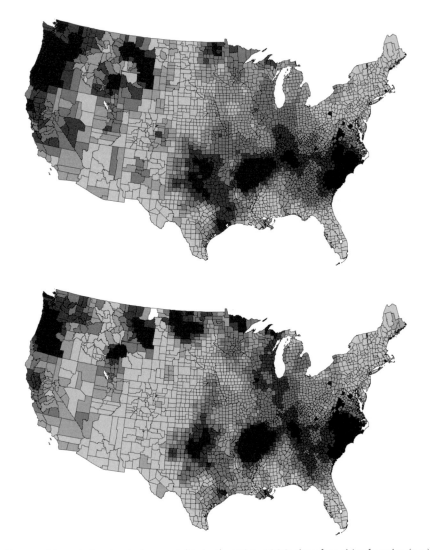

Figure 7 Geographic variation in stroke mortality in the USA, 1996; data for white females (top) and white males (bottom) have been smoothed, and data are displayed with the top 10% of counties in the darkest shade, counties between the 75th and 90th percentile in the next darkest, between the 50th and 75th percentile in the next darkest, between the 25th and the 50th percentile in the second lightest, and below the 25th percentile as the lightest shading. Reproduced with permission from Howard *et al.*, *Stroke* 2001;32:2213–20

remarkable 60% decline in stroke mortality[2]. Over this same period it has been noted that the geographic regions with the highest stroke mortality have tended to shift, raising the possibility that the stroke belt may be moving[17]. One possible reason for this 'migration' is that regions have differentially participated in the decline in stroke mortality[18]. Recently published data, however, show that despite these migrations, the stroke belt appears to be persistent[18]. The geographic variations in stroke mortality are shown in Figure 7[18], and analyses suggest that recent 'migrations' of the stroke belt have led to: (1) the continued high stroke

Table 2 Relative risk of stroke mortality for blacks and whites in states with sufficient African-American population for reliable estimation (age-adjusted rates); 1996–1998. Data from reference 22

State	B/W Relative risk for stroke
New York	1.06
Indiana	1.17
Oklahoma	1.18
Connecticut	1.24
Massachusetts	1.24
Illinois	1.24
Missouri	1.25
Kentucky	1.25
Pennsylvania	1.31
Ohio	1.32
Arkansas	1.32
Maryland	1.33
Michigan	1.34
Louisiana	1.35
California	1.41
Georgia	1.41
Texas	1.45
New Jersey	1.47
Wisconsin	1.48
Mississippi	1.49
Virginia	1.49
Alabama	1.49
North Carolina	1.51
Tennessee	1.55
South Carolina	1.56
Florida	1.92

mortality rates for the buckle of the belt, (2) the emergence of the Pacific Northwest as a new region of high stroke mortality, (3) a decline in stroke mortality in the deep south states of Mississippi and Alabama, and (4) the continued very low stroke mortality in New York City and southern Florida[18].

The reasons for existence of the stroke belt are poorly understood. At the most fundamental level it is not known whether the excess stroke mortality in the southeast is attributable to a higher incidence or higher case fatality. Although the data are, at best, mixed to support any specific hypothesis as the cause for the stroke belt, there is a wealth of hypothesized reasons including geographic differences in

major stroke risk factors (hypertension, diabetes, etc), lifestyle choices (including diet, exercise and smoking habits), the micronutrient content of soil or water, the genetic prevalence of stroke genes or genes for stroke risk factors, prevalence of chronic infections or inflammations, quality of health care and socioeconomic status[19,20].

The existence of the stroke belt has been clearly demonstrated for both the African-American and white populations. However, there are substantial differences in the African-American to white mortality ratios reported at the state level, showing a possible synergism between the impact of geographic and racial factors on stroke mortality (Table 2)[21,22]. In 26 states, the African-American population is sufficiently large to calculate the African-American to white stroke mortality ratio reliably. While the overall African-American to white mortality ratio for stroke was 1.42, there was considerable variation in the ratio for each of these 26 states. The seven states with the highest African-American to white mortality ratio were all in the southeastern US, and all had mortalities with at least a 16% relative increase in the black-to-white ratio. At the other end of the risk spectrum, African-Americans living in NY were at only a 6% increased risk compared to whites also living in NY. The reasons for this discrepancy are poorly understood.

CONCLUSIONS

Clearly, the factors of age, race, sex and geography are associated with substantial differences in stroke risk. The elderly, men, African-Americans and those living in the southeastern US are all at increased risk of stroke death (and probable increased risk of incident stroke events). It is tempting, and certainly easy, to assume that these factors represent 'nonmodifiable' risk factors. However, taking such an approach does not provide the opportunity to understand the underlying reasons why these substantial differences exist, and to develop interventions to reduce these health disparities. For example, few would assume that the difference in stroke risk between African-Americans and whites is solely attributable to genetics, but rather is more probably attributable to a wide spectrum of forces including socioeconomic status, racism, John Henryism (prolonged, high effort coping with difficult social and economic stressors[23]) and macrosocietal factors. A better understanding of how these factors work to increase risk should be the foundation of an understanding of how to reduce the racial disparities in stroke risk. It is of equal importance to understand and potentially intervene in the underlying causes of the health disparities in stroke mortality defined by sex, age, or geographic region. Efforts should be redoubled to establish the foundation for these differences attributable to 'nonmodifiable' risk factors with the goal of identifying aspects to address with active clinical or societal interventions.

References

1. Centers for Disease Control. National Center for Health Statistics. Death rates for 72 selected causes by 5-year age groups, race, and sex: United States, 1979–1998. Http://www.cdc.gov/nchs/datawh/statab/unpubd/mortabs/gmwk291.htm. Date accessed, October 24, 2001

2. American Heart Association. *2001 Heart and Stroke Statistical Update*. Dallas, Texas: American Heart Association, 2000

3. Wolf PA, D'Agostino RB, Belanger AJ, Kannel WB. Probability of stroke: a risk profile from the Framingham Study. *Stroke* 1991;22:312–18

4. Manolio TA, Kronmal RA, Burke GL, et al. Short term predictors of incident stroke in older adults: the Cardiovascular Health Study. *Stroke* 1996;27:1479–86

5. Adams PF, Hendershot GE, Marano MA. Current estimates from the National Health Interview Survey, 1996. National Center for Health Statistics. *Vital Health Stat* 1999;10(200):

6. Centers for Disease Control. National Center for Health Statistics. Data warehouse. Mortality Tables. http://www.cdc.gov/nchswww/datawh/statab/unpubd/mortabs.htm, Table: GMWK51 (293)

7. Centers for Disease Control. Age-specific excess deaths associated with stroke among racial/ethnic minority populations – United States, 1997. *Morbid Mortal Weekly Rep* 2000;49:94–7

8. Cooper ES. Cardiovascular diseases and stroke in African-Americans: a call for action. *J Natl Med Assoc* 1993;85:97–100

9. Howard G, Anderson R, Sorlie P, et al. Ethnic differences in stroke mortality between non-Hispanic whites, Hispanic whites, and blacks: the National Longitudinal Mortality Study. *Stroke* 1994;25:2120–5

10. Gillum RF, Ingram DD. Relation between residence in the southeast region of the United States and stroke incidence: the NHANES I Epidemiologic Follow-up Study. *Am J Epidemiol* 1996;144:665–73

11. Woo D, Gebel J, Miller R, et al. Incidence rates of first-ever ischemic stroke subtypes among blacks: a population-based study. *Stroke* 1999;30:2517–22

12. Borhani NO. Changes and geographic distribution of mortality from cerebrovascular disease. *Am J Public Health* 1965;55:673–81

13. Lanska DJ. Geographic distribution of stroke mortality in the United States: 1939–1941 to 1979 to 1981. *Neurology* 1993;43:1839–51

14. Howard G, Anderson R, Johnson NJ, et al. Evaluation of social status as a contributing factor to the stroke belt of the United States. *Stroke* 1997;28:936–40

15. Cooper R, Sempos C, Hsieh SC, Kovar MG. Slowdown in the decline of stroke mortality in the United States, 1978–1986. *Stroke* 1990;21:1274–9

16. Shahar E, McGovern PG, Pankow JS, et al. Stroke rates during the 1980s. The Minnesota Stroke Survey. *Stroke* 1997;28:275–9

17. Gillum RF, Sempos CT. The end of the long-term decline in stroke mortality in the United States? *Stroke* 1997;28:1527–9

18. Casper ML, Wing S, Anda RF, *et al*. The shifting stroke belt: changes in the geographic pattern of stroke mortality in the United States, 1962 to 1988. *Stroke* 1995;26:755–60

19. Howard G, Howard VJ, Katholi C, *et al*. Decline in US stroke mortality: an analysis of temporal patterns by sex, race, and geographic region. *Stroke* 2001;32:2213–20

20. Perry HM, Roccella EJ. Conference report on stroke mortality in the Southeastern United States. *Hypertension* 1998;31:1205–15

21. Howard G. Why do we have a stroke belt in the Southeastern United States? A review of unlikely and uninvestigated potential causes. *Am J Med Sci* 1999;317:160–7

22. Howard G, Howard VJ. Ethnic disparities in stroke: the scope of the problem. *Ethnic Dis* 2002, in press

23. James SA, Hartnett SA, Kalsbeek WD. John Henryism and blood pressure differences among black men. *J Behav Med* 1983;6: 259–78

Modifiable risk factors for stroke: hypertension, diabetes mellitus, lipids, tobacco use, physical inactivity, and alcohol

Bernadette Boden-Albala, MD, and Ralph L. Sacco, MD

INTRODUCTION

Various biological and lifestyle factors have been associated with increasing the risk of stroke. These include hypertension, diabetes, hyperlipidemias, physical inactivity, smoking and consumption of excess alcohol. Strategies for effective modification of these factors include risk factor identification, goal attainment for risk factor control, compliance strategies and continued follow-up. While each of these lifestyle factors is a unique and important independent risk factor, they frequently occur in combination in the same individual and together represent a heavy burden of increased stroke risk.

Both the consensus statement 'Guidelines for the Prevention of First Stroke' supported by the National Stroke Association (NSA)[1] and the American Heart Association (AHA) scientific statement 'Primary Prevention of Ischemic Stroke' provide evidence-based recommendations for decreasing stroke risk that act as a template for risk factor reduction (Table 1)[2]. Lifestyle modifications to reduce stroke risk may present a great challenge in that social, behavioral and cultural factors increase the complexity of the risk reduction strategy. It must remain the priority of health professionals to define and promote a lifestyle conducive to reducing blood pressure, controlling blood glucose, elevating high-density lipoprotein-cholesterol, increasing physical activity, evaluating alcohol use and promoting the cessation of cigarette smoking.

HYPERTENSION

Hypertension is the most powerful and potentially modifiable risk factor for stroke. It is prevalent in both men and women, and is of even greater significance in African-Americans. Stroke risk rises proportionately with increasing blood pressure. In the Framingham Study the age-adjusted relative risk of stroke among those with definite hypertension (blood pressure > 160/95) was 3.1 for men and 2.9 for women[3]. Even among borderline hypertensives, the relative risk was 1.5 compared to normotensives. Components of blood pressure such as isolated systolic hypertension may also

Table 1 Modifiable risk factors, prevalence, relative risk, and management recommendations for stroke

Risk factor	Estimated prevalence (%)	Estimated relative risk	Management recommendations
Hypertension[1,2,9]	20–65	2.0–5.0	Promote BP measurement every 2 years, weight control, limit salt intake. If BP > 140/90 mmHg after 3 months or BP > 180/100 use antihypertensive agents
Diabetes[1,2,9]	4–20	1.5–3.0	Tight glucose control through diet, oral hyperglycemics and insulin. Strict regulation of BP if hypertensive
Hyperlipidemia[1,2,9]	6–40	1.0–2.0	Lipoprotein analysis, and dietary modification, if TC 200–239 mg/dl, HDL ≥ 40 and < 2 CHD risk factors. Use of drug therapy including statin agents recommended if TC ≥ 240 mg/dl or LDL ≥ 160 mg/dl, or LDL ≥ 130 and 2 CHD risk factors, or LDL ≥ 100 mg/dl and definite CHD or atherosclerotic disease
Smoking[1,2,9]	20–40	1.5–2.5	Smoking cessation
Physical inactivity[1,2,9]	25–50	2.0–3.5	Moderate exercise including brisk walking
Excess alcohol (≥ 5 drinks per day)[1,2,131]	2–5	1.0–2.0	Up to two drinks per day

BP, blood pressure; CHD, coronary heart disease; TC, total cholesterol

contribute to an increased risk of stroke. The prevalence of systolic hypertension increases with age and the risk of stroke is increased 2- to 4-fold even after controlling for age and diastolic blood pressure[4–7]. In the British Regional Heart Study, men with systolic blood pressures (SBPs) between 160 and 180 mmHg had about four times the risk of stroke compared with men with SBPs below 160 mmHg[8]. Individuals with SBPs above 180 mmHg had a six-fold greater stroke risk. In the Northern Manhattan Stroke Study (NOMASS) hypertension was a strong, independent stroke risk factor for whites (OR 1.8), blacks (OR 2.0) and Hispanics (OR 2.1) living in the same community. The increased prevalence of hypertension among blacks and Hispanics led to an elevated etiologic fraction for these two race-ethnic groups (Figure 1)[9].

Reduction of both systolic and diastolic pressure in hypertensive patients substantially reduces stroke risk. Prospective studies and clinical trials have consistently shown a decreased risk of stroke with control of mild, moderate and severe hypertension in all age groups. In a meta-analysis of nine prospective studies following 420 000 individuals over 10 years, stroke risk increased by 46% for every 7.5-mmHg increase in diastolic blood pressure (DBP)[10]. This analysis suggests that a graded relationship exists between blood pressure and stroke risk with no lower threshold, a relationship that has been confirmed by another meta-analysis of 14 treatment trials including 37 000 unconfounded, randomized individuals followed for a mean of 5 years[11,12]. This meta-analysis demonstrated that a mean reduction in DBP of 5–6 mmHg corresponded to a 35–40% reduction in stroke incidence. The reduction in stroke risk was identified regardless of the level of the index DBP. Other meta-analyses have documented benefits among various subgroups[13]. These data suggest that antihypertensive therapy is critical in stroke

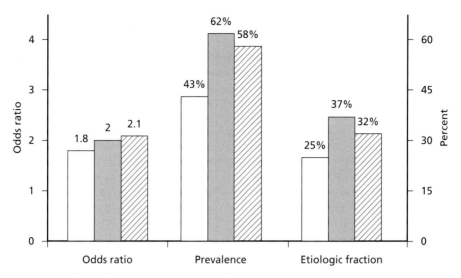

Figure 1 Effect of hypertension on risk of stroke: odds ratio, prevalence and etiologic fraction matched for age, gender and ethnicity and adjusted for diabetes mellitus, atrial fibrillation, coronary artery disease, no physical activity and education. Data from the Northern Manhattan Stroke Study. □, white; ■, black; ▨, Hispanic

prevention and should be prescribed for all hypertensives. In addition, as no low threshold for risk was found with DBP, antihypertensive therapy may also be considered for those defined as 'normotensive' by conventional criteria who are otherwise at high stroke risk[14].

A number of individual trials have also provided important information about the relationship between control of hypertension and stroke risk particularly in elderly populations. The STOP-Hypertension program (Swedish Trial in Old Patients with Hypertension) followed over 1600 randomized hypertensive patients aged 70–84 years for an average of 25 months[15]. This study found a significant decline in stroke morbidity and mortality, as well as in total mortality, indicating the importance of managing hypertension in the elderly. The SHEP (Systolic Hypertension in the Elderly Program) trial randomized 4736 individuals over 60 years of age with isolated systolic hypertension (SBP > 160 mmHg with DBP < 90 mmHg) and followed them for 4.5 years[16]. The resulting 36% reduction in total stroke

incidence confirmed the significance of managing isolated systolic hypertension, a condition affecting two-thirds of elderly hypertensives[14]. The Syst-Eur trial demonstrated that treatment of older patients with isolated systolic hypertension led to a 42% reduction in stroke risk with no significant decline in overall mortality[17]. In absolute terms, these trials indicate that treating only 10–20 patients for five years will prevent one major cardiovascular event[17]. Results from the STOP-2 trial, which compared rates of cardiovascular outcomes and stroke by type of antihypertensive agent, found similar stroke rates for conventional antihypertensive agents (22%), angiotensin-converting enzyme (ACE) inhibitors (20%), and calcium antagonists (20%)[18].

A risk factor profile based on the Framingham cohort has been developed that included SBP and the use of antihypertensive treatment, as well as other stroke risk factors[6]. The relative risk of stroke for a 10-mmHg increase in SBP was 1.9 for men and 1.7 for women, after controlling for other known stroke risk factors. Current guidelines for the treatment of hypertension have been published by the Joint National Committee on Prevention, Detection, Evaluation and Treatment of High Blood Pressure[19]. Definitions of hypertension have been broadened to include individuals who were once considered 'borderline hypertensive'. Normotensive is now defined as systolic BP < 140 and diastolic BP < 85 mmHg. Since the attributable stroke risk for hypertension (proportion of strokes explained by hypertension) ranges from 35 to 50% depending on age, even a slight improvement in the control of hypertension could translate into a substantial reduction in stroke frequency[7].

The National Stroke Association recommends three strategies for hypertensive individuals to help decrease the risk of a first stroke: (1) blood pressure should be controlled in patients with hypertension who are most likely to develop stroke; (2) physicians should check the blood pressure of all their patients at every visit; and (3) patients with hypertension should monitor their blood pressure at home[1]. AHA guidelines suggest that antihypertensive agents be given to individuals if initial BP is greater than 180/100 mmHg or if BP remains higher than 140/90 after three months of lifestyle modification[2]. Numerous efficacious treatments exist which reduce BP, and clinical trials have demonstrated that hypertension can be lowered, leading to a dramatic reduction in stroke risk[20,21]. Despite these facts, the control of blood pressure among different populations is poor[22]; it is estimated that only between 6% and 50% of hypertensive patients are controlled[23–26]. Data suggest that within the community, awareness of the importance of the level of hypertension and BP control is suboptimal[27].

Much effort is now being focused on the reduction of elevated BP. Research has moved beyond treatment modalities to focus on barriers to risk reduction including educational disparities, compliance, access to care and lack of support services. Socioeconomic conditions are powerful predictors of mortality and morbidity[28–36] and pilot studies have been undertaken to develop methodologies identifying social conditions successful in reducing blood pressure[37–41]. Studies have demonstrated that education about risk factors alone, or combined with free antihypertensive medication, was related to a significant decrease in BP[37,38]. A number of pilot studies are underway utilizing religious activity, as well as mobilization, cultural relevance and partnership in the management of blood pressure among African-Americans[39–41].

DIABETES MELLITUS

There is clear evidence that diabetes is an important risk factor for stroke, with relative risks ranging from 1.5 to 3.0 depending on the type and severity. Moreover, mortality from cerebrovascular disease is greatly increased among subjects with elevated blood glucose values[42]. In a study of British men, the mean serum glucose level was significantly higher in those who developed stroke, but lacked significance after adjusting for age and hypertension[8]. The impact of diabetes was more pronounced in the Framingham Study, which found diabetes associated with increased stroke risk in both men and women that was independent of age and hypertension[3]. In the Copenhagen City Heart Study, diabetes had a marked independent effect on stroke risk[43]. Likewise, diabetes was associated with increased stroke risk during an 8-year prospective stroke study in rural Sicily[44]. Diabetes was associated with a two-fold increased adjusted risk of thromboembolic stroke among Japanese men living in Hawaii[45] and in men and women in Rancho Bernardo, CA[46]. Overall, in the Northern Manhattan Stroke Study diabetes was associated with an odds ratio of 1.7 (95% CI, 11.3–2.2) after adjusting for other risk factors.

This study found that the prevalence of diabetes may be as high as 22% and 20% among elderly blacks and Hispanics, respectively, with corresponding attributable risks of stroke of 13% and 20%[9]. The prevalence of type 2 diabetes in the USA is projected to increase from an estimated 124 million at present to 221 million by the year 2010[47].

Intensive treatment of both type 1 and type 2 diabetes, aimed at maintaining near normal levels of blood glucose, can substantially reduce the risk of microvascular complications such as retinopathy, nephropathy and neuropathy, but has not been conclusively shown to reduce macrovascular complications including stroke[48–50]. However, aggressive treatment of hypertension in patients with type 2 diabetes will significantly reduce the risk of stroke. The UK Prospective Diabetes Study group reported that active control of blood pressure (< 150/85 mmHg) among type 2 diabetics helped significantly to reduce the risk of stroke, by 44%[51]. The use of ACE inhibitors in hypertensive diabetics may be even more beneficial in the prevention of stroke. Results of the Heart Outcomes Prevention Evaluation (HOPE) study and MICRO-HOPE sub-study investigated whether the ACE inhibitor ramipril would lower the risk of stroke and other cardiac outcomes in diabetics. Ramipril lowered the risk of stroke by 33%. Even after adjustment for blood pressure measurements, this ACE inhibitor was found to reduce the risk of the combined endpoint of myocardial infarction (MI), stroke or cardiovascular death by 25%[52].

The prevention of stroke through control of diabetes yields important results[53]. The NSA recommends rigorous comprehensive control of blood sugar levels for compliant patients with type 1 and type 2 diabetes to prevent microvascular complications[1]. The AHA scientific statement recommends rigorous control of hypertension in addition to improved glucose control[2]. Guidelines for the management of diabetes have been published by the American Diabetes Association and have lowered the target fasting blood glucose level to 126 mg/dl. However, despite solid evidence regarding the increased risk of stroke associated with diabetes, glycemic control is inadequate for between 30 and 50% of the diabetic population[54]. Better control of blood sugar and more aggressive treatment of other risk factors, such as hypertension, among diabetics is certainly needed.

LIPIDS

Many studies have provided strong evidence that serum lipids including triglycerides, cholesterol, low-density lipoprotein (LDL) and high-density lipoprotein (HDL) are important modifiable risk factors for coronary artery disease[55]. There is a direct relationship between cholesterol and LDL and the incidence of heart disease, while an inverse relationship has been documented between HDL and cardiac disease. The cholesterol–stroke association has been less consistently documented. Mortality rates from ischemic stroke were greater among men with high cholesterol levels in the Multiple Risk Factor Intervention Trial[56]. The Honolulu Heart Program demonstrated a continuous and progressive increase in both CHD and thromboembolic stroke rates with increasing levels of cholesterol, with a relative risk of 1.4 comparing highest and lowest quartiles[57]. Meta-analyses among prospective studies have been less conclusive with regard to elevated cholesterol levels and stroke risk[58, 59]. It is possible that the absence of a consistent significant relationship between cholesterol and stroke may be due to the heterogeneity of stroke subtypes, which are not all atherosclerotic in origin. Additionally, most prospective studies were done among younger populations and focused on cardiac outcomes, and lipoprotein fractions were not always evaluated separately from total cholesterol.

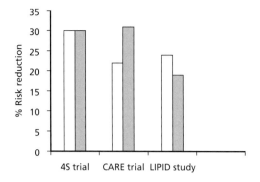

Figure 2 Reduction of risk of cardiovascular disease mortality (□) and risk of stroke (▣) by statin agents as shown by the Scandinavian Simvastatin Survival Study (4S)[67], the Cholesterol and Recurrent Events (CARE) trial[68] and the Long-term Intervention with Pravastatin in Ischemic Disease (LIPID) study[69]

When lipid sub-fractions have been measured and analyzed separately, a protective association between HDL and ischemic stroke has emerged[42]. The Oxfordshire community study demonstrated a dose-dependent, inverse relationship between HDL and risk of transient ischemic attacks (TIAs) or minor stroke. Stroke risk was attenuated by nearly one-third in those with higher HDL levels[60]. In Northern Manhattan, a significant protective dose–response relationship was found between HDL and ischemic stroke[61]. This relationship was seen in the elderly and among different race-ethnic groups, including whites, blacks and Hispanics. The degree and progression of carotid atherosclerosis are also directly related to cholesterol and LDL levels and inversely related to HDL levels[62,63]. Other lipid markers, such as a high level of serum lipoprotein(a), have been found to be risk factors in a group of patients with early onset of cerebral infarction[64].

Before the introduction of statin agents, clinical trials analyzing the relationship of lipid-lowering strategies and stroke found no benefits[65]. The MRFIT study showed a paradoxical increase in hemorrhagic stroke risk with very low cholesterol levels[66]. Clinical trials analyzing the efficacy of lipid lowering strategies with statin agents have demonstrated impressive reductions in stroke risk in various high-risk populations with cardiac disease. In these studies stroke was either a secondary endpoint or a non-specified endpoint determined on the basis of *post-hoc* analyses[67]. Two large trials in which stroke was pre-specified as a secondary endpoint have also shown significant reductions with pravastatin among subjects with coronary artery disease and normal to borderline elevations of cholesterol[68,69]. Meta-analyses that included some of these trials have found a 29% reduced risk of stroke and a 22% reduction in overall mortality[70,71]. Secondary prevention trials showed a 32% reduction in stroke risk and primary trials demonstrated a 20% reduction (Figure 2). Using serial carotid ultrasound measurements, some clinical trials have also demonstrated carotid plaque regression with statins[72–76].

Both observational and clinical trial data have provided support for the role of lipoproteins as precursors of carotid atherosclerosis and ischemic stroke. These data likewise suggest the benefits of lowering cholesterol as a stroke reduction strategy. Individuals with cholesterol levels above 200 mg/dl and cardiovascular risk factors should have a complete lipid analysis (total cholesterol, LDL, HDL, triglycerides) and most probably would benefit from cholesterol-lowering regimens including statins[1,2]. The second report of the National Cholesterol Education Program (NCEP) recommended the addition of HDL to initial cholesterol testing, the designation of high HDL as a protective factor, and an increased emphasis on physical activity and weight loss as components of the dietary therapy of high levels of blood cholesterol. In the third report of the NCEP, the level of HDL cholesterol has been changed to 40 mg/dl (1.03 mmol/l) and the goal for LDL cholesterol lowering therapy has been modified for those with low levels of HDL cholesterol[77]. Guidelines for both the AHA and the NSA recommend the use of statin agents for individuals with high cholesterol and atherosclerotic cardiac disease[1,2].

TOBACCO USE

Tobacco use, most frequently cigarette smoking, is a major public health problem. It is estimated that tobacco is responsible for the deaths of 434 000 American smokers and 53 000 non-smokers (from passive exposure) annually[78]. Recent reports suggest that there has been no decrease in the prevalence of cigarette smoking over the last 20 years. Despite these dire health statistics, almost 50 million Americans continue to smoke and the majority of adolescents at least experiment with cigarettes. The problem is widespread. Worldwide, tobacco is estimated to cause about 3 million deaths each year[79]. Smoking, especially current smoking, is an extremely modifiable, independent determinant of stroke[80]. In case–control studies the effect of cigarette smoking remained significant after adjustment for other factors, and a dose–response relationship became apparent. In cohort studies, cigarette smoking was found to be an independent predictor of ischemic stroke. A meta-analysis showed that the relative risk (RR) of stroke was 1.9[81]. Furthermore, a dose–response effect and an interaction with age was noted, with the average risk being relatively greater among younger persons. Women smokers were at slightly higher risk than men who smoke. The association between cigarette smoking and ischemic stroke has been consistent among major cohort studies such as the Framingham Study and the Nurses' Health Study[82,83]. Additionally, smoking is highly associated with the development of carotid atherosclerosis[84]. Potential biological effects of smoking that can induce stroke include increased blood viscosity, hypercoagulability, elevated fibrinogen levels, enhanced platelet aggregation and elevation of blood pressure[85]. For different stroke types, the stroke risk attributed to cigarette smoking was greatest for subarachnoid hemorrhage, intermediate for cerebral infarction, and lowest for cerebral hemorrhage.

There is ample evidence from observational epidemiologic studies that smoking cessation leads to a reduction in stroke risk; several studies have shown that a substantial reduction in risk occurs within 2–5 years. In a prospective study of 177 006 female registered nurses, the excess risk of ischemic stroke for former smokers disappeared two years after cessation[86]. These reductions were found regardless of the number of cigarettes smoked, age at starting and other stroke risk factors. Data from the Framingham Study confirm that the risk of stroke for former smokers approaches the risk for those who never smoked within five years of giving up[87]. An intervention program randomizing 1445 British men found that after ten years the intervention group had 53% less smoking than the controls[88]. While stroke mortality was not measured, the reduction was associated with an 18% reduction in mortality due to coronary heart disease (CHD). Data also suggest an increased risk of stroke among non-smokers and long-term ex-smokers exposed to environmental tobacco smoke[89].

Data from prospective cohort studies have demonstrated convincingly that cessation of cigarette smoking can reduce the risk of stroke. Targeted community interventions for smoking cessation have resulted in modest gains among light-to-moderate smokers, but little change in heavy smokers, when recent secular trends for smoking are considered[90]. Counseling, health incentives and the various nicotine substitutes (e.g., patches, gum) have shown modest success over time. Physicians have been criticized for not taking an active role in educating their own patients on the importance of smoking cessation. It has been estimated that if cigarette smoking in the United States were eliminated, the number of strokes occurring each year could be reduced by 61 500 and the nation would save 3.08 billion in stroke-related health-care dollars[91]. National guidelines recommend the cessation of smoking as a stroke prevention measure, in accordance with guidelines by the Agency for Health Care Policy and Research. This guideline addresses various topics including screening for tobacco use, advice to quit, interventions, smoking cessation pharmacotherapy, motivation to quit and prevention of relapse[1,2]. Public health education programs, economic measures and individual counseling should be continued and expanded to discourage initial smoking behavior and encourage smoking cessation.

PHYSICAL INACTIVITY

Physical inactivity is an important and under-emphasized, potentially modifiable stroke risk factor. Guidelines endorsed by the Centers for Disease Control and Prevention and the National Institutes of Health recommend that people should exercise for at least 30 minutes and perform moderately intense physical activity on most, and preferably all, days of the week[92,93]. Regular physical activity has well established benefits for reducing the risk of premature death and cardiovascular disease. Moderate and heavy levels of physical activity have been associated with reduced CHD incidence when those who exercise are compared with inactive persons, although there is no evidence that heavy physical activity conferred any more benefit than a moderate level[94,95]. In recent years evidence has been accumulating that supports a protective effect of moderate physical activity on stroke incidence in men and women. For stroke, the benefits are apparent even for light–moderate activities, such as walking, and the data support the inference that additional benefits are to be gained from

increasing the level and duration of one's recreational physical activity[94–105]. Other studies that have shown a protective effect of physical activity for men include the Honolulu Heart Program, the Framingham Study and the Oslo Study[97–99]. In Framingham, physical activity in subjects with a mean age of 65 years was associated with a reduced stroke incidence. In men, the relative risk was 0.41 after accounting for the effects of potential confounders, although there was no evidence of a protective effect of physical activity on the risk of stroke in women[98]. However, both the Copenhagen City Heart Study and the Nurses' Health Study have demonstrated an inverse association between level of physical activity and the incidence of stroke among women[100,105]. The protective effects of leisure-time physical activity have also been found for blacks and Hispanics in the National Health and Nutrition Examination Survey I follow-up study and the Northern Manhattan Stroke Study[101,102]. Dose–response relationships have sometimes been difficult to demonstrate although few deleterious effects from vigorous physical activity compared to lower levels of physical activity have been demonstrated[103,104]. In the Northern Manhattan Stroke Study, heavy forms of physical activity actually provided additional benefits compared to light–moderate activities, and additional protection was observed with increasing duration of exercise. However, the prevalence of such activities in the elderly was quite low[102]. The benefits of leisure-time physical activity were noted for all age, gender and race-ethnic subgroups (Figure 3). The large prospective cohort of the Atherosclerosis Risk in Communities (ARIC) Study also reported a modest protective effect of different types of physical activity on the risk of ischemic stroke[106].

The protective effect of physical activity may be partly mediated through its role in controlling various known risk factors for stroke such as hypertension[107], cardiovascular

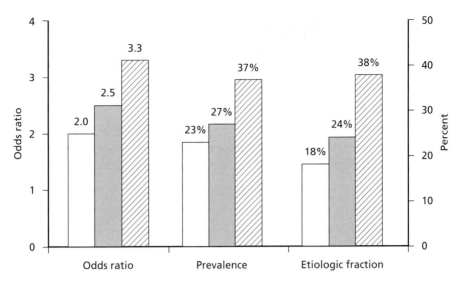

Figure 3 Effect of hypertension on risk of stroke: odds ratio, prevalence and etiologic fraction matched for age, gender and ethnicity and adjusted for hypertension, diabetes mellitus, atrial fibrillation, coronary artery disease and education. Data from the Northern Manhattan Stroke Study. □ white; ■ black; ▨ Hispanic

disease[108], diabetes[109] and body weight. Other biological mechanisms are also associated with physical activity, including reductions in plasma fibrinogen and platelet activity, elevations in plasma tissue plasminogen activator activity and HDL concentrations, as well as reductions in homocysteine levels[110–115].

Physical activity is a modifiable behavior that requires greater emphasis in stroke prevention campaigns. The 1994 Behavioral Risk Factor Surveillance Survey found that 60% of adults did not achieve the recommended amount of physical activity, and people with the lowest incomes and less than 12th grade education are more likely to be sedentary. Moreover, 70 to 80% of older women report levels less than the recommended amount of physical activity[116]. Public health goals are to increase the proportion of people who engage in regular physical activity and reduce the proportion of those who engage in no leisure-time physical activity, particularly among people aged 65 and over[117]. Leisure-time

physical activity could translate into a cost-effective means of decreasing the public health burden of stroke and other cardiovascular diseases among the USA's rapidly aging population[1].

ALCOHOL USE

Alcohol is consumed in substantial quantities by large numbers of Americans annually and excess consumption poses a major health threat. There are an estimated 107 800 alcohol-related deaths each year in the USA[118]. These include, but are not restricted to, deaths due to traffic accidents, various cancers, accidental deaths, suicides and homicides. The economic cost of alcohol abuse and dependence is estimated to be $100 billion per annum. Although the health risks of excess alcohol consumption are well known, moderate drinking may reduce cardiovascular disease risk and total mortality.

The effect of alcohol as a stroke risk factor is controversial and probably dependent on dose. For hemorrhagic stroke, prospective cohort studies have shown that alcohol consumption has a direct dose-dependent effect[119–121]. For cerebral infarction, chronic heavy drinking and acute intoxication have been associated with an increased risk among young adults[122]. In older adults, studies have shown an increased risk among male heavy-drinkers with no effects among women after controlling for other confounding risk factors[123–125] and a protective effect for moderate alcohol consumption[126–129].

Epidemiologic studies have shown a U-shaped curve for alcohol consumption and coronary heart disease mortality, with low to moderate alcohol consumption associated with lower overall mortality[130]. In an overview analysis of stroke studies, a J-shaped association curve was suggested for the relation of moderate customary alcohol consumption and ischemic stroke[129]. As for coronary heart disease, alcohol could be protective for ischemic stroke if consumed in moderation. Protection against ischemic stroke has been most consistently observed in white populations but little if any benefit has been demonstrated in Japanese or possibly in black populations. In Northern Manhattan, moderate alcohol consumption was protective among a largely black and Hispanic population, while drinking in excess of five drinks per day increased the risk of ischemic stroke (Figure 4)[131]. A large prospective cohort of male physicians has confirmed the protective effects of light to moderate alcohol consumption for ischemic stroke. This study found an overall relative risk of 0.79 (95% CI, 0.66–0.94) for all strokes and an RR of 0.77 (95% CI, 0.63–0.94) for ischemic stroke in a study of over 22 000 male physicians during 12 years of follow-up[132].

The dose-dependent relationship between alcohol and stroke is consistent with the observed deleterious and beneficial effects of alcohol. The deleterious effects of alcohol for stroke may operate through various

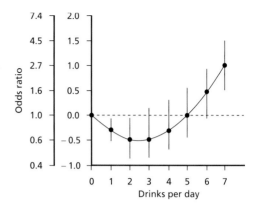

Figure 4 The relationship between alcohol consumption and the risk of ischemic stroke; data from the Northern Manhattan Stroke Study[131]

mechanisms that include increasing hypertension, hypercoagulable states and cardiac arrhythmias, and reducing cerebral blood flow. However, there is also evidence that light to moderate drinking can reduce the risk of coronary artery disease, increase HDL cholesterol and endogenous tissue plasminogen activator, improve endothelial function, stabilize plaque and have antithrombotic properties[133]. Numerous studies have also attempted to clarify whether the protective effect of alcohol was actually limited to wine versus beer and other hard alcohols, such as gin or vodka. It has been suggested that polyphenolic compounds found in red wine, white wine, grape juice and beer act as antioxidants, actually reducing the atherogenicity connected with LDL[134].

No trials of the relationship between modification of alcohol use and stroke risk have been performed. Such studies will be difficult because of the non-linear dose–response relationship between alcohol and stroke, as well as for ethical concerns. Elimination of heavy drinking may reduce the incidence of stroke. Since some ingestion of alcohol, perhaps up to two drinks per day, may actually help reduce the risk of stroke, drinking in moderation should not be discouraged for most of the public[1,2]. While it is difficult to consider recommending alcohol to those who are non-drinkers, elimination of heavy drinking and reduction to moderate levels of alcohol intake, e.g. to no more than two drinks per day, for those who are currently drinking could be expected to reduce the incidence of stroke. Based on alcohol-related longevity and cardiac risk data, public health policy for stroke prevention in alcohol users could be adopted, similar to that for cardiac disease. In the US, this would conform to a recommendation of no more than two standard drinks of beer, wine or liquor per day in those who wish to drink and do not have a contraindication to alcohol use.

SUMMARY

Data from numerous epidemiological studies confirm that hypertension, diabetes and lipids are among the most important biological risk factors for stroke. Likewise, there is compelling evidence that lifestyle factors including smoking, alcohol consumption and physical inactivity are significant factors for stroke risk. What is equally important is that related biological and lifestyle factors are all modifiable. Modification of these risk factors may require the use of anti-hypertensive agents and statins. Additionally, lifestyle changes require continued support and encouragement. Strategies such as goal attainment may be effective in changing certain behaviors such as increasing physical activity; other behaviors, including smoking, may require broader social and political interventions. Despite the obstacles to modification of lifestyle factors, health professionals should be encouraged to continue to identify such factors to help prevent stroke.

References

1. Gorelick PB, Sacco RL, Smith DB, *et al*. Prevention of a first stroke: a review of guidelines and a multidisciplinary consensus statement from the National Stroke Association. *J Am Med Assoc* 1999;281:1112–20
2. Goldstein LB, Adams R, Becker MD, *et al*. Primary prevention of ischemic stroke. A statement for healthcare professionals from the stroke council of the American Heart Association. *Stroke* 2001;32:280–99
3. Wolf PA, Cobb JL, D'Agostino RB. Epidemiology of stroke. In Barnett HJM, Mohr JP, Stein BM, Yatsu FM, eds. *Stroke – Pathophysiology, Diagnosis, and Managment*. New York: Churchill Livingstone, 1992:3–27
4. Joseph L, Kase CS, Beiser AS, Wolf PA. Mild blood pressure elevation and stroke: the Framingham Study. *Stroke* 1998;29:277
5. Davis PH, Dambrosia JM, Schoenberg BS, *et al*. Risk factors for ischemic stroke: a prospective study in Rochester, Minnesota. *Ann Neurol* 1987;22:319–27
6. Wolf PA, D'Agostino RB, Belanger AJ, Kannel WB. Probability of stroke: a risk profile fron the Framingham Study. *Stroke* 1991;22:312–18
7. MacMahon S, Rodgers A. The epidemiological association between blood pressure and stroke: implications for primary and secondary prevention. *Hypertens Res* 1994;17:S23–S32
8. Shaper AG, Phillips AN, Pocock SJ, *et al*. Risk factors for stroke in middle aged British men. *Br Med J* 1991;302:1111–15
9. Sacco RL. Boden-Albala B, Abel G, *et al*. Race-ethnic disparities in the impact of stroke risk factors: the northern Manhattan stroke study. *Stroke* 2001;32:1725–31
10. MacMahon S, Peto R, Cutler J, *et al*. Blood pressure, stroke, and coronary heart disease. Part 1: Prolonged differences in blood pressure: prospective observational studies corrected for the regression dilution bias. *Lancet* 1990;335:765–74

11. Collins R, Peto R, MacMahon S, *et al.* Blood pressure, stroke, and coronary heart disease. Part 2: Short-term reductions in blood pressure: overview of randomised drug trials in their epidemiological context. *Lancet* 1990;335: 827–38

12. MacMahon S, Peto R, Cutler J, Stamler J. Antihypertensive drug treatment: potential, expected, and observed effects on stroke and on coronary heart disease. *Hypertension* 1989; 13(Suppl I):I45–I50

13. Hebert PR, Moser M, Mayer J, *et al.* Recent evidence on drug therapy of mild to moderate hypertension and decreased risk of coronary heart disease. *Arch Intern Med* 1993;153: 578–81

14. Dunabibin DW, Sandercock PAG. Preventing stroke by the modification of risk factors. *Stroke* 1990;21(Suppl IV):IV36–IV39

15. Dahlöf B, Linholm L, Hansson L, *et al.* Morbidity and mortality in the Swedish Trial in Old Patients with Hypertension (STOP–Hypertension). *Lancet* 1991;338:1281–5

16. SHEP Cooperative Research Group. Prevention of stroke by antihypertensive drug treatment in older persons with isolated systolic hypertension: final results of the Systolic Hypertension in the Elderly Program (SHEP). *J Am Med Assoc* 1991;265(24):3255–64

17. Staessen JA, Fagard R, Thijs L, *et al.* Randomized double-blind comparison of placebo and active treatment for older patients with isolated systolic hypertension. *Lancet* 1997;350:757–64

18. Hansson L, Lindholm LH, Ekbom T, *et al.* Randomised trial of old and new antihypertensive drugs in elderly patients: cardiovascular mortality and morbidity; the Swedish Trial in Old patients with Hypertension-2 study. *Lancet* 2000;354:1744–5

19. The Sixth Report of the Joint National Committee on Prevention, Detection, Evaluation, and Treatment of High Blood Pressure. *Arch Intern Med* 1997;157:2413–46

20. Cushman WC, Black HR, Probstiful JL, *et al.* Blood pressure control in the antihypertensive and lipid lowering treatment to prevent heart attack trial. *Am J Hypertens* 1998;11:17A

21. Hypertension Detection and Follow-up Program Cooperative Group. Five-year findings of the hypertension detection and follow-up. I: Reduction in mortality of persons with high blood pressure, including mild hypertension. *J Am Med Assoc* 1979;242:2562–71

22. Black HR. Optimal blood pressure: how low should we go? *Am J Hypertens* 1999;12: 113–20

23. Joffres MR, Ghadrian P, Fodod JG, *et al.* Awareness, treatment and control of hypertension in Canada. *Am J Hypertens* 1997;10: 1097–102

24. Colhoun HM, Dong W, Poulter NR. Blood pressure screening, management and control in England: results from the health survey for England 1994. *J Hypertens* 1998;16:747–52

25. Chamontin B, Poggi L, Lang T, *et al.* Prevalence, treatment, and control of hypertension in the French population: data from a survey on high blood pressure in general practice, 1994. *Am J Hypertens* 1998;11:759–62

26. Marques-Vidal P, Tuomilehto J. Hypertension awareness, treatment and control in the community: is the "rule of halves" still valid? *J Hum Hypertens* 1997;11:213–20

27. Whisnant JP. Effectiveness versus efficacy of treatment of hypertension for stroke prevention. *Neurrology* 1996;46:301–7

28. Marmot MG, Shipley MJ, Rose G. Inequalities in death – specific explanations of a general pattern? *Lancet* 1984;1:1003–6

29. Meissmer I, Whisnant JP, Sheps SG, *et al.* Detection and control of high blood pressure in the community: do we need a wake-up call? *Hypertension* 1999;34:466–71

30. House JS, James M, Lepkowski JM, *et al.* Age, socioeconomic status and health. *The Millbank Memorial Fund* 1990;63:383–411.

31. Sorlie PD, Backlund MS, Keller JB. US mortality by economic, demographic and social demographics: the national longitudinal mortality study. *Am J Public Health* 1995;85:949–56

32. Pappas G, Queen S, Hadden W, *et al.* The increasing disparity in mortality between socioeconomic groups in the United States, 1960–1986. *N Engl J Med* 1993;329:103–9

33. Lantz PM, House JS, Lepkowski JM, *et al.* Socioeconomic factors, health behaviors and mortality: results from a nationally-representative prospective study of U.S. adults. *J Am Med Assoc* 1998;279:1703–8

34. Lui K, Cedres LB, Stamler J, *et al.* Relationship of education to major risk factors and death from coronary heart disease, cardiovascular diseases and all causes. Findings of three Chicago epidemiologic studies. *Circulation* 1982;66:1308–14

35. Lynch JW, Kaplan GA, Cohen RD, *et al.* Do cardiovascular risk factors explain the relation

between socioeconomic status, risk of all-cause mortality, cardiovascular mortality, and acute myocardial infarction? *Am J Epidemiol* 1996; 144:934–42

36. Vogt TM, Mullooly JP, Ernst D, *et al*. Social networks as predictors of ischemic heart disease, cancer, stroke and hypertension: incidence, survival and mortality. *J Clin Epidemiol* 1992;45:659–66

37. Applegate BW, Ames SC, Mehan DJ, *et al*. Maximizing medication adherence in low-income hypertensives: a pilot study. *J Louisiana State Med Soc* 2000;152:349–56

38. Wang CY, Abbott LJ. Development of a community-based diabetes and hypertension preventative program. *Public Health Nurs* 1998;15:406–14

39. Brown CM. Exploring the role of religiosity in hypertension management among African-Americans. *J Health Care Poor and Underserved* 2000;11:19–32

40. Gerber JC, Stewart DL. Prevention and control of hypertension and diabetes in an underserved population through community detection and disease management: a plan of action. *J Assoc Academic Minority Physicians* 1998;9:48–52

41. Ward HJ, Morisky DE, Lees NB, Fong R. A clinic- and community-based approach to hypertension control for an underserved minority population: design and methods. *Am J Hypertens* 2000;13:177–83

42. Balkau B, Shipley M, Jarrett RJ, *et al*. High blood glucose concentration is a risk factor for mortality in middle-aged nondiabetic men. 20-year follow-up in the Whitehall Study, the Paris Prospective Study, and the Helsinki Policemen Study. *Diabetes Care* 1998;21(3): 360–7

43. Boysen G, Nyboe J, Appleyard M, *et al*. Stroke incidence and risk factors for stroke in Copenhagen, Denmark. *Stroke* 1988;19: 1345–53

44. Noto D, Barbagallo CM, Cavera G, *et al*. Leukocyte count, diabetes mellitus and age are strong predictors of stroke in a rural population in southern Italy: an 8-year follow-up. *Atherosclerosis* 2001;17:225–31

45. Abbott RD, Donahue RP, MacMahon SW, *et al*. Diabetes and the risk of stroke: the Honolulu Heart Program. *J Am Med Assoc* 1987;257:949–52

46. Barrett-Connor E, Khaw K. Diabetes mellitus: an independent risk factor for stroke. *Am J Epidemiol* 1988;128:116–24

47. Watkins PJ, Thomas PK. Diabetes mellitus and the nervous system. *J Neurol Neurosurg Psychiatry* 1998;65(5):620–32

48. Effect of intensive diabetes management on macrovascular events and risk factors in the Diabetes Control and Complications Trial. *Am J Cardiol* 1995;75:894–903

49. UK Prospective Diabetes Study Group. Intensive blood-glucose control with sulphonylureas or insulin compared with conventional treatment and risk of complications in patients with type 2 diabetes: UKPDS 33. *Lancet* 1998;352:837–53

50. The Diabetes Control and Complications Trial Research Group. The effect of intensive treatment of diabetes on the development and progression of long-term complications in insulin-dependent diabetes mellitus. *N Engl J Med* 1993;329(14):977–86

51. UK Prospective Diabetes Study Group. Tight blood pressure control and risk of macrovascular and microvascular complications in type 2 diabetes: UK PDS38. *Br Med J* 1998; 317:703–13

52. Heart Outcomes Prevention Evaluation Study Investigators. Effects of ramipril on cardiovascular and microvascular outcomes in people with diabetes mellitus: results of the HOPE study and MICRO-HOPE substudy. *Lancet* 2000;355:253–9

53. American Diabetes Association. Clinical practice recommendations 1998. *Diabetes Care* 1998;21(Suppl 1):S1–S89

54. Lantion-Ang LC. Epidemiology of diabetes in Western Pacific region: focus on Philippines. *Diabetes Res Clin Pres* 2000;50:S29–S34

55. Smith GD, Shipley MJ, Marmot MG, Rose G. Plasma cholesterol concentration and mortality. *J Am Med Assoc* 1992;267:70–6

56. Iso H, Jacobs DR, Wentworth D, *et al*. Serum cholesterol levels and six-year mortality from stroke in 350,977 men screened for the Multiple Risk Factor Intervention Trial. *N Engl J Med* 1989;320:904–10

57. Benfante R, Yano K, Hwang LJ, *et al*. Elevated serum cholesterol is a risk factor for both coronary heart disease and thromboembolic stroke in Hawaiian Japanese men: implications of shared risk. *Stroke* 1994;25: 814–20

58. Prospective Studies Collaboration. Cholesterol, diastolic blood pressure, and stroke: 13,000 strokes in 450,000 people in 45 prospective cohorts. *Lancet* 1995;346:1647–53

59. Qizilbash N, Duffy SW, Warlow C, Mann J. Lipids are risk factors for ischemic stroke – overview and review. *Cerebrovasc Dis* 1992;2: 127–36

60. Qizilbash N, Jones L, Warlow C, Mann J. Fibrinogen and lipid concentrations as risk factors for transient ischaemic attacks and minor ischaemic strokes. *Br Med J* 1991;303:605–9

61. Sacco RL, Benson RT, Kargman DE, *et al.* High-density lipoprotein cholesterol and ischemic stroke in the elderly: the Northern Manhattan Stroke Study. *J Am Med Assoc* 2001;285:2729–35

62. O'Leary DH, Anderson KM, Wolf PA, *et al.* Cholesterol and carotid atherosclerosis in older persons: the Framingham Study. *Ann Epidemiol* 1992;2:147–53

63. Salonen R, Seppanen K, Rauramaa R, Salonen JT. Prevalence of carotid atherosclerosis and serum cholesterol levels in eastern Finland. *Atherosclerosis* 1988;8:788–92

64. Shintani S, Kikuchi S, Hamaguchi H, Shiigai T. High serum lipoprotein(a) levels are an independent risk factor for cerebral infarction. *Stroke* 1993;24:965–9

65. Atkins D, Pstay B, Koepsell T, *et al.* Cholesterol reduction and the risk factors for stroke in men: a meta-analysis of randomized, controlled trials. *Ann Intern Med* 1993;119:136–45

66. Iso H, Jacobs D, Wentworth D, *et al.* Serum cholesterol levels and six-years mortality from stroke in 350,977 men screened for the Multiple Risk Factor Intervention Trial. *N Engl J Med* 1989;320:904–10

67. Scandinavian Simvastatin Survival Study Group. Randomized trial of cholesterol lowering in 4,444 patients with coronary heart disease: The Scandinavian Simvastatin Survival Study (4S). *Lancet* 1994;344:1383–9

68. Sacks FM, Pfeffer MA, Moye LA, *et al*, for the Cholesterol and Recurrent Events Trial Investigators. The effects of pravastatin on coronary events after myocardial infarction in patients with average cholesterol levels. *N Engl J Med* 1996;335:1001–9

69. The Long-Term Intervention with Pravastatin in Ischemic Disease (LIPID) Study Group. Prevention of cardiovascular events and death with pravastatin in patients with coronary heart disease and a broad range of initial cholesterol levels. *N Engl J Med* 1998;339: 1349–57

70. Hebert PR, Gaziano JM, Chan KS, Hennekens CH. Cholesterol lowering with statin drugs, risk of stroke, and total mortality. An overview of randomized trials. *J Am Med Assoc* 1997;278:313–21

71. Blauw GJ, Lagaay AM, Smelt AHM, Westendorp RGJ. Stroke, statins, and cholesterol: a meta-analysis of randomized, placebo-controlled, double-blind trials with HMG-CoA reductase inhibitors. *Stroke* 1997; 28:946–50

72. Blakenhorn DH, Selzer RH, Crawford DW, *et al.* Beneficial effects of colestipol-niacin therapy on the common carotid artery. Two- and four-year reduction of intimal-media thickness measured by ultrasound. *Circulation* 1993;88:20–8

73. Furberg CD, Adams HP, Applegate WB, *et al.*, for the Asymptomatic Carotid Artery Progression Study (ACAPS) Research Group. Effects of lovastatin on early carotid atherosclerosis and cardiovascular events. *Circulation* 1994;90:1679–87

74. Crouse JR, Byington RP, Bond MA, *et al.* Pravastatin, Lipids, and Atherosclerosis in the Carotid Arteries (PLAC-II). *Am J Cardiol* 1995;75:455–9

75. Salonen R, Nyyssonen K, Porkkala E, *et al.* Kuopio Atherosclerosis Prevention Study (KAPS): a population-based primary prevention trial of the effect of LDL lowering on atherosclerotic progression in carotid and femoral arteries. *Circulation* 1995;92:1758–64

76. Hodis HN, Mack WJ, LaBree L, *et al.* Reduction in carotid arterial wall thickness using lovostatin and dietary therapy: a randomized, controlled clinical trial. *Ann Intern Med* 1996;124:548–56

77. Executive summary of the third report of the National Cholesterol Education Program (NCEP) expert panel on detection, evaluation, and treatment of high blood cholesterol in adults (Adult Treatment Panel III). *J Am Med Assoc* 2001;285:2486–97

78. Centers for Disease Control: Smoking-attributable 1991 mortality and years of potential life lost – United States, 1988. *Morbid Mortal Weekly Rep* 1991;40(4):62, 69–71

79. Peto R, Lopez AD, Boreham J, *et al.* Mortality from tobacco in developed countries: indirect estimation from national statistics. *Lancet* 1992;339;1268–78

80. Donan GE, Adena MA, O'Malley HM, *et al.* Smoking as a risk factor for cerebral ischaemia. *Lancet* 1989;2:643–7

81. Shinton R, Beevers G. Meta-analysis of relation between cigarette smoking and stroke. *Br Med J* 1989;298:789–94

82. Kawachi I, Colditz GA, Stampfer MJ, *et al.* Smoking cessation and decreased risk of stroke in women. *J Am Med Assoc* 1993;269:232–6

83. Wolf PA, D'Agostino RB, Kannel WB, *et al.* Cigarette smoking as a risk factor for stroke. The Framingham study. *J Am Med Assoc* 1988;259:1025–9

84. Sacco RL, Roberts JK, Boden-Albala B, *et al.* Race-ethnicity and determinants of carotid atherosclerosis in a multi-ethnic population: the Northern Manhattan Stroke Study. *Stroke* 1997;27:929–35

85. Wolf PA. Cigarettes, alcohol and stroke. *N Engl J Med* 1986;315:1087–9

86. Kawachi I, Colditz G, Stampfer M, *et al.* Smoking cessation and decreased risk of stroke in women. *J Am Med Assoc* 1993;269(2): 232–6

87. Wolf PA, Belanger AJ, D'Agostino RB. Management of risk factors. *Neurol Clin* 1992;10:177–91

88. Rose G, Hamilton PJS, Colwell L, Shipley MJ. A randomised controlled trial of anti-smoking advice: 10 year results. *J Epidemiol Comm Health* 1982;36:102–8

89. Bonita R, Duncan J, Truelson T, *et al.* Passive smoking as well as active smoking increases the risk of acute stroke. *Tob Control* 1999;8: 156–60

90. The COMMIT Research Group: Community Intervention Trial for Smoking Cessation (COMMIT). I. Cohort results from a four-year community intervention and II. Changes in adult cigarette smoking prevalence. *Am J Public Health* 1995;85:183–92, 193–200

91. Gorelick PB. Stroke prevention: windows of opportunity and failed expectations – a discussion of modifiable cardiovascular risk factors and a prevention proposal. *Neuroepidemiology* 1997;16:163–73

92. Pate RR, Pratt M, Blair SN, *et al.* Physical activity and public health: a recommendation from the Centers for Disease Control and Prevention and the American College of Sports Medicine. *J Am Med Assoc* 1995;273: 402–7

93. NIH Consensus Development Panel on Physical Activity and Cardiovascular Health. Physical activity and cardiovascular health. *J Am Med Assoc* 1996;276:241–6

94. Manson JE, Stampfer MJ, Willett WC, *et al.* Physical activity and incidence of coronary heart disease and stroke in women. *Circulation* 1995;91(suppl):5

95. Fischer HG. Koenig W. Physical activity and coronary heart disease. *Cardiologia* 1998; 43(10):1027–35

96. Fletcher GF. Exercise in the prevention of stroke. *Health Reports* 1994;6:106–10

97. Abbott RD, Rodriguez BL, Burchfiel CM, Curb JD. Physical activity in older middle-aged men and reduced risk of stroke: the Honolulu Heart Program. *Am J Epidemiol* 1994;139:881–93

98. Kiely DK, Wolf PA, Cupples LA, *et al.* Physical activity and stroke risk: the Framingham Study. *Am J Epidemiol* 1994;140:608–20

99. Haheim LL, Holme I, Hjermann I, Leren P. Risk factors of stroke incidence and mortality. A 12-year follow-up of the Oslo Study. *Stroke* 1993;24:1484–9

100. Lindenstrom E, Boysen G, Nyboe J. Lifestyle factors and risk of cerebrovascular disease in women. The Copenhagen City Heart Study. *Stroke* 1993;24:1468–72

101. Gillum RF, Mussolino ME, Ingram DD. Physical activity and stroke incidence in women and men – The NHANES I Epidemiologic Follow-up Study. *Am J Epidemiol* 1996;143:860–9

102. Sacco RL, Gan R, Boden-Albala B, *et al.* Leisure-time physical activity and ischemic stroke risk: the Northern Manhattan Stroke Study. *Stroke* 1998;29:380–7

103. Wannamethee G, Shaper AG. Physical activity and stroke in British middle aged men. *Br Med J* 1992;304:597–601

104. Shinton R, Sagar G. Lifelong exercise and stroke. *Br Med J* 1993;307:231–4

105. Hu FB, Stampfer MJ, Colditz G, *et al.* Physical activity and risk of stroke in women. *J Am Med Assoc* 2000;283:2961–7

106. Evenson KR, Rosamond WD, Cai J, *et al.* Physical activity and ischemic stroke risk. The atherosclerotic risk in communities study. *Stroke* 1999;30(7):1333–9

107. Kokkinos PF, Narayan P, Colleran JA, *et al.* Effects of regular exercise on blood

pressure and left ventricular hypertrophy in African-American men with severe hypertension. *N Engl J Med* 1995;333:1462–7

108. Blair SN, Kampert JB, Kohl HW III, *et al.* Influences of cardiorespiratory fitness and other precursors on cardiovascular disease and all-cause mortality in men and women. *J Am Med Assoc* 1996;276:205–10

109. Manson JE, Rimm EB, Stampfer MJ, *et al.* A prospective study of physical activity and incidence of non-insulin-dependent diabetes mellitus in women. *Lancet* 1991;338:774–8

110. Lakka TA, Salonen JT. Moderate to high intensity conditioning leisure time physical activity and high cardiorespiratory fitness are associated with reduced plasma fibrinogen in eastern Finnish men. *J Clin Epidemiol* 1993;46:1119–27

111. Wang JS, Jen CJ, Chen HI. Effects of exercise training and deconditioning on platelet function in men. *Arterioscler Thromb Vasc Biol* 1995;15:1668–74

112. Rangemark C, Hedner JA, Carlson JT, *et al.* Platelet function and fibrinolytic activity in hypertensive and normotensive sleep apnea patients. *Sleep* 1995;18:188–94

113. Lee IM, Hennekens CH, Berger K, *et al.* Exercise and risk of stroke in male physicians. *Stroke* 1999;30:1–6

114. Williams PT. High-density lipoprotein cholesterol and other risk factors for coronary heart disease in female runners. *N Engl J Med* 1996;334:1298–303

115. Nygard O, Vollset SE, Refsum H, *et al.* Total plasma homocysteine and cardiovascular risk profile – the Hordaland Homocysteine Study. *J Am Med Assoc* 1995;274:1526–33

116. US Department of Health and Human Services. *Physical Activity and Health: A Report of the Surgeon General.* Atlanta, GA: US Department of Health and Human Services, Center for Disease Control and Prevention, National Center for Chronic Disease Prevention and Health Promotion, 1996

117. Department of Health and Human Services. *Healthy People 2000: National Health Promotion and Disease Prevention Objectives.* Washington, DC: Department of Health and Human Services, 1991: DHHS publication no. (PHS) 91-50213

118. Archer L, Grant BF, Dawson DA. What if Americans drank less? The potential effect on the prevalence of alcohol abuse and dependence. *Am J Public Health* 1995; 85:61–6

119. Donahue RP, Abbott RD, Reed DM, Yano K. Alcohol and hemorrhagic stroke: the Honolulu Heart Study. *J Am Med Assoc* 1986;255:2311–14

120. Stampfer MJ, Colditz GA, Willett WA, *et al.* A prospective study of moderate alcohol consumption and the risk of coronary disease and stroke in women. *N Engl J Med* 1988;319: 267–73

121. Tanaka H, Ueda Y, Hayashi M, *et al.* Risk factors for cerebral hemorrhage and cerebral infarction in a Japanese rural community. *Stroke* 1982;13:62–73

122. Hillbom M, Kaste M. Does ethanol intoxication promote brain infarction in young adults? *Lancet* 1978;2:1181–3

123. Gorelick PB. The status of alcohol as a risk factor for stroke. *Stroke* 1989;20:1607–10

124. Gorelick PB, Rodin MB, Lagenberg P, *et al.* Is acute alcohol ingestion a risk factor for ischemic stroke? Results of a controlled study in middle-aged and elderly stroke patients at three urban medical centers. *Stroke* 1987;18: 359–64

125. Boysen G, Nyboe J, Appleyard M, *et al.* Stroke incidence and risk factors for stroke in Copenhagen, Denmark. *Stroke* 1988;19: 1345–53

126. Klatsky AL, Armstrong MA, Friedman GD. Alcohol use and subsequent cerebrovascular disease hospitalizations. *Stroke* 1989;20: 741–6

127. Palomäki H, Kaste M. Regular light-to-moderate intake of alcohol and the risk of ischemic stroke: is there a beneficial effect? *Stroke* 1993;24:1828–32

128. Klatsky AL, Friedman GD. Annotation: alcohol and longevity. *Am J Public Health* 1995; 85:16–18

129. Camargo CA. Moderate alcohol consumption and stroke: the epidemiologic evidence. *Stroke* 1989;20:1611–26

130. Gill JS, Zezulka AV, Shipley MJ, *et al.* Stroke and alcohol consumption. *N Engl J Med* 1996;315:1041–6

131. Sacco RL, Elkind ME, Boden-Albala B. The protective effect of moderate alcohol consumption on ischemic stroke. *J Am Med Assoc* 1999;281:53–60

132. Berger K, Ajani UA, Kase CS, *et al.* Light to moderate alcohol consumption and the risk of stroke among U.S. male physicians. *N Engl J Med* 1999;341:1557–64

133. Thornton J, Symes C, Heaton K. Moderate alcohol intake reduces bile cholesterol saturation and raises HDL cholesterol. *Lancet* 1983;2:819–22

134 Puddey IB, Croft KD, Abdu-Amsha Caccetta R, Beilin LJ. Alcohol, free radicals and antioxidants. *Novartis Foundation Symposium* 1998;216:51–62

Chapter 4

Cardiac disease and risk of ischemic stroke

Richard F. Gillum, MD

INTRODUCTION

Ischemic stroke is a preventable cause of major morbidity and mortality in the US and worldwide[1–10]. In 1998 stroke was the underlying cause of 158 448 deaths in the US, following only heart disease and cancer as a leading cause of death[3]. An estimated 700 000 first strokes occur each year and there are an estimated 4.4 million stroke survivors[1]. The American Heart Association estimated the economic burden of stroke at $51 billion in 1999[1]. It is possible to identify persons at high risk for stroke for specific interventions, for example persons with certain forms of heart disease constitute one such group[1,3,5,7,10]. An estimated 20% of ischemic strokes are due to cardioembolism[1]. Table 1 shows the estimated number of US hospital discharges with diagnoses of cerebral embolism, necessarily an underestimate of case numbers since many cases may receive less specific diagnoses. Further, atherosclerosis in cardiac and cerebral arteries is highly correlated, sharing several

risk factors[1]. Thus, improved cardiac treatment modalities and survival and an aging population provide an increasing pool of persons at risk for ischemic stroke[1,3–9]. In the US in 1996, there were an estimated 20.7 million persons living with heart disease[5]. This chapter will discuss the epidemiology and potential for prevention of stroke in such persons.

ATRIAL FIBRILLATION

Prevalence and incidence

Heart disease, especially atrial fibrillation (AF), is an established risk factor for ischemic stroke[1,5,7,10–14]. Mechanisms of cerebral embolism of cardiac origin have been discussed at length elsewhere[12,13], as has the epidemiology of atrial fibrillation[5,11,15–20]. The prevalence of AF increases with age[11]. Among 244 blacks aged 65 and over in the Cardiovascular Health Study,

Table 1 Estimated number of hospital discharges (thousands) with cerebral embolism as the primary or secondary diagnosis in the USA, 1989–98

Year	1989	1990	1991	1992	1993	1994	1995	1996	1997	1998
Number	33	29	40	44	46	44	47	55	54	46

Source: National Hospital Discharge Survey

Table 2 Estimated number of hospital discharges (thousands) with atrial fibrillation as the primary or secondary diagnosis in the USA, 1989–98

Year	1989	1990	1991	1992	1993	1994	1995	1996	1997	1998
Number	1050	1103	1241	1360	1455	1586	1618	1814	2011	2101

Source: National Hospital Discharge Survey

1.5% of men and 3.6% of women had ever been told by a doctor they had AF[18]. Among 4926 whites, rates were 6.0% in men and 4.8% in women. AF diagnosed by electrocardiogram (ECG) was reported in 1.1% of black men and 0.7% of black women compared to 4.0% and 2.7%, respectively, in whites (non-significant racial difference). The prevalence of abnormal left atrial size ranged from 13.9% in black women to 21.4% in white men. In one large US study, whites were more likely than blacks to have AF at ages over 50 years (prevalence in whites 2.2%, in blacks 1.5%, $p < 0.001$)[19]. Among patients with acute myocardial infarction (AMI) in a clinical trial, the frequency of atrial fibrillation prior to randomization was 1.8% in blacks and 6.7% in whites[21].

In the US in 1998, there were 2 101 000 hospital discharges with any diagnosis of atrial fibrillation[20], a doubling of the number per annum since 1989 (Table 2)[17,20]. One report of AF incidence is from the Cardiovascular Health Study. In persons aged 65 and over, the incidence was higher with advancing age, in males, among whites, those with a history of cardiac disease, those using diuretics, those not using beta blockers, and those with higher systolic blood pressure, fasting glucose levels, ECG cardiac injury score and left atrial size[22]. Thus, in the US, the number of elderly persons with AF is large and increasing[19].

Association of AF with ischemic stroke

AF is a potent risk factor for stroke[1,10]. The annual risk of stroke in patients with non-valvular AF ranges from 3 to 5%[1]. Silent cerebral infarcts occur in another 1 to 2%, which may account for the increased risk of dementia and cognitive dysfunction in patients with AF[7]. AF is estimated to be responsible for 50% of thromboembolic strokes[1], and about two-thirds of stroke in patients with AF are thromboembolic[1]. A study of 4 million Medicare recipients followed for four years revealed that compared to those without AF black men and women with AF had 1.4 and 1.7 times the risk for non-embolic stroke and 4.3 and 7.3 times the risk for embolic stroke, respectively[23]. Four-year risks were highest in black women with AF (21.3% for non-embolic and 3.28% for embolic stroke). The association was similar in whites. In a series of 430 hospitalized stroke patients with acute ischemic stroke in New York City, atrial fibrillation was less prevalent in blacks (11%) than whites (29%); the mean age was 70 in blacks and 80 in whites; age-adjusted results were not presented[24]. Within the population of patients with AF, the highest risk for thromboembolic stroke has been observed with advancing age, among females over 75 years, among those with prior stroke or transient ischemic attack (TIA) or systemic embolism, systolic hypertension, impaired left ventricular function, prosthetic heart valve, rheumatic mitral valve disease or diabetes mellitus[1,7].

Prevention of stroke

Numerous clinical trials have demonstrated the effectiveness of antithrombotic and antiplatelet therapy in reducing the risk of stroke in AF[1,7,25-29]. Five placebo-controlled trials of the efficacy of warfarin in the primary prevention of stroke in patients with AF were combined for analysis of data, showing that treatment with adjusted-dose warfarin reduced the risk of thromboembolic stroke by 68% compared with placebo[1,27,28]. Aspirin alone has been advocated for the prevention of stroke in younger AF patients with none of the risk factors for thromboembolic stroke listed above[1,7]. Aspirin may primarily prevent non-embolic cerebral infarction in AF[7,29]. Prevention of chronic or intermittent AF will also contribute to the prevention of stroke, hence the importance of using beta blockers and ACE inhibitors when indicated, blood pressure and blood glucose control, and vigorous management of predisposing diseases[7,16,22]. Also important are drug therapy and cardioversion of new onset AF to maintain the sinus rhythm, and treatment of underlying cardiac disease[7,16].

CORONARY HEART DISEASE

Prevalence and incidence

In developed countries such as the US, coronary heart disease (CHD) is the leading cause of death in whites and blacks, with age-adjusted death rates of blacks now exceeding those of whites in both women and men using the 1940 age standard[2-5,30-33]. In 1998 in the US, there were 783 000 hospital discharges with the diagnosis of acute myocardial infarction (AMI)[20]. An estimated 12.4 million Americans have a history of CHD (myocardial infarction, angina pectoris or both)[32]. Patterns of incidence are well described[4,5,30,32].

Association of CHD with ischemic stroke

Ischemic cerebral infarction has long been recognized as a complication of acute myocardial infarction[5,10,13,31,34]. Even in the subset of cases of AMI patients receiving recombinant tissue plasminogen activator (rt-PA) and heparin, cerebral infarction still occurs in about one percent within four weeks, as reported in the Thrombolysis in Myocardial Infarction II (TIMI-II) clinical trial[34]. In the Framingham Study 8% of men and 11% of women had a stroke within six years following AMI[1]. In analyses of the risk of cerebral infarction in the National Health and Nutrition Examination Survey (NHANES) I Epidemiologic Follow-up Study[35], there was a significant interaction of race with history of heart disease ($p = 0.01$), indicating a different effect on risk in blacks than whites. Blacks with and without a history of heart disease had a similar risk for cerebral infarction, while whites with a history of heart disease had a much greater risk than those without[24,35]. Thus, CHD and AMI are risk factors for ischemic stroke, and prevention of ischemic stroke remains an objective of the management of CHD and AMI[31].

Prevention

Antithrombotic therapy with aspirin is advocated for patients with CHD for prevention of both recurrent AMI and ischemic stroke. Ventricular thrombus in the setting of AMI is an indication for anticoagulation[31]. Primary prevention of CHD remains of vital importance[32,33].

Post-hoc analyses of data from clinical trials of secondary and primary prevention of CHD with hydroxy methylglutaryl coenzyme A reductase (HMG-Co-A) inhibitors or 'statins' have led to a re-examination of the role of lipid lowering in stroke prevention. Such therapy has been shown to lower the risk of ischemic stroke by up to 51% in several clinical trials[1,36]. Secondary and primary stroke prevention trials of statin therapy are now under way. Meanwhile there is already persuasive evidence for prescribing statin treatment for ischemic stroke patients with prior AMI or hyperlipidemia. Data from ongoing trials will clarify the role of statin drugs for other subgroups of ischemic stroke patients and for primary prevention of stroke.

CONGESTIVE HEART FAILURE

Prevalence and incidence

In the US an estimated 4.8 million persons have congestive heart failure[37]. Prevalence rates increase from 2% at age 40–59 to 10% at age 70 and over. In persons over 65, echocardiograms show an enlarged left ventricle (LV) in 16.7% of white men and 6.8% of white women and abnormal LV ejection fraction (EF) in 14.1% of white men and 5.1% of white women[18]. Myocardial disease and congestive heart failure (CHF) are more common in men than women and blacks than whites in the US[37–49]. Prevalence rates increased at each age between national surveys done in 1976–80 and 1988–91. Hospital discharge rates increased steadily, tripling between 1970 and 1995[37]. In 1998 there were 3.3 million discharges with diagnoses of CHF[20], and an estimated 550 000 new cases occur annually[32]. The incidence of heart failure increases with age, hypertension, and a history of AMI[4]. The epidemiology of hypertension and hypertensive heart disease, both more common in blacks than whites, has been reviewed at length elsewhere[4,41–43].

Association of heart failure with ischemic stroke

Severe CHF due to idiopathic dilated cardiomyopathy, ischemia, hypertension or other causes increases the risk of thromboembolic stroke[1]. However, data quantifying the risk are relatively few[23,24]. In a large Medicare cohort, patients with CHF had increased risk over four years of follow-up of both non-embolic (relative risk (RR) 1.40) and embolic (RR 1.69) stroke[23]. An analysis of data from heart failure trials suggests an incidence of arterial thromboembolism ranging from 0.9 to 5.5 events per 100 patient-years[45]. Based on these data, an association of CHF with stroke is likely[1,13].

Prevention of stroke

Supervening AF is an indication for antithrombotic therapy as described above[44,45]. Other clinical indicators of high risk for thromboembolism such as LV EF less than 20–25% are sometimes managed with anticoagulants, but evidence from clinical trials is needed in such patients[45,46].

OTHER CARDIAC AND VASCULAR CAUSES OF ISCHEMIC STROKE

Valvular heart disease

Studies have linked valvular heart disease to an increased risk of ischemic stroke[10–13,23,50–55]. Rheumatic heart disease and infective endocarditis remain serious problems, especially in less developed nations[12,50]. In hospitalized medicare patients free of stroke, rheumatic heart disease affected 24% of those with AF and 0.4% of those without AF[23]. Mitral valve prolapse reportedly occurs with substantial frequency in the US[51–54]. Mobile, filamentous strands on the mitral or aortic valve were associated with stroke in a case–control study (odds ratio 2.0, CI 0.4–9.3) with large numbers taking part[55]. Thus, persons with these conditions are probably at increased risk for embolic stroke. Appropriate antithrombotic therapy with warfarin for high-risk and aspirin for low-risk patients, in combination with treatment of the underlying condition, may be indicated for the prevention of stroke[1].

Other causes

The relationship of left ventricular hypertrophy (LVH) to stroke has been little studied.

Table 3 Estimated number of coronary revascularization procedures performed in persons aged 65 years and over in the USA, 1989–98

Year	1989	1990	1991	1992	1993	1994	1995	1996	1997	1998
CABG	137 768	142 902	140 452	174 146	169 129	172 043	208 576	210 469	209 503	189 502
PTCA	107 047	115 000	142 599	191 907	183 118	202 736	208 539	321 780	339 876	456 157

CABG, coronary artery bypass graft; PTCA, percutaneous transluminal coronary angioplasty
Source: National Hospital Discharge Survey

Table 4 US health promotion and disease prevention goals and objectives for the year 2010: heart disease

Goals
Increase quality and years of healthy life
Eliminate health disparities
Improve cardiovascular health and quality of life through the prevention, detection, and treatment of
   risk factors; early identification and treatment of heart attacks and strokes; and prevention of
   recurrent cardiovascular events

Objectives
Reduce coronary heart disease deaths
Increase the proportion of adults aged 20 years and older who are aware of the early warning
   symptoms and signs of a heart attack and the importance of accessing rapid emergency
   care by calling 911
Increase the proportion of eligible patients with heart attacks who receive artery-opening
   therapy within an hour of symptom onset
Increase the proportion of adults aged 20 years and older who call 911 and administer
   cardiopulmonary resuscitation (CPR) when they witness an out-of-hospital cardiac arrest
Increase the proportion of persons with witnessed out-of-hospital cardiac arrest who are
   eligible and receive their first therapeutic electrical shock within 6 minutes after collapse recognition
Reduce hospitalizations of older adults with heart failure as the principal diagnosis

Source: Healthy People 2010 Conference Edition, CD-ROM, US Dept of Health and Human Services, 2000. (Detailed information also available at http://www.health.gov/healthypeople)

In the North Manhattan population-based study, LVH determined by ECG was more frequent in black (20%) than white (9%) stroke victims[24]. Antecedent electrocardiographic abnormalities were associated with a marked increased risk for stroke only in white men in the Evans County, Georgia, study[49]. Approximate age-adjusted relative risks were 1.3 for black men, 1.9 for white men, 1.3 for black women and 1.3 for white women. Also associated with stroke is sick sinus syndrome[13] and possible associations of other cardiac rhythm disorders with embolic stroke have been discussed elsewhere[12]. Global cerebral ischemia and focal deficits occur in some survivors of cardiac arrest[13,56,57].

Dissecting aortic aneurysm, and carotid artery dissection may also cause ischemic stroke[13,58] while proximal aortic atheromas occurred with increased frequency in stroke cases in a study by Di Tullio *et al.*[59]. Intracardiac congenital defects may increase the risk of stroke[1,12,13]; for example, in one study, patent foramen ovale was a risk factor for ischemic stroke in whites and Hispanics though not in blacks[60].

Coronary bypass surgery (CABG) and open heart surgery are common procedures that are associated with a 1 to 7% risk of perioperative stroke[1,61–65]. In 1998, 336 000 coronary bypass procedures (CABG) in all ages were performed in the US[20]. Table 3 shows the rise in the number of CABG and percutaneous transluminal coronary angioplasty (PTCA) procedures performed in the US on persons aged 65 and over during the last decade. Data from the Society of Thoracic Surgery National Cardiac Surgery Database revealed that in 1996–7 2.4% of men and 3.8% of women undergoing any cardiac surgery suffered postoperative stroke, transient ischemic attack and/or coma[66]. The risk of perioperative stroke is highest in patients with a prior stroke, advanced age, diabetes, AF, proximal aortic atherosclerosis, valve surgery and long duration of cardiopulmonary bypass[1,61,64–66]. Thus, measures for the prevention of early and late stroke after cardiac surgery are indicated – as discussed at length in cardiology and surgery texts. These include antithrombotic therapy, increased use of percutaneous angioplasty and the development of new techniques that do not require cardiopulmonary bypass. The drop in the number of CABG procedures in 1998 suggests that the increasing frequency of angioplasty may lead to a decrease in the number of CABG procedures and perioperative strokes in the future (Table 3).

RESEARCH, HEALTH PROMOTION AND DISEASE PREVENTION NEEDS

The role of cardiac disease in slowing the rate of decline in stroke mortality in the 1990s should be investigated[32]. Both the decline of a competing cause of mortality and the increase in the prevalence of a stroke risk factor should be considered as mechanisms. Case–control studies should be performed to estimate the relative odds of ischemic stroke associated with CHF without AF and less common types of heart disease discussed above. The larger population-based cohort studies may also be able to provide data on the risk associated with LVH by echocardiography or electrocardiogram. Data from national registries of AMI, other diseases, and cardiac surgery and from Medicare may also be valuable resources for analysis of the elderly American population. Meta-analyses should continue to be performed of all studies of anticoagulation and antiplatelet therapy in the setting of heart disease in population subgroups. Safer and more effective antiarrhythmic and antithrombotic agents are needed. As mentioned above, further research is needed to clarify and possibly expand the role of statins in the secondary and primary prevention of stroke[1,36,67–69]. New techniques, procedures and strategies for preventing perioperative stroke associated with cardiac surgery should be tested in clinical trials. Improved intervention strategies should be sought to implement programs to attain the US health promotion and disease prevention goals and objectives for heart disease by the year 2010 (Table 4)[8,9,32].

References

1. Goldstein LB, Adams R, Becker K, *et al*. Primary prevention of ischemic stroke: a statement for healthcare professionals from the Stroke Council of the American Heart Association. *Circulation* 2001;103:163–82
2. Murray CJ, Lopez AD. Mortality by cause for eight regions of the world: Global Burden of Disease Study. *Lancet* 1997;349(9061):1269–76
3. National Center for Health Statistics. *Health, United States, 2000 with adolescent health chartbook*. Hyattsville, Maryland, 2000.
4. Gillum RF, Feinleib M. Cardiovascular disease in the United States: Mortality, prevalence, and incidence. In Kapoor AS, Singh BN, eds. *Prognosis and Risk Assessment in Cardiovascular Disease*. New York: Churchill Livingston Inc., 1993:49–59

5. Gillum RF, Thomas J, Curry CL. Atrial fibrillation, heart disease, and ischemic stroke in blacks. In Gillum RF, Gorelick PB, Cooper ES, eds. *Stroke in Blacks*. Basel: Karger, 1999: 129–41

6. Gillum RF. The epidemiology of stroke in blacks. In Gillum RF, Gorelick PB, Cooper ES, eds. *Stroke in Blacks*. Basel: Karger, 1999:83–93

7. Ezekowitz MD, Levine JA. Preventing stroke in patients with atrial fibrillation. *J Am Med Assoc* 1999;281:1830–5

8. US Department of Health and Human Services. *Healthy People 2010: understanding and improving health*. Washington, DC: US Department of Health and Human Services, Government Printing Office, 2000

9. US Department of Health and Human Services. *Healthy People 2010: objectives for improving health*. Washington, DC: US Department of Health and Human Services, Government Printing Office, 2000

10. Sacco RL. Ischemic stroke. In Gorelick PB, Alter M, eds. *Handbook of neuroepidemiology*. New York: Marcel Dekker, Inc., 1994: 77–119

11. Kannel WB, Abbott DR, Savage DD, McNamara PM. Epidemiologic features of chronic atrial fibrillation. *N Engl J Med* 1982; 306:1018–22

12. Salgado ED, Furlan AJ, Conomy JP. Cardioembolic sources of stroke. In Furlan AJ, ed. *The Heart and Stroke. Exploring mutual cerebrovascular and cardiovascular issues*. London: Springer-Verlag, 1987:47–61

13. Caplan LR. *Stroke: a Clinical Approach*. Boston: Butterworth-Heinemann, 1993

14. Gillum RF. Stroke in blacks. *Stroke* 1988; 19:1–9

15. Camm AJ, Obel OA. Epidemiology and mechanism of atrial fibrillation and atrial flutter. *Am J Cardiol* 1996;78(8A):3–11

16. Allessie MA, Boyden PA, Camm J, *et al.* Pathophysiology and prevention of atrial fibrillation. *Circulation* 2001;103:769–77

17. Wolf PA, Benjamin EJ, Belanger AJ, *et al.* Secular trends in the prevalence of atrial fibrillation: The Framingham Study. *Am Heart J* 1996;131(4):790–5

18. Manolio TA, Burke GL, Psaty BM, *et al.* Black–white differences in subclinical cardiovascular disease among older adults: the Cardiovascular Health Study. *J Clin Epidemiol* 1995;48: 1141–52

19. Go AS, Hylek EM, Phillips KA, *et al.* Prevalence of diagnosed atrial fibrillation in adults. National implications for rhythm management and stroke prevention: the AnTicoagulation and Risk Factors in Atrial Fibrillation (ATRIA) Study. *J Am Med Assoc* 2001;285:2370–5

20. Popovic JR, Kozak LJ, Graves EJ. National Hospital Discharge Survey: Annual Summary, 1998. National Center for Health Statistics. *Vital Health Stat* 2000;13(148):1–42

21. Haywood LJ. Coronary heart disease mortality/ morbidity and risk in blacks. I: Clinical manifestations and diagnostic criteria: the experience with the Beta Blocker Heart Attack Trial. *Am Heart J* 1984;108:787–93

22. Psaty BM, Manolio TA, Kuller LH, *et al.* Incidence of and risk factors for atrial fibrillation in older adults. *Circulation* 1997;96: 2455–61

23. Yuan Z, Bowlin S, Einstadter D, *et al.* Atrial fibrillation as a risk factor for stroke: a retrospective cohort study of hospitalized Medicare beneficiaries. *Am J Public Health* 1998;88: 395–400

24. Sacco RL, Kargman DE, Zamanillo M. Race-ethnic differences in stroke risk – factors among hospitalized patients with cerebral infarction – the Northern Manhattan Stroke Study. *Neurology* 1995;45:659–63

25. Laupacis A, Albers G, Dalen J. Antithrombotic therapy in atrial fibrillation. *Chest* 1998; 114(Suppl):579S–589S

26. Stroke Prevention in Atrial Fibrillation Investigators. Stroke Prevention in Atrial Fibrillation Study: final results. *Circulation* 1991;84:527–39

27. The Atrial Fibrillation Investigators. Risk factors for stroke and efficacy of antithrombotic therapy in atrial fibrillation: analysis of pooled data from five randomized controlled trials. *Arch Intern Med* 1994;154:1449–57

28. Hart RG, Benavente O, McBride R, Pearce LA. Antithrombotic therapy to prevent stroke in patients with atrial fibrillation: a meta-analysis. *Ann Intern Med* 1999;131:492–501

29. Hart RG, Pearce LA, Miller VT, *et al.* Cardioembolic vs. noncardioembolic strokes in atrial fibrillation: frequency and effect of antithrombotic agents in stroke prevention in atrial fibrillation studies. *Cerebrovasc Dis* 2000;10:39–43

30. Gillum RF, Mussolino ME, Madans JH. Coronary heart disease incidence and survival

in African-American women and men: The NHANES I Epidemiologic Follow-up Study. *Ann Intern Med* 1997;127:111–18

31. Ryan TJ, Anderson JL, Antman EM, *et al.* ACC/AHA guidelines for the management of patients with acute myocardial infarction. A report of the American College of Cardiology/American Heart Association Task Force on Practice Guidelines (Committee on Management of Acute Myocardial Infarction). *J Am Coll Cardiol* 1996;28:1328–428

32. Cooper R, Cutler J, Desvigne-Nickens P, *et al.* Trends and disparities in coronary heart disease, stroke, and other cardiovascular diseases in the United States. Findings of the National Conference on Cardiovascular Disease Prevention. *Circulation* 2000;102:3137–47

33. Pearson TA, Criqui MH, Luepker RV, *et al.* *Primer in Preventive Cardiology.* Dallas, Texas: American Heart Association, 1994

34. Sloan MA, Price TR, Terrin ML, *et al.* Ischemic cerebral infarction after rt-PA and heparin therapy for acute myocardial infarction. The TIMI-II pilot and randomized clinical trial combined experience. *Stroke* 1997;28:1107–14

35. Giles WH, Kittner SJ, Heble JR, *et al.* Determinants of black-white differences in the risk for cerebral infarction: the National Health and Nutrition Examination Survey Epidemiologic Follow-up Study. *Arch Intern Med* 1995; 155:1319–24

36. Byington RP, Davis BR, Plehn JF, *et al.* Reduction of stroke events with pravastatin. The Prospective Pravastatin Pooling (PPP) Project. *Circulation* 2001;103:387–92

37. Congestive heart failure in the United States: a new epidemic. Bethesda, Md: National Heart, Lung, and Blood Institute, 1996:1–6

38. Gillum RF. Epidemiology of heart failure in the United States. *Am Heart J* 1993;126:1042–7

39. Gillum RF. Idiopathic cardiomyopathy in the United States, 1970–1982. *Am Heart J* 1986; 111:752–5

40. Gillum RF. The epidemiology of cardiomyopathy in the United States. *Prog Cardiol* 1989; 2:11–21

41. Flack JM, Wiist WH. Epidemiology of hypertension and hypertensive target-organ damage in the United States. *J Assoc Acad Minor Phys* 1991;2(4):143–50

42. Cooper ES, Caplan LR. Cerebrovascular disease in hypertensive blacks. *Cardiovasc Clin* 1991;21(3):145–55

43. Thomas J, Semenya K, Thomas DJ, *et al.* Precursors of hypertension in black compared to white medical students. *J Chron Dis* 1987; 40:721–7

44. Gomberg-Maitland M, Baran DA, Fuster V. Treatment of congestive heart failure: guidelines for the primary care physician and the heart failure specialist. *Arch Intern Med* 2001;161:342–52

45. Guidelines for the evaluation and management of heart failure. Report of the American College of Cardiology/American Heart Association Task Force on Practice Guidelines (Committee on Evaluation and Management of Heart Failure). *J Am Coll Cardiol* 1995;26: 1376–98

46. Pullicino PM, Halperin JL, Thompson JLP. Stroke in patients with heart failure and reduced left ventricular ejection fraction. *Neurology* 2000;54:288–94

47. Aronow WS, Ahn C, Kronzon I, Koenigsberg M. Congestive heart failure, coronary events, and atherothrombotic brain infarction in elderly blacks and whites with systemic hypertension and with and without echocardiographic and electrocardiographic evidence of left ventricular hypertrophy. *Am J Cardiol* 1991;67:295–9

48. Bonner LL, Kanter DS, Manson JE. Primary prevention of stroke. *N Engl J Med* 1995;333: 1392–400

49. Heyman A, Karp HR, Heyden S, *et al.* Cerebrovascular disease in the bi-racial population of Evans County, Georgia. *Stroke* 1971;2: 509–18

50. Gillum RF. Trends in acute rheumatic fever and chronic rheumatic heart disease – a national perspective. *Am Heart J* 1986;111:430–2

51. Savage DD, Devereux RB, Donahue R. Mitral valve prolapse in blacks. *J Natl Med Assoc* 1982;74:895–900

52. Savage DD, Garrison RJ, Castelli WP, *et al.* Prevalence of submitral (annular) calcium and its correlates in a general population-based sample (The Framingham Study). *Am J Cardiol* 1983;51:1375–8

53. Lauzier S, Barnett HJM. Cerebral ischemia with mitral valve prolapse and mitral annulus calcification. In Furlan AJ, ed. *The Heart and Stroke. Exploring mutual cerebrovascular and cardiovascular issues.* London: Springer-Verlag, 1987:63–100

54. Petty GW, Khandheria BK, Whisnant JP, *et al.* Predictors of cerebrovascular events and death

among patients with valvular heart disease: a population-based study. *Stroke* 2000;31: 2628–35

55. Roberts JK, Omarali I, Di Tullio MR, *et al.* Valvular strands and cerebral ischemia: effect of demographics and strand characteristics. *Stroke* 1997;28:2185–8

56. Gillum RF. Sudden coronary death in the United States, 1980–1985. *Circulation* 1989; 79:756–65

57. Gillum RF. Sudden cardiac death in Hispanic Americans and African Americans. *Am J Public Health* 1997;87:1461–6

58. Gillum RF. Epidemiology of aortic aneurysm in the United States. *J Clin Epidemiol* 1995;48: 1289–98

59. Di Tullio MR, Sacco RL, Gersony D, *et al.* Aortic atheromas and acute ischemic stroke: a transesophageal echocardiographic study in an ethnically mixed population. *Neurology* 1996;46:1560–6

60. Di Tullio MR, Sacco RL, Sciacca R, *et al.* Patent foramen ovale as a risk factor for ischemic stroke in a multiethnic population. *Stroke* 1998;29:277

61. Hogue CW Jr, Murphy SF, Schectman KB, Davila-Roman VG. Risk factors for early or delayed stroke after cardiac surgery. *Circulation* 1999;100:642–7

62. Gillum RF, Gillum BS, Francis CK. Coronary revascularization and cardiac catheterization in the United States: trends in racial differences. *J Am Coll Cardiol* 1997;29:1557–62

63. Gillum RF. Coronary artery bypass surgery and coronary angiography in the United States, 1979–1983. *Am Heart J* 1987;113:1255–60

64. Furlan AJ, Jones SC. Central nervous system complications related to open heart surgery. In Furlan AJ, ed. *The Heart and Stroke. Exploring mutual cerebrovascular and cardiovascular issues.* London: Springer-Verlag, 1987:287–304

65. Roach GW, Kanchuger M, Mangano CM, *et al.* Adverse cerebral outcomes after coronary bypass surgery: Multicenter Study of Perioperative Ischemic Research Group and the Ischemia Research and Education Foundation Investigators. *N Engl J Med* 1996;335:1857–63

66. Hogue CW Jr, Barzilai B, Pieper KS, *et al.* Sex differences in neurological outcomes and mortality after cardiac surgery. A Society of Thoracic Surgery National Database Report. *Circulation* 2001;103:2133–7

67. DiMascio R, Marchioli R, Tognoni G. Cholesterol reduction and stroke occurrence: an overview of randomized clinical trials. *Cerebrovasc Dis* 2000;10:85–92

68. Futterman LG, Lemberg L. Stroke risk, cholesterol and statins. *Am J Crit Care* 2000;9:416–19

69. Rosenson RS. Biological basis for statin therapy in stroke prevention. *Curr Opin Neurol* 2000;13:57–62

Chapter 5

Inflammation, infection and homocysteine in atherosclerosis

Thomas J. DeGraba, MD

INTRODUCTION

For years, emphasis on the pathophysiology and management of atherosclerosis had focused on the deposition of cholesterol in the subintimal ground space of the large arteries. Treatment of elevated LDL levels, hypertension, diabetes and smoking had led to a reduction in strokes and heart attacks from the 1960s through the mid-1990s. However, since the mid-1990s the incidence of stroke has been on the rise in the USA[1]. This trend is believed to be due in part to the aging of the population and suboptimal management of the major stroke risk factors[2]. However, data are now emerging that demonstrate that atherosclerosis is not just a cholesterol disease but is more accurately characterized as a chronic inflammatory disease[3,4]. In addition to the aggressive modification of the major conventional risk factors, further understanding of the pathophysiologic mechanisms that are dependent upon the inflammatory and immune pathways in atherosclerosis is necessary to make advances in the reduction of atherothrombotic stroke. Attention is now focused on the inflammatory factors that lead to the development of 'unstable' or 'vulnerable' plaque, which is believed to be linked to acute coronary syndromes and thrombo-embolic stroke.

This chapter will review the current understanding of the role of inflammation in the pathophysiology of atherosclerosis, examine the role of putative inflammatory factors such as infection and elevated homocysteine levels in the initiation, progression and activation of atherosclerotic disease, briefly discuss the contribution of the conventional risk factors to the inflammatory state, identify novel biological markers such as C-reactive protein and soluble interleukin (IL)-6 and intercellular adhesion molecule-1 (ICAM-1) which may indicate increased stroke risk, and discuss therapeutic strategies that are directed at reducing the inflammatory characteristics of atherosclerotic plaque.

INFLAMMATION: CELLULAR AND MOLECULAR MECHANISMS

Response to injury

The initiation and formation of atherosclerotic plaque represents a complex interplay of environmental factors and genetic susceptibility that results in a chronic inflammatory process eventually leading to stroke (and myocardial infarction). Evidence indicates that exposure of the endothelial surfaces to a variety of stimuli such as the shear stress forces of hypertension, hyperglycemia, oxidized LDL, toxins from cigarette smoke, infections and other inflammatory compounds results in the deposition and accumulation of lipids in the subintimal ground space of the large arteries. This process results in the expression of surface adhesion molecules such as ICAM-1, vascular cell adhesion molecule-1 (VCAM-1), and P-selectin. Expression of these adhesion molecules results in the migration of circulating monocytes and T-lymphocytes into the wall of the vessel. The monocyte-derived macrophages become filled with lipid (foam cell formation) and contribute to the release of a number of inflammatory mediators, which perpetuates the inflammatory and chemotactic state of the growing atherosclerotic plaque. The atherogenic process also results in the production of transforming growth factor beta (TGF-β) and platelet derived growth factor (PDGF) that results in a proliferation of smooth muscle cells and fibroblasts that leads to the deposition of an interstitial fibrous matrix. The extracellular matrix – consisting of collagen, elastin, proteoglycans and other proteins including fibronectin and thrombospondin, among others – serves to form a fibrous cap that constitutes the key to plaque stabilization of the underlying inflammatory and necrotic lipid core (Figure 1).

Mechanism of intraluminal thrombosis

Given the evolution of a chronic inflammatory state within the atherosclerotic plaque, there are two major pathways by which intraluminal thrombus formation are thought to occur that result in thrombo-embolic stroke (and myocardial infarction).

The first pathway involves the release of pro-inflammatory cytokines such as tumor necrosis factor-α (TNF-α) and IL-1β from activated macrophages, which results in the conversion of the endothelium over the plaque to a pro-thrombotic state[5–10]. This conversion is characterized by a reduction of tissue plasminogen activator (tPA) and protein-S synthesis, along with an increased production of plasminogen activator inhibitor-1 (PAI-1), platelet activating factor (PAF), leukocyte adhesion molecules such as ICAM-1, VCAM-1, P-selectin and E-selectin, chemotactic factors such as IL-8 and monocyte chemotactic protein-1 (MCP-1), and endothelin-1 (ET-1: a potent vasospastic agent). These changes are brought about by activation of transcription factors such as nuclear factor κB (NFκB). In addition, T-cell interaction of CD40L with CD40 receptors on macrophages results in the release of tissue factor, a key initiating co-factor in the coagulation pathway. These events promote platelet aggregation and clot formation. Recent studies support the concept that a pro-inflammatory, pro-thrombotic state is associated with symptomatic carotid disease. Studies in human carotid atherosclerotic plaque reveal a significant elevation in endothelial surface ICAM-1 expression, VCAM-1 expression, tissue factor expression, and human leukocyte antigen (HLA) DR2 antigen in symptomatic individuals[11–13].

The second pathway involves plaque instability, which is enhanced by a thinning of the fibrous matrix that maintains a 'cover' over the necrotic lipid core. Breakdown of the fibrous matrix by matrix metalloproteinases (MMPs) released from activated macrophages via CD40 exposure and exposure to soluble cytokines such as IL-1 and TNF-α causes the degradation of the collagen and elastin fibers. T-lymphocyte activation of the macrophages, resulting in the production of collagenases, gelatinase-B (MMP-9), stromelysin (MMP-3) and gelatinase-A (MMP-2), causes degradation of the matrix. In addition, when T-lymphocytes are activated they produce interferon gamma (IFN-γ), that reduces the synthesis of collagen material normally produced by smooth muscle

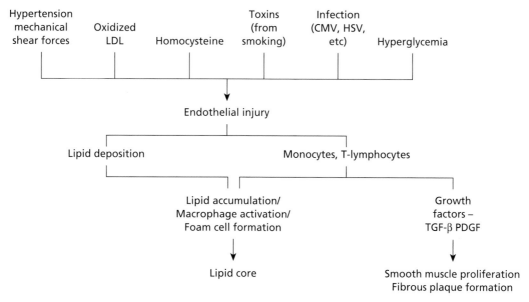

Figure 1 Endothelial injury model of atherosclerosis initiation; TGF-β, transforming growth factor-β; PDGF, platelet derived growth factor

cells. IFN-γ can also result in the apoptosis of smooth muscle cells thus reducing both the cellular component and the stabilizing constituents of the extracellular matrix. This phenomenon results in the potential for plaque rupture and extrusion of lipid and collagen material into the lumen of the vessel, leading to fibrin clot formation and either arterial occlusion at the site or thrombo-embolic events.

THE ROLE OF INFECTION IN ATHEROSCLEROSIS

Infection has been strongly associated with the formation, progression and activation of atherosclerotic disease[14–16]. Studies have demonstrated that the presence of viruses such as herpes simplex virus (HSV) and cytomegalo-virus (CMV) has been associated with early atherosclerotic plaque and fatty streak development[17]. Injury to the vessel wall, resulting in the migration of inflammatory cells as well as the release of pro-inflammatory cytokines (TH-1 helper cytokines) and growth factors, has been attributed to infectious agents. In addition, memory T-lymphocytes for specific infectious agents, with or without the presence of the organism, have been identified in athero-sclerotic plaques of all ages. This suggests that infection may initiate plaque formation that may progress without the infection neces-sarily being chronic. Evidence indicates that T-lymphocytes are recruited non-specifically to the site of inflammatory tissue in atherosclerotic plaques. These T-lymphocytes represent popu-lations of T-cells that are known as memory T-cells (approximately 90%) and are generally in an inactivated state in the atherosclerotic plaque. Potential activators of the resting T-cells can come from several sources. First, plaques with T-cells that have been previously sensitized to infectious agents can be activated by the reinfection of the plaque with those organisms. A recent study revealed that in patients with *Chlamydia pneumoniae* identified in symptomatic carotid atherosclerotic plaque the organism was associated with a significant increase in all T-lymphocyte subtypes including MHC-I restricted CD8+ T-cells. This strongly suggests antigen activation by an inflammatory event[18]. Re-exposure of the T-cell through the MHC-I and MHC-II pathways causes T-cell proliferation and activation of inflammatory cytokines that activate macrophages as well as affecting smooth muscle cells. Additionally, T-cell receptors can respond to endogenous peptides and antigens from the atherosclerotic plaque that mimic sensitizing organisms. Finally, arterial walls may have been previously infected early in life with agents such as CMV that resulted in the deposition of T-cells sensitized to that organism. Even with the clearing of the infection, memory T-cells may persist in tissue for 30 years or more and may be reactivated at a later time by a recurrent infection or an antigen that mimics the infection. Thereafter, activation of the T-cells can result in an escalation of the inflammatory cascade leading to enhanced thrombogenicity and/or plaque rupture.

Additionally, recent data reveal a temporal association between acute infection and the incidence of ischemic stroke[19-22]. It is believed that increased levels of systemic inflammatory products from inflammatory cells, circulating immune complexes and activated platelets interact with the pro-inflammatory, pro-thrombotic endothelial surface of a plaque site, which could potentially create a rapid escalation in the formation of platelet aggregates and thrombus.

It has been suggested that several specific types of infectious agent are causally related to atherosclerosis on the basis of further epidemiological and pathological studies. These agents include CMV and other herpes viruses[23,24], *Helicobacter pylori*[25-27], chronic periodontal disease with Gram-negative organisms[28], and *C. pneumoniae*. While the causal relationship between any of these infections

and atherosclerosis remains unproven, the accumulated data regarding the plausible role of *C. pneumoniae* in common forms of chronic vascular disease are the most convincing. The sections below will review the data on each of these organisms and the pathogenetic mechanisms and potential clinical implications of the data for each.

Herpes viruses

Data have long been available that support the premise that a viral infection can initiate atherogenesis. Studies show that the smooth muscle cells involved in human atherosclerotic plaque are monoclonal, suggesting a viral or other mutagenic process[29]. Herpes viruses were shown many years ago to induce atherosclerosis-like changes in animal models[30,31]. An avian herpes virus was found to cause atherosclerosis similar to that seen in human beings in both normal and hypercholesterolemic chickens. However, without the avian herpes virus infection, even hypercholesterolemic chickens do not develop atherosclerosis[32,33]. Herpes simplex virus has been found in early aortic atherosclerotic lesions[34].

Cytomegalovirus (CMV)

Human serologic evidence of cytomegalovirus (CMV) infection is more common in patients with coronary artery disease than in normal controls[35]. A cross-sectional study of serologies in patients showed a higher proportion of CMV seropositivity in patients with angiographically documented stenosis[36], though recent studies have been less definitive about the role of CMV in atherosclerosis[37-39]. In the Intermountain Heart Study, however, both C-reactive protein and CMV seropositivity were associated with long-term mortality in patients with angiographically verified coronary artery disease (CAD). Restenosis after coronary angioplasty also occurs more frequently in patients positive for CMV[40,41]. CMV has also been detected by polymerase chain reaction (PCR) techniques in atherosclerotic plaques in those with coronary disease more frequently than in those without atherosclerosis[42]. These findings represent associations only. An attempt to demonstrate causality has led to experiments in animals and *in vitro* human tissue of CMV infection which reveal that CMV increases the expression of platelet-derived growth factor and transforming growth factor in rat aortic allografts[43] and regulates IL-2, IL-2r, TNF-α[44] and NF-κB, a pro-inflammatory transcription factor[45]. CMV promotes human vascular smooth muscle cell proliferation and migration *in vitro*[46] and *in vivo*[47], promotes the coagulation cascade[48–50], and facilitates adherence of leukocytes to endothelial cells[17,51,52].

Chlamydia pneumoniae

C. pneumoniae has been widely identified in coronary and carotid atherosclerotic plaque. Additionally, elevated IgA levels have been strongly associated with symptomatic atherosclerotic disease[53]. A number of factors make *C. pneumoniae* an attractive candidate as a potential mediator of plaque activation. *C. pneumoniae* is an obligate intracellular parasite that commonly infects mononuclear phagocytes. Macrophages derived from monocytes are characteristically localized in human atherosclerotic plaque and provide a mechanism for entry of the organism into the vessel wall[54]. Infection with *Chlamydia* may also create a persistent non-lethal infection which can lead to a chronic inflammatory state[55].

There are multiple mechanisms by which chronic infection can contribute to an inflammatory state in atherosclerosis. Endotoxin release and heat shock protein-60 (HSP-60) from *Chlamydia* have been associated with an increase of TNF-α and matrix metalloproteinase from macrophages[56,57]. *Chlamydia*

HSP-60 causes oxidation of low-density lipoprotein (LDL), which alters LDL to its highly atherogenic form[58] and converts macrophages into foam cells[59]. HSP-60 induces peripheral blood monocytes to produce TNF-α, IL-1β, IL-6, and IFN-γ[60]. *C. pneumoniae* increases C-reactive protein[61], tissue factor, TNF-α and PAI-1 and can cause a hypersensitivity reaction on re-exposure to the organism[62,63]. In addition, autoimmune mechanisms may play a role[64–66]. These factors demonstrate propensity and ability of this agent to reach the atherosclerotic plaque and exacerbate, if not initiate, the atherosclerotic inflammatory process. Animal studies have demonstrated an association between inoculation with *C. pneumoniae* and the development of atherosclerotic disease in New Zealand white rabbits[67,68]. The atherosclerotic process has also been shown to accelerate in apo-E deficient mice after injection of *C. pneumoniae*[69].

Numerous studies have been reported showing an association of chlamydial infection by immunohistochemical staining, PCR and serologic positive studies with coronary artery disease[70–72] and, more recently, with cerebrovascular events[66,73–75]. Despite the association, no definitive proof exists that the presence of *Chlamydia* or other infectious agents can cause the initiation of atherosclerosis or the progression of the atherosclerotic plaque in humans. Despite the lack of such proof, antibiotic therapy may be employed in the future to reduce the risk of heart attack and stroke. However, attempts to date to use antibiotic therapy in the reduction of heart attacks have met with mixed results. Theoretically, the reduction of inflammatory effects based on potential infectious organisms holds great promise given the known mechanisms of inflammation. For example, reduction of myocardial infarction (MI) has been associated with a history of prior use of tetracycline antibiotics[76]. Among 3315 patients 75 years and younger with MI, and 13 139 matched controls, cases were significantly less likely to have taken tetracycline or quinolone antibiotics, though no beneficial effect was found for macrolides, sulfonamides, penicillins, or cephalosporins[76]. However, conflicting prospective studies reveal that a reduction of cardiovascular events was not observed with antibiotic use in a two-year follow-up study[77]. At present, the data do not support the use of antibiotic therapy for patients with symptomatic atherosclerotic disease, despite an association with elevated immunoglobulin levels for some known organisms. Accurate identification of infected plaque, duration of antibiotic therapy and the need for recurrent antibiotic therapy remain to be delineated for testing this potential treatment.

Helicobacter pylori

Helicobacter pylori (H. pylori) is another organism postulated to initiate or affect the pathophysiology of atherosclerosis. Identification of *H. pylori* (chronic infectious state) as an etiology of gastritis and peptic ulcer disease[78–80] has sparked interest in the possibility of this organism being involved in other potentially chronic inflammatory disease processes such as atherosclerosis. Several retrospective epidemiological studies have suggested an association between the presence of *H. pylori* and coronary disease by identifying a higher antibody titer in patients who have experienced a coronary event. Most of these studies are small and flawed, for example, by not adjusting for other risk factors. Several prospective studies have been unable to confirm the association when correcting for other risk factors[25,81–86]. In addition, studies to date have been unable to identify *H. pylori* in atherosclerotic plaques, in contrast to positive studies with other organisms such as *Chlamydia*[87].

It has been suggested that virulence factors among the different subtypes of *H. pylori* may have led to inconsistency of the data. The *H. pylori* strain carrying the virulence factor cytotoxin-associated gene A and producing cytotoxin-associated protein A was found in some studies to be associated with an increase in cytokine expression[88,89], but this finding has not been confirmed in subsequent studies[81]. Because of the nature of *H. pylori* and its association with chronic inflammatory process, *H. pylori* will continue to be studied as a potential causative factor of atherosclerosis.

Periodontal disease

Periodontal disease is a chronic progressive infection of the gingiva, connective tissue and alveolar bone that could potentially contribute to atherosclerosis by way of chronic systemic inflammation. The prevalence of advanced periodontitis has been estimated at approximately 15% in patients aged 60–64[90], and as high as 45% in patients over the age of 65[91]. There is an increased prevalence of periodontitis among African-Americans[92,93], Mexican-Americans, and other Hispanic groups, each of which has an increased risk of stroke compared with whites. In addition, periodontal disease is expected to increase with aging of the population. Given the high prevalence of periodontal disease, any increased association with it in the risk of atherosclerosis could have a substantial adverse clinical impact on health in the US.

Prospective cohort studies have had conflicting results with regard to the relationship between periodontal disease and vascular disease. The differences are believed to be related to differences in the populations studied and the different methodologies used to assess and define periodontal disease. The National Health and Nutrition Examination Survey I (NHANES I) demonstrated that periodontitis was associated with a 25% increased risk for coronary heart disease, the association being particularly strong in those under the age of 50. Analysis suggests that poor periodontal status may be a proxy for poor health rather than being the etiology of the increased mortality. However, more recent studies with rigorous adjustment for other confounding factors have demonstrated an association between periodontal disease and stroke[94], but not heart disease[95], suggesting that stroke and coronary artery disease may differ in their relationship to periodontal disease. After adjustment for other risk factors, there was a statistically significant increased relative risk of 2.1 for ischemic stroke in those with periodontitis compared to the risk in those without it.

While over 300 types of bacteria may live in the oral cavity, only a minority cause periodontal disease. Gram-positive organisms commonly colonize healthy teeth while Gram-negative organisms are associated with gingivitis and periodontitis. Gram-negative organisms may induce pathogenic effects that contribute to atherosclerosis. For example, lipopolysaccharides (LPS) produced by the Gram-negative organisms can activate macrophages to produce pro-inflammatory cytokines such as TNF-α and IL-1β. These cytokines can upregulate the pro-coagulant state of the endothelium as well as platelet activation fibrinogen and von Willebrand factor. In addition, periodontal infections can elevate leukocyte and fibrinogen counts causing the atherosclerotic plaques to become pro-thrombotic.

Research continues to attempt to determine whether there is a significant relationship between periodontitis, stroke and atherosclerosis but is confounded in a number of ways: there are varying ways to measure periodontal infection; many different pathogenic and non-pathogenic organisms exist in the oral cavity; genetic and race/ethnic differences may affect susceptibility to the atherogenic properties of infections; and factors such as smoking and diet may play a role.

HOMOCYSTEINE AND OTHER RISK FACTORS AND MARKERS

Hyperhomocysteinemia

Hyperhomocysteinemia has been reported to have both a pro-atherogenic as well as pro-thrombotic effect on blood vessels[96–98]. Homocysteine is a highly reactive amino acid which is toxic to vascular endothelium and can potentiate the auto-oxidation of LDL. It has been shown to be an independent risk factor for vascular disease[99,100], and is emerging as a potentially modifiable risk factor for atherosclerosis.

Antioxidant vitamins

The utilization of the antioxidant B vitamin complex has been hypothesized to be a potentially useful therapy for the reduction of homocysteine levels and prevention of the development of atherosclerosis. The potential theoretical benefit has been related to the reduction of LDL levels and a positive influence on the inflammatory characteristics of plaque. However, to date, the data on antioxidant vitamins have been mixed with respect to efficacy in stroke prevention. The utilization of the B vitamin complex (B_{12}, B_6 and folate) has been positively associated with a reduction of homocysteine levels[101] and an association with a reduction of carotid atherosclerotic plaque progression[102]. The data suggest that treatment of levels as low as 9 μM is beneficial in patients with atherosclerotic disease. Studies that may demonstrate significant benefit in stroke reduction with the utilization of the B complex are on-going. The Vitamin Intervention in Stroke Prevention Trial (VISP) is currently enrolling 3600 subjects with a recent cerebral ischemic event(s) and elevated homocysteine levels (men > 9.5 mg/dl; women > 8.5 mg/dl). Subjects will be randomized to a high-dose or low-dose B complex vitamin regimen. The analysis of the primary endpoint of cerebral ischemic event and secondary endpoint of MI or fatal coronary heart disease will help identify a potential therapeutic dose[103].

The case for the utilization of other vitamins such as vitamin E and vitamin C is, as yet, unclear. Data suggest that vitamin E therapy is enhanced by concomitant use of vitamin C[104], that potentially helps regenerate vitamin E (α-tocopherol)[105]. The doses of these vitamins necessary for clinically relevant effects on atherosclerosis remain to be determined.

Hypertension

Mechanical forces such as those caused by hypertension result in endothelial changes and injury that promote the formation of atherosclerosis. Hypertension activates shear stress response elements in endothelial cells, resulting in the upregulation of genes for leukocyte adhesion molecules such as ICAM-1[106], and reduce elements, such as thrombomodulin, essential for the normal anticoagulant state of the endothelium[107].

ACE inhibitors

Recently, angiotensin converting enzyme (ACE) inhibitors have been shown to reduce the risk of heart attack and stroke in the atherosclerotic[108]. Benefits appear to be, in part, independent of their effects on hypertension, with the Heart Outcomes Prevention Evaluation (HOPE) study revealing that even patients who did not have a reduction in blood pressure had a significant reduction in stroke (and heart attack). The effect of ACE inhibitors[109] on athero-thrombotic events is thought to be related to their effects on inflammation. Blockade of angiotensin-II results in the reduction of oxygen free radicals, transcription factors, adhesion molecules expression, inflammatory cytokines and smooth muscle proliferation[110]. These data suggest a future role for monitoring inflammatory markers with the use of ACE inhibitors in patients with atherosclerosis.

Beta blockers

Beta blockers have been clearly shown to reduce the incidence of sudden death following

MI and may have a positive, beneficial effect on the reduction of inflammation by reducing adrenergic effects in the blood vessels[111].

Oxidized LDL

Vessel exposure to oxidized LDL results in increased atherogenicity[112], expression of adhesion molecules and permeability and deposition of lipid into the subintimal ground space. Macrophages accumulate lipid and become foam cells, forming the fatty streak. In addition, oxidized LDL can be presented by macrophages to T-cells as a foreign antigen causing the proliferation of T-cells and release of inflammatory cytokines.

The hydroxymethyl glutaryl coenzyme A (HMG Co-A) reductase inhibitors (statins)

In addition to the clinically beneficial effects of LDL reduction[113], statins are reported to have anti-inflammatory effects[114] that are believed to play a role in the reduction of vascular events. Clinical and pre-clinical studies have demonstrated that statins reduce levels of C-reactive protein[115], and adhesion molecules, as well as cytokine and chemokine expression by TNF-α, IL-1β, monocyte chemotactic protein (MCP)-1 and IL-8[116–118]. Additionally, statins reduce the oxidation of LDL and improve vaso-reactivity by increasing levels of endothelial nitric oxide synthase (eNOS)[119].

A recent study that examined symptomatic atherosclerotic plaque in patients undergoing carotid endarterectomy revealed that patients treated with pravastatin 40 mg/day for three months tended to have a less inflammatory profile than patients on placebo. Morphologic analysis of plaque in patients treated with statins had significantly lower LDL content and matrix metalloproteinases, 50% fewer macrophages, 40% fewer lymphocytes and an increase in collagen and tissue inhibitors of metalloproteinases compared to placebo-treated patients[120]. These data suggest not only a long-term benefit of statins with respect to plaque progression but also more immediate effects of plaque stabilization.

Cigarette smoking

Cigarette smoking has been strongly associated with a pro-atherogenic and pro-thrombotic condition[121–126]. The active compounds from cigarette smoke, including nicotine and carbon monoxide as well as other active agents, have an adverse effect on endothelial function, vascular tone, hemostasis, lipid profile and inflammatory cells[127,128]. The action of oxidizing and toxic glycation products present in cigarette smoke is believed to be the principal mediator. Smoking is also associated with increased platelet aggregation (owing to increased thromboxane A_2) and fibrinogen levels when cigarette smoke is inhaled that is not seen when a nicotine patch is used[129].

Hyperglycemia

Hyperglycemia, secondary to diabetes, potentiates atherosclerosis. In addition to its effects on lipids, hyperglycemia causes a potentially modifiable pro-inflammatory profile. Patients with NIDDM have a significant increase in circulating activated monocytes compared to non-diabetics[130], and elevation in plasma glucose levels is associated with a rise in ICAM-1 levels that are reduced with insulin therapy[131].

Biological markers

Given the possibility that atherosclerosis may represent an inflammatory disease, the question arises 'Are there biological markers to follow that would indicate the efficacy of existing or new therapies in reducing the overall inflammatory state in the body?' To date, numerous systemic indicators have been identified that are associated with active atherosclerotic disease,

including elevated levels of C-reactive protein[132], IL-6, ICAM-1,[11,133] TNF-α, VCAM-1, and fibrinogen[114,134,135]. Of these, C-reactive protein has been shown to be reduced with the use of statins as well as with acetyl salicylic acid (ASA)[136,137]. Additional studies need to be done to verify the usefulness of following C-reactive protein levels when therapies designed to reduce stroke (and heart attack) are used. The difficulty of utilizing markers in the circulation is directly related to their potential non-specificity in atherosclerotic disease.

Genetic contribution to inflammation

Many of the genes that regulate inflammatory cytokines and adhesion molecules have been found to be polymorphic in nature. Specific alleles for cytokines such as TNF-α and IL-1β have been identified that are associated with an increased frequency of inflammatory diseases such as lupus, chronic inflammatory bowel disease and multiple sclerosis.

The concept of susceptibility

In processes influenced by inflammatory and infectious factors such as atherosclerosis, the concept of genetic susceptibility is well established. Particular HLA types are recognized as increasing the risk for auto-immune diseases, and the role of host genetic factors in both susceptibility and resistance to infections has been previously reported[138,139].

The evolutionary perspective

Particular genetic profiles may have provided an advantage to our ancestors that may now confer a selective disadvantage, particularly as the average life span increases and the types of stressors to which the human body is exposed change. An evolutionary advantage for a pro-inflammatory genotype (or high cytokine expression) may improve wound healing and eradication of infection during periods of nutritional deprivation. However, with the advent of an ample westernized diet and westernized lifestyle, this genetic profile may now put humans at a disadvantage, potentially leading to atherosclerotic disease[140]. Although predominantly hypothetical in nature, this theory may suggest a high prevalence of particularly potent pro-inflammatory gene polymorphisms. Continuing research is needed using linkage analysis techniques as well as studies of genetic influences associated with atherosclerosis in relation to risk factor exposure.

Therapeutic interventions

With each advance in knowledge in the pathogenesis of atherosclerosis, the possibility for novel therapeutic approaches arises. Pharmacological intervention could affect immune modulation that might block atherosclerosis in susceptible individuals. Gene delivery through a variety of vectors could introduce a critical wild type protein to atherosclerotic lesions to prevent progression of the process, promote regression, stimulate collateral formation or stabilize the atherosclerotic plaque. Drugs that cause immune modulation have revealed that the local transfection of specific genes down-regulates inflammatory factors that may be useful in reducing inflammation in atherosclerotic plaques[141] without affecting the general immune system that is necessary for health. One example of gene transfection that is currently being explored is the use of vascular endothelial growth factor (VEGF), which has been used in coronary artery disease[142]. As with any genetic therapeutic strategy, patient selection, route of delivery and vector selection are critical to future success.

CONCLUSIONS

The modification of genetic expression holds promise for future therapy in regulating the inflammatory cascade that can cause the progression and activation of atherosclerosis. Additional research and increased understanding of the pathogenesis and the effects of genes may allow modification of both the genetic expression and the influence of environmental exposures that influence the atherosclerotic process.

In summary, atherosclerosis is now regarded as a chronic inflammatory disease, which opens the possibility for improvement of stroke (and heart attack) prevention by the modification of immuno-modulatory therapy. Emerging evidence suggests that blockage of pro-inflammatory cytokines[143] or enhancement of anti-inflammatory cytokines may be beneficial in treating chronic inflammatory processes such as atherosclerosis. Future use of theses agents holds promise for reduction in plaque development[144,145]. Utilization of newer techniques may provide advances over the next several years that could rapidly translate into a significant reduction in the incidence of stroke in the population.

References

1. Gillum RF, Sempas CT. The end of the long-term decline in stroke mortality in the United States? *Stroke* 1997;28:1527–9
2. Gorelick PB. Stroke prevention. *Arch Neurol* 1995;52(4):347–55
3. Libby P. Coronary artery injury and the biology of atherosclerosis: inflammation, thrombosis, and stabilization. *Am J Cardiol* 2000;86(suppl): 3J–9J
4. Ross R. The pathogenesis of atherosclerosis: a perspective for the 1990s. *Nature* 1993;362: 801–9
5. Benveniste EN. Inflammatory cytokines within the central nervous system: source, function, and

mechanism of action. *Am J Physiol* 1992;263: C1–C16

6. Hallenbeck JM. Inflammatory reactions at the blood–endothelial interface in acute stroke. *Adv Neurol* 1996;71:281–300

7. Rothwell NJ, Loddick SA, Stroemer P. Interleukins and cerebral ischemia. *Int Rev Neurobiol* 1997;40:281–98

8. Bevilacqua MP, Pober JS, Majeau GR, *et al*. Interleukin-1 (IL-1) induces biosynthesis and cell surface expression of pro-coagulant activity in human vascular endothelial cells. *J Exp Med* 1984;160:618–23

9. Nawroth PP, Handley DA, Esmon CT, *et al*. Interleukin-1 induces endothelial cell procoagulant while suppressing cell-surface anticoagulant activity. *Proc Natl Acad Sci USA* 1986;83:3460–4

10. Nawroth PP, Stern DM. Modulation of endothelial cell hemostatic properties by tumor necrosis factor. *J Exp Med* 1986;163:740–5

11. DeGraba TJ, Sirén A-L, Penix LaRoy, *et al*. Increased endothelial expression of intercellular adhesion molecule-1 (ICAM-1) in symptomatic vs asymptomatic human atherosclerotic plaque. *Stroke* 1998;29(7):1405–10

12. Jander S, Sitzer M, Schumann R, *et al*. Inflammation in high-grade carotid stenosis: a possible role for macrophages and T-cells in plaque destabilization. *Stroke* 1998;29: 1625–30

13. van der Wal AC, Becker AE, van de Loos CM, Das PK. Site of intimal rupture or erosion of thrombosed coronary atherosclerotic plaques is characterized by an inflammatory process irrespective of the dominant plaque morphology. *Circulation* 1994;89:36–44

14. Libby P, Egan D, Skarlatos S. Roles of infectious agents in atherosclerosis and re-stenosis: an assessment of the evidence and need for future research. *Circulation* 1997;96:4095–103

15. Epstein SE, Zhou YF, Zhu J. Infection and atherosclerosis: emerging mechanistic paradigms. *Circulation* 1999;100:E20–E28

16. Vercellotti G. Infectious agents that play a role in atherosclerosis and vasculopathies. What are they? What do we do about them? *Can J Cardiol* 1999;15(SupplB):13B–15B

17. Span AH, vam Dam-Mieras MC, Mullers W, *et al*. The effect of virus infection on the adherence of leukocytes or platelets to endothelial cells. *Eur J Clin Invest* 1991;21:331–8

18. Nadareishvili Z, Szekely B, Koziol D, *et al*. Increased CD8+ T-cells associated with

Chlamydia pneumoniae in symptomatic carotid plaque. *Stroke* 2001;32:1966–72

19. Syrjanen J, Valtonen VV, Iivanainen M, *et al*. Preceding infection as an important risk factor for ischaemic brain infarction in young and middle aged patients. *Br Med J* 1988;296: 1156–60

20. Grau AJ, Buggle F, Becher H, *et al*. Recent bacterial and viral infection is a risk factor for cerebrovascular ischemia. *Neurology* 1998;50: 196–203

21. Macko R, Ameriso SF, Gruber FA, *et al*. Impairment of the protein C system and fibrinolysis in infection-associated stroke. *Stroke* 1996;27:2005

22. Grau AJ, Buggle F, Ziegler C, *et al*. Association between acute cerebrovascular ischemia and chronic or recurrent infection. *Stroke* 1997;28: 1724–9

23. Nieto FJ, Adam E, Sorlie P, *et al*. Cohort study of cytomegalovirus infection as a risk factor for carotid intimal-medial thickening, a measure of subclinical atherosclerosis. *Circulation* 1996;94: 922–7

24. Sorlie PD, Adam E, Melnick SL, *et al*. Cytomegalovirus/herpes virus and carotid atherosclerosis: the ARIC Study. *J Med Virol* 1994;42(1):33–7

25. Whincup PH, Mendall MA, Perry IJ, *et al*. Prospective relations between *Helicobacter pylori* infection, coronary heart disease, and stroke in middle-aged men. *Heart* 1996;75: 568–72

26. Patel P, Mendall MA, Carrington D, *et al*. Association of *Helicobacter pylori* and *Chlamydia pneumoniae* infections with coronary heart disease and cardiovascular risk factors. *Br Med J* 1995;311:711–14

27. Ponzetto A, La Rovere MT, Sanseverino P, Bazzoli F. Association of *Helicobacter pylori* with coronary heart disease. Study confirms previous findings. *Br Med J* 1996;312:251

28. Beck J, Garcia R, Heiss G, *et al*. Periodontal disease and cardiovascular disease. *J Periodontol* 1996;67:1123–37

29. Benditt EP, Benditt JM. Evidence for a monoclonal origin of human atherosclerotic plaque. *Proc Natl Acad Sci USA* 1973;70:1753–6

30. Hajjar DP. Viral pathogenesis of atherosclerosis. *Am J Pathol* 1991;139:1195–211

31. Minick CR, Fabricant CG, Fabricant J, Litrenta MM. Atheroarteriosclerosis induced by infection with a herpes virus. *Am J Pathol* 1979;96:673–700

32. Fabricant CG, Fabricant J, Minick CR, Litrenta MM. Herpes virus-induced atherosclerosis in chickens. *Fed Proc* 1983;42:2476–9

33. Fabricant CG, Fabricant J, Litrenta MM, Minick CR. Virus-induced atherosclerosis. *J Exp Med* 1978;148:335–40

34. Benditt EP, Barrett T, McDougall JK. Viruses in the etiology of atherosclerosis. *Proc Natl Acad Sci USA* 1983;80:6386–9

35. Melnick JL, Adam E, Debakey ME. Possible role of cytomegalovirus in atherogenesis. *J Am Med Assoc* 1990;263:2204–7

36. Zhu J, Quyyumi AA, Norman JE, *et al.* Cytomegalovirus in the pathogenesis of atherosclerosis: the role of inflammation as reflected by elevated C-reactive protein levels. *J Am Coll Cardiol* 1999;34:1738–43

37. Ridker PM, Hennekens CH, Stampfer MJ, *et al.* Prospective study of herpes simplex virus, cytomegalovirus, and the risk of future myocardial infarction and stroke. *Circulation* 1998;98:2796–9

38. Ridker PM, Hennekesn CH, Roitman-Jolanson B, *et al.* Plasma concentration of soluble ICAM-1 and risk of future myocardial infarction in apparently healthy men. *Lancet* 1998;351:88–92

39. Fagerberg B, Gnarpe J, Gnarpe H, *et al.* *Chlamydia pneumoniae* but not cytomegalovirus antibodies are associated with future risk of stroke and cardiovascular disease. *Stroke* 1999;30:299–305

40. Speir E, Modali R, Huang ES, *et al.* Potential role of human cytomegalovirus and p53 interaction in coronary restenosis. *Science* 1994; 265:391–4

41. Zhou YF, Leon MB, Waclawiw MA, *et al.* Association between prior cytomegalovirus infection and the risk of restenosis after coronary atherectomy. *N Engl J Med* 1996;335: 624–30

42. Hendricks MG, Salimans MM, van Boven CP, Bruggeman CA. High prevalence of latently present cytomegalovirus in arterial walls of patients suffering from grade III atherosclerosis. *Am J Pathol* 1990;136:23–8

43. Lemstrom KB, Aho PT, Bruggeman CA, Hayry PJ. Cytomegalovirus infection enhances mRNA expression of platelet-derived growth factor-BB and transforming growth factor-beta-1 in rat aortic allografts: possible mechanism for cytomegalovirus-enhanced graft arteriosclerosis. *Arterioscler Thromb* 1994;14:2043–52

44. Geist LJ, Monick MM, Stinski MF, Hunninghake GW. The immediate early genes of human cytomegalovirus upregulate tumor necrosis factor-alpha gene expression. *J Clin Invest* 1994;93:474–8

45. Kowalik TF, Wing B, Haskill JS, *et al.* Multiple mechanisms are implicated in the regulation of NF-β activity during human cytomegalovirus infection. *Proc Natl Acad Sci USA* 1993;90: 1107–11

46. Zhou YF, Yu ZX, Wanishsawad C, *et al.* The immediate early gene products of human cytomegalovirus increase vascular smooth muscle cell migration, proliferation, and expression of PDGF beta-receptor. *Biochem Biophys Res Commun* 1999;256:608–13

47. Yonemitsu Y, Kaneda Y, Komori K, *et al.* The immediate early gene of human cytomegalovirus stimulates vascular smooth muscle cell proliferation *in vitro* and *in vivo*. *Biochem Biophys Res Commun* 1997;231: 447–51

48. Van Dam-Mieras MCE, Muller AD, van Hinsbergh VWM, *et al.* The procoagulant response of cytomegalovirus infected endothelial cells. *Thromb Haemost* 1992;68:364–70

49. Eingen OR, Silverstein RL, Friedman HM, Hajjar DP. Viral activation of the coagulation cascade: molecular interactions at the surface of infected endothelial cells. *Cell* 1990;61: 657–62

50. Pryzdial ELG, Wright JF. Prothrombinase assembly on an enveloped virus: evidence that the cytomegalovirus surface contains procoagulant phospholipid. *Blood* 1994;84:3749–57

51. Grundy JE, Downes KL. Up-regulation of LFA-3 and ICAM-1 on the surface of fibroblasts infected with cytomegalovirus. *Immunology* 1993;78:405–12

52. Span AH, Mullers W, Miltenberg AM, Bruggeman CA. Cytomegalovirus induced PMN adherence in relation to an ELAM-1 antigen present on infected endothelial cell monolayers. *Immunology* 1991;72:355–60

53. LaBiche R, Koziol D, Quinn T, *et al.* Presence of *Chlamydia pneumoniae* in human symptomatic and asymptomatic carotid atherosclerotic plaque. *Stroke* 2001;32:855–60

54. Gaydos CA, Summersgill JT, Sahne NN, *et al.* Replication of *Chlamydia pneumoniae in vitro* in human macrophages, endothelial cells, and aortic artery smooth muscle cells. *Infect Immunol* 1996;64:1614–20

55. Beatty WL, Byrne GI, Morrison RP. Repeated and persistent infection with *Chlamydia* and the development of chronic inflammation and disease. *Trends Microbiol* 1994;2:94–8

56. Kol A, Sukhova GK, Lichtman AH, Libby P. Chlamydial heat shock protein 60 localizes in human atheroma and regulates macrophage tumor necrosis factor-α and matrix metalloproteinase expression. *Circulation* 1998;98:300–7

57. Rothermel CD, Schachter J, Lavrich P, *et al.* *Chlamydia trachomatis*-induced production of interleukin-1 by human monocytes. *Infect Immunol* 1989;57:2705–11

58. Kalayoglu MV, Hoerneman B, La Verda D, *et al.* Cellular oxidation of low density lipoprotein by *Chlamydia pneumoniae. J Infect Dis* 1999;180:780–90

59. Kalayoglu MV, Byrne BI. Induction of macrophage foam cell formation by *Chlamydia pneumoniae. J Infect Dis* 1998;177(3):725–9

60. Kaukoranta-Tolvanen SSE, Teppo AM, Laitinen K, *et al.* Growth of *Chlamydia pneumoniae* in cultured human peripheral blood mononuclear cells and induction of a cytokine response. *Microbiol Pathogen* 1996;21:215–21

61. Papanicolaou DA, Wilder RL, Manolagas SC, Chrousos GP. The pathophysiologic roles of interleukin-6 in human disease. *Ann Intern Med* 1998;128:127–37

62. Watkins NG, Hadlow WJ, Moos AB, Caldwell HD. Ocular delayed hypersensitivity: apathogenetic mechanism of chlamydial conjunctivitis in guinea pigs. *Proc Natl Acad Sci USA* 1986;83:7480–7

63. Morrison RP, Belland RJ, Lyng K, Caldwell HD. Chlamydial disease pathogenesis. The 57-kD chlamydial hypersensitivity antigen is a stress response protein. *J Exp Med* 1989;170:1271–83

64. Puolakkaien M, Linnanmäki E, Leinonen M, *et al.* Circulating immune complexes containing chlamydial lipopolysaccharide in pelvic inflammatory disease. In Bowie WR, Caldwell HD, Jones RP eds. *Chlamydial Infections.* Cambridge University Press, 1990:319–22

65. Linnanmäki E, Leinonen M, Ekman M-R, *et al.* *Chlamydia pneumoniae* specific circulating immune complexes in chronic coronary heart disease. *Circulation* 1993;87:1130–4

66. Wimmer MLJ, Sandmann-Strupp R, Saikku P, Haberl RL. Association of chlamydial infection with cerebrovascular disease. *Stroke* 1996;27:2207–10

67. Laitinen K, Aluria A, Pyhala L, *et al.* *Chlamydia pneumoniae* infection induces inflammatory changes in the aorta of rabbits. *Infect Immunol* 1997;65:4832–5

68. Fong IW, Chiu B, Viira E, *et al.* Rabbit model for *Chlamydia pneumoniae* infection. *J Clin Microbiol* 1997;35(1):48–52

69. Moazed TC, Campbell LA, Rosenfeld ME, *et al.* *Chlamydia pneumoniae* accelerates the progression of atherosclerosis in apolipoprotein E deficient mice. *J Infect Dis* 1999;180:238–41

70. Nieto FJ, Folsom AR, Sorley PD, *et al.* *Chlamydia pneumoniae* infection and incident coronary heart disease: the Atherosclerosis Risk in Communities Study. *Am J Epidemiol* 1999;150:149–56

71. Kuo CC, Shor A, Campbell LA, *et al.* Demonstration of *Chlamydia pneumoniae* in atherosclerotic lesions of coronary arteries. *J Infect Dis* 1993;167:841–9

72. Kuo CC, Gown AM, Benditt EP, Grayston JT. Detection of *Chlamydia pneumoniae* in aortic lesions of atherosclerosis by immunocytochemical staining. *Arterioscler Thromb* 1993; 13:1501–4

73. Maass M, Krause E, Engel PM, Kruger S. Endovascular presence of *Chlamydia pneumoniae* in patients with hemodynamically effective carotid artery stenosis. *Angiology* 1997;48:699–706

74. Grayston JT, Kuo CC, Coulson AS, *et al.* *Chlamydia pneumoniae* (TWAR) in atherosclerosis of the carotid artery. *Circulation* 1995;92:3397–400

75. Jackson LA, Campbell LA, Kuo CC, *et al.* Isolation of *Chlamydia pneumoniae* from a carotid endarterectomy specimen. *J Infect Dis* 1997;176:292–5

76. Meier CR, Derby LE, Jick SS, *et al.* Antibiotics and risk of subsequent first-time acute myocardial infarction. *J Am Med Assoc* 1999;281: 427–31

77. Anderson JL, Muhlestein JB, Carlquist J, *et al.* Randomized secondary prevention trial of azithromycin in patients with coronary artery disease and serological evidence for *Chlamydia pneumoniae* infection: the Azithromycin in Coronary Artery Disease: Elimination of Myocardial Infection with *Chlamydia* (ACADEMIC) study. *Circulation* 1999;99:1540–7

78. Veldhyuzen van Zanten SJO, Sherman PM. *Helicobacter pylori* infection as a cause of gastritis, duodenal ulcer, gastric cancer and

nonulcer dyspepsia: a systemic overview. *Can Med Assoc J* 1994;150(2):177–85

79. Sipponen P, Seppala K, Aarynen M, *et al.* Chronic gastritis and gastroduodenal ulcer: a case control study on risk of coexisting duodenal or gastric ulcer in patients with gastritis. *Gut* 1989;30(7):922–9

80. Cullen DJE, Collins BJ, Christiansen KJ, *et al.* Long term risk of peptic ulcer disease in people with *Helicobacter pylori* infection – a community based study. *Gastroenterology* 1993;104(4):A60

81. Koenig W, Rothenbacher D, Hoffmeister A, *et al.* Infection with *Helicobacter pylori* is not a major independent risk factor for stable coronary heart disease. *Circulation* 1999;100: 2326–31

82. Strandberg TE, Tilvis RS, Vuoristo M, *et al.* Prospective study of *Helicobacter pylori* seropositivity and cardiovascular diseases in a general elderly population. *Br Med J* 1997;314: 317–18

83. Wald NJ, Law MR, Morris JK, Bagnall AM. *Helicobacter pylori* infection and mortality from ischaemic heart disease: negative result from a large, prospective study. *Br Med J* 1997;315:1199–201

84. Folsom AR, Nieto JF, Sorlie P, *et al.*, for the Atherosclerosis Risk in Communities (ARIC) study investigators. *Helicobacter pylori* seropositivity and coronary heart disease incidence. *Circulation* 1998;98:845–50

85. Strachan DP, Mendall MA, Carrington D, *et al.* Relation of *Helicobacter pylori* infection to 13-year mortality and incident ischemic heart disease in the Caerphilly Prospective Heart Disease Study. *Circulation* 1998;98:1286–90

86. Danesh J, Peto R. Risk factors for coronary heart disease and infection with *Helicobacter pylori*: meta-analysis of 18 studies. *Br Med J* 1998;316:1130–2

87. Blasi F, Denti F, Erba M, *et al.* Detection of *Chlamydia pneumoniae* but not *Helicobacter pylori* in atherosclerotic plaques of aortic aneurysms. *J Clin Microbiol* 1996;34:2766–9

88. Pasceri V, Cammarota G, Patti G, *et al.* Association of virulent *Helicobacter pylori* strains with ischemic heart disease. *Circulation* 1998;97:1675–9

89. Peek RM, Miller G, Tham KT, *et al.* Heightened inflammatory response and cytokine expression *in vivo* to CagA+ *Helicobacter pylori* strains. *Lab Invest* 1995;71: 760–70

90. Williams RC. Periodontal disease. *N Engl J Med* 1990;322(6):373–82

91. Brown LJ, Brunelle JA, Kingman A. Periodontal status in the United States, 1988–9: prevalence, extent, and demographic variation. *J Dent Res* 1996;75:672

92. Beck JD, Koch GG, Rozier RG, Tudor GE. Prevalence and risk indicators for periodontal attachment loss in a population of old community-dwelling blacks and whites. *J Periodontol* 1991;61:520

93. Alpagot T, Smith QT, Tran SD. Risk indicators for periodontal disease in a racially diverse urban population. *J Clin Periodontol* 1996; 23:982

94. Wu T, Trevisan M, Genco RJ, *et al.* Periodontal disease and risk of cerebrovascular disease: the first national health and nutrition examination survey and its follow-up study. *Arch Intern Med* 2000;160(18): 2749–55

95. Hujoel PP, Drangsholt M, Spiekerman C, DeRouen TA. Periodontal disease and coronary heart disease risk. *J Am Med Assoc* 2000;284:1406–10

96. Voutilainen S, Morrow JD, Roberts JR II, *et al.* Enhanced *in vivo* lipid peroxidation at elevated plasma total homocysteine levels. *Arterioscler Thromb Vasc Biol* 1999;19: 1263–6

97. Jakubowski H, Zhang L, Bardeguez A, Aviv A. Homocysteine thiolactone and protein homocysteinylation in human endothelial cells: implications for atherosclerosis. *Circ Res* 2000;87:45–51

98. Duan J, Murohara T, Ikeda H, *et al.* Hyperhomocysteinemia impairs angiogenesis in response to hindlimb ischemia. *Arterioscler Thromb Vasc Biol* 2000;20:2579–85

99. Clarke R, Daly L, Robinson K, *et al.* Hyperhomocysteinemia: an independent risk factor for vascular disease. *N Engl J Med* 1999;324(17):1149–55

100. Spence JD, Malinow MR, Barnett PA, *et al.* Plasma homocysteine concentration, but not MTHFR genotype, is associated with variation in carotid plaque area. *Stroke* 1999;30: 969–73

101. Woodside JV, Yarnell JW, McMaster D, *et al.* Effect of B-group vitamins and antioxidant vitamins on hyperhomocysteinemia: a double-blind, randomized, factorial-design, controlled trial. *Am J Clin Nutr* 1998;67(5):858–66

102. Hackam DG, Peterson JC, Spence JD. What level of plasma homocysteine should be treated? Effects of vitamin therapy on progression of carotid atherosclerosis in patients with homocysteine levels above and below 14 μmol/L. *Am J Hypertens* 2000;13:105–10

103. Spence JD, Howard VJ, Chambless LE, *et al.* Vitamin Intervention for Stroke Prevention (VISP) trial: rationale and design. *Neuroepidemiology* 2001;20(1):16–25

104. Liao K, Yin M. Individual and combined antioxidant effects of seven phenolic agents in human erythrocyte membrane ghosts and phosphatidylcholine liposome systems: importance of the partition coefficient. *J Agric Food Chem* 2000;48:2266–70

105. Hamilton IMJ, Gilmore WS, Benzie IFF, *et al.* Interactions between vitamins C and E in human subjects. *Br J Nutr* 2000;84:261–7

106. Morigi M, Zoja C, Figliuzzi M, *et al.* Fluid shear stress modulates surface expression of adhesion molecules by endothelial cells. *Blood* 1995;85:1696–703

107. Malek AM, Jackman R, Rosenberg RD, Izumo S. Endothelial expression of thrombomodulin is reversibly regulated by fluid shear stress. *Circ Res* 1994;74(5):852–60

108. The Heart Outcomes Prevention Evaluation study investigators. Effects of an angiotensin-converting-enzyme inhibitor, ramipril, on cardiovascular events in high-risk patients. *N Engl J Med* 2000;342(3):145–53

109. Fukuhara M, Geary RL, Diz DI, *et al.* Angiotensin-converting enzyme expression in human carotid artery atherosclerosis. *Hypertension* 2000;35(part 2):353–9

110. Dzau VJ. Mechanism of protective effects of ACE inhibition on coronary artery disease. *Eur Heart J* 1998;19(Suppl J):J2–J6

111. Fitzgerald JD. By what means might beta-blockers prolong life after acute myocardial infarction? *Eur Heart J* 1987;3:945–51

112. Steinberg D, Parthasarathy S, Carew TE, *et al.* Beyond cholesterol: modifications of low-density lipoprotein that increase its atherogenicity. *N Engl J Med* 1989;320(14):915–24

113. Scandinavian simvastatin study group. Randomised trial of cholesterol lowering in 4444 patients with coronary heart disease: the Scandinavian Simvastatin Survival Study (4S). *Lancet* 1994;344:1383–9

114. Sacks FM, Pfeffer MA, Moye LA, *et al.*, for the recurrent events trial investigators. The effect of pravastatin on coronary events after myocardial infarction in patients with average cholesterol levels. *N Engl J Med* 1996; 335(14):1001–9

115. Ridker PM, Rifai N, Pfeffer MA, *et al.*, for the Cholesterol and Recurrent Events (CARE) investigators. *Circulation* 1998;98:839–44

116. Romano M, Diomede L, Sironi M, *et al.* Inhibition of monocyte chemotactic protein-1 synthesis by statins. *Lab Invest* 2000;80: 1095–100

117. Bustos C, Hernandez-Presa MA, Orgego M, *et al.* HMG-CoA reductase inhibition by atorvastatin reduces neointimal inflammation in a rabbit model of atherosclerosis. *J Am Coll Cardiol* 1998;32(7):2057–64

118. Kothe H, Dalhoff K, Rupp J, Hydroxymethylglutaryl coenzyme-A reductase inhibitors modify the inflammatory response of human macrophages and endothelial cells infected with *Chlamydia pneumoniae*. *Circulation* 2000;101:1760–3

119. Vaughan CJ, Gotto AM Jr, Basson CT. The evolving role of statins in the management of atherosclerosis. *J Am Coll Cardiol* 2000;35: 1–10

120. Crisby J, Nordin-Fredriksson G, Shah PK, *et al.* Pravastatin treatment increases collagen content and decreases lipid content, inflammation, metalloproteinases, and cell death in human carotid plaques. *Circulation* 2001; 103:926–33

121. Zhu B, Sun Y, Sievers RE, *et al.* Passive smoking increases experimental atherosclerosis in cholesterol-fed rabbits. *J Am Coll Cardiol* 1993;21:225–32

122. Miller GJ, Bauer KA, Cooper JA, Rosenberg RD. Activation of the coagulant pathway in cigarette smokers. *Thromb Haemost* 1998;79: 549–53

123. Newby DE, Wright RA, Labinjoh C, *et al.* Endothelial dysfunction, impaired endogenous fibrinolysis, and cigarette smoking. *Circulation* 1999;99:1411–15

124. Zidovetzki R, Chen P, Fisher M, Hofman FM. Nicotine increases plasminogen activator inhibitor-1 production by human brain endothelial cells via protein kinase C-associated pathway. *Stroke* 1999;30:651–5

125. Markovitz JH, Tolbert L, Winders SE. Increased serotonin receptor density and platelet GPIIb/IIIa activation among smokers. *Arterioscler Thromb Vasc Biol* 1999;19:762–6

126. Matetzky S, Tani S, Kangavari S, *et al.* Smoking increases tissue factor expression in atherosclerotic plaques: implications for plaque thrombogenicity. *Circulation* 2000; 102:602–4

127. Celermajer DS, Adams MR, Clarkson P, *et al.* Passive smoking and impaired endothelium-dependent arterial dilatation in healthy young adults. *N Engl J Med* 1996;334(3): 150–4

128. Hutchison SJ, Sudhir K, Sievers RE, *et al.* Effects of L-arginine on atherogenesis and endothelial dysfunction due to secondhand smoke. *Hypertension* 1999;34:44–50

129. Benowitz NL, Fitzgerald GA, Wilson M, Zhang Q. Nicotine effects on eicosanoid formation and hemostatic function: comparison of transdermal nicotine and cigarette smoking. *J Am Coll Cardiol* 1993;22:1159–67

130. Patiño R, Ibarra J, Rodriguez A, *et al.* Circulating monocytes in patients with diabetes mellitus, arterial disease, and increased CD14 expression. *Am J Cardiol* 2000;85: 1288–91

131. Marfella R, Esposito K, Giunta R, *et al.* Circulating adhesion molecules in humans: role of hyperglycemia and hyperinsulinemia. *Circulation* 2000;101:2247–51

132. Tataru MC, Heinrich J, Junker R, *et al.* C-reactive protein and the severity of atherosclerosis in myocardial infarction patients with stable angina pectoris. *Eur Heart J* 2000 21(12):1000–8

133. Rohde LE, Lee RT, Rivero J, *et al.* Circulating cell adhesion molecules are correlated with ultrasound-based assessment of carotid atherosclerosis. *Arterioscler Thromb Vasc Biol* 1998;18:1765–70

134. Ridker PM, Rifai N, Pfeffer M, *et al.* Elevation of TNF-α and increased risk of recurrent coronary events after myocardial infarction. *Circulation* 2000;101:2149–53

135. Hwang SJ, Ballantyne CM, Sharrett AR, *et al.* Circulating adhesion molecules VCAM-1, ICAM-1 and E-selectin in carotid atherosclerosis and incident coronary heart disease cases: the atherosclerosis risk in communities (ARIC) study. *Circulation* 1997;96:4219–25

136. Ridker PM, Rifai N, Pfeffer MA, *et al.*, for the cholesterol and recurrent events (CARE) investigators. Long-term effects of pravastatin on plasma concentration of C-reactive protein. *Circulation* 1999;100:230–5

137. Ridker PM, Cushman M, Stampfer MJ, *et al.* Inflammation, aspirin, and the risk of cardiovascular disease in apparently healthy men. *N Engl J Med* 1997;336(14):973–9

138. Kokkotou E, Philippon V, Gueye-Ndiaye A, *et al.* Role of the CCR5 delta 32 allele in resistance to HIV-1 infection in west Africa. *J Hum Virol* 1998;1(7):469–74

139. Taylor ML, Perez-Mejia A, Yamamoto-Furusho JK, Granados J. Immunologic, genetic and social human risk factors associated to histoplasmosis: studies in the state of Guerrero, Mexico. *Mycopathologia* 1997; 138(3):137–42

140. Fernandez-Real JM, Ricart W. Insulin resistance and inflammation in an evolutionary perspective: the contribution of cytokine genotype/phenotype to thriftiness. *Diabetologia* 1999;42(11):1367–74

141. Laukkanen J, Lehtolainen P, Gough P, *et al.* Adenovirus-mediated gene transfer of a secreted form of human macrophage scavenger receptor inhibits modified low-density lipoprotein degradation and foam-cell formation in macrophages. *Circulation* 2000;101: 1091–6

142. Inoue M, Itoh H, Ueda M, *et al.* Vascular endothelial growth factor (VEGF) expression in human coronary atherosclerotic lesions: possible pathophysiological significance of VEGF in progression of atherosclerosis. *Circulation* 1998;98(20):2108–16

143. Elhage R, Maret A, Pieraggi M-T, *et al.* Differential effects of interleukin-1 receptor antagonist and tumor necrosis factor binding protein on fatty-streak formation in apolipoprotein E-deficient mice. *Circulation* 1998;97: 242–4

144. Young JL, Sukhova GK, Foster D, *et al.* The serpin proteinase inhibitor 9 is an endogenous inhibitor of interleukin 1β-converting enzyme (caspase-1) activity in human vascular smooth muscle cells. *J Exp Med* 2000;191(9): 1535–44

145. Charles P, Elliott MJ, Davis D, *et al.* Regulation of cytokines, cytokine inhibitors, and acute-phase proteins following anti-TNF-α therapy in rheumatoid arthritis. *J Immunol* 1999;163:1521–8

Chapter 6

Stroke in sickle cell disease

Sung B. Lee, MD, and Robert J. Adams, MS, MD

INTRODUCTION

Sickle cell disease (SCD) is an autosomal recessive hemoglobinopathy characterized by the production of structurally abnormal hemoglobin, causing a pathologic sickle shape in the erythrocyte. The clinical manifestations of SCD had been recognized for centuries in Africa before the etiology of this disease was known[1,2]. In 1910, Herrick published the first clinical case of an African-American with severe anemia associated with the occurrence of a 'large number of thin, elongated, sickle-shaped and crescent-shaped forms' in stained and wet smears of blood (Figure 1)[3]. He stated 'Whether the blood picture represents merely a freakish poikilocytosis or is dependent on some peculiar physical or chemical condition of the blood, or is characteristic of some particular disease, I cannot at present answer'. Five years later Cook and Myers considered this sickling disorder of the blood to be a familial clinical entity[4]. It was not until 1922 that Mason used the term sickle cell anemia for the first time[5]. In 1923, Sydenstricker and colleagues published the first description of hemiplegia and seizure secondary to SCD in a five-year-old boy[2]. Since that time SCD has been a well-recognized risk factor for neurologic complications of a wide clinical spectrum, ranging from cognitive deficits to stroke. However, among the complications of SCD it is stroke that represents the most catastrophic sequela and the leading cause of death in both children[6] and adults[7] with the disease.

EPIDEMIOLOGY OF SCD

About one in every 500 births in the African-American population is identified by neonatal testing to be homozygous for the sickle hemoglobin gene (HbS) and thus, by definition, to have SCD. However, the prevalence among adults is reduced by early mortality. Approximately 8% of African-Americans are heterozygous for HbS, also referred to as sickle cell trait, while in western Africa the prevalence is as high as 25%–30%[8–10]. Worldwide, the HbS gene is found not only in black Africans but also among non-blacks in Mediterranean countries, India and Saudi Arabia. The gene of the Mediterranean SCD is of an African haplotype, while the gene in India and Saudi Arabia is another haplotype possibly representing an independent mutation[10]. Owing in part to the genetic programming which determines the degree to which normal fetal hemoglobin (HbF) continues to be synthesized during adult life, people of African lineage have the most severe clinical course. In contrast, those from Saudi Arabia tend to have a relatively benign form of the disease.

The high prevalence of sickle trait in western Africa represents a balanced polymorphism between a genetically disadvantageous condition and the environmental advantages of the diseased state[1]. In areas hyperendemic for *Falciparum malaria*, the increased stable frequency of the sickle gene was the result of balanced gene exclusion from early death of

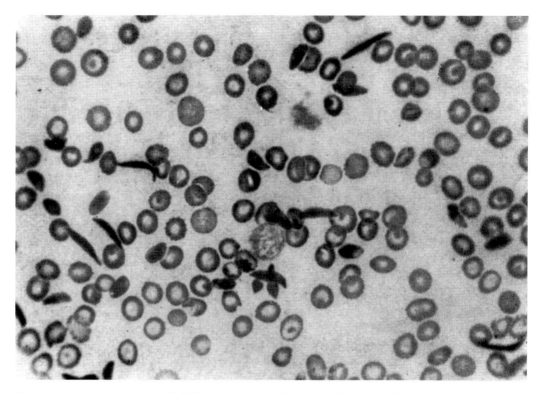

Figure 1 Photomicrograph of sickled erythrocytes from Herrick's report of 1910. Figure reproduced with permission from *Arch Intern Med* 1910;6:517–24. © 1910, American Medical Association

homozygotes and gene selection from protection of heterozygotes against death by malaria. Owing to its unique environmental fitness, the worldwide distribution of SCD mirrors the 'malaria belt'.

In addition to the simple heterozygous state, there exists a large population of compound heterozygotes in which HbS is combined with a second abnormal hemoglobin, leading to a sickling disorder of varying severity. Common examples are HbSC (HbS/HbC) and HbS-thalassemia (HbS/β^0, HbS/β^+, HbS α-/$\alpha\alpha$, HbS α-/α-)[8,9]. Among African-Americans, the frequencies of the HbC gene and the β-thalassemia gene, compared to that of the HbS gene, are approximately 25% and 10%, respectively. The α-thalassemia gene deletion occurs in up to 30% of the African-American population[11]. Anemia due to HbSC is milder than that of HbSS disease. The clinical nature of HbS/β^+

is more benign than that of HbS/β^0. The α-thalassemia trait may be beneficial in SCD because there is a lower intracellular hemoglobin concentration and reduced polymerization of HbS and less severe anemia[11].

PATHOPHYSIOLOGY OF SCD

Hemoglobin is a tetramer of four globin chains comprised of two pairs of similar chains, each with its own heme group. Hemoglobin in the adult is composed of 96% HbA ($\alpha_2\beta_2$), 3% HbA$_2$ ($\alpha_2\delta_2$), and 1% HbF ($\alpha_2\gamma_2$). In 1957, Ingram showed that SCD results from a point mutation that leads to the substitution of valine for glutamic acid at the sixth position of the β-globin chain (β6Glut →Val)[12]. The resultant hemoglobin, HbS, behaves like HbA during oxygenated states. However, during deoxygenation the HbS molecules undergo aggregation and polymerization. This change converts hemoglobin from a freely flowing liquid to a viscous para-crystalline gel that forms rigid polymers and leads to red cells of abnormal or frankly sickled configurations of higher density. Initially, sickling is reversible upon reoxygenation, but with each subsequent deoxygenation and polymerization reversibility is decreased. The tendency of an erythrocyte containing HbSS to sickle is influenced primarily by deoxygenation, intracellular Hb concentration, and the intracellular concentration of HbF[1,7,9,13]. Therefore, this sickling produces a clinical picture that can be divided into three different categories: (1) the effects of hemolysis, (2) constitutional sequela, and (3) vaso-occlusive phenomena[14]. The systemic effects of SCD are complex and beyond the scope of this chapter. However, it is important to consider the mechanisms of anemia and vaso-occlusion in relation to cerebrovascular complications in this disease.

Anemia from hemolysis is a reflection of the overall severity of SCD. Sickle erythrocyte survival time in the circulation is greatly shortened as compared to that of normal erythrocytes. The HbSS cell is predisposed to hemolysis by oxidative damage of the cell membrane caused by sickling that, in turn, causes a chain of events: (1) first, immune uptake of damaged cells fixed by IgG and complement, (2) trapping of these sickled cells in extravascular space, and (3) lysis of the cell. This hemolysis results in severe anemia and the stimulation of erythropoiesis. It has been suggested that the compensatory increase in cerebral blood flow due to severe anemia may cause flow disturbances that may lead to cerebrovascular damage[15].

The so-called 'vaso-occlusive crisis' is a dramatic clinical complication of SCD, manifesting as, for example, pain crisis or acute chest syndrome. However, studies have shown that vaso-occlusive events cannot be explained simply by mechanical clogging of postcapillary venules by sickled cells. Thus, other mechanisms must be at play. At body temperature, the solubility of deoxy-HbS is only about half that of normal HbA or oxy-HbS. Yet an equal mix of HbS and HbF has twice the solubility of HbS alone, owing to HbF's unique ability to block polymerization[16]. The inhibitory effect of HbF on HbS sickling is due to the differences in the surface hydrophobicities of HbS and HbF. In addition, polymer formation that is sufficiently extensive to cause sickling requires a certain amount of time to develop, and is designated delay time (T_d). Fortunately, micro-circulatory transit times *in vivo* are usually shorter than T_d; thus, at least 80% of cells escape sickling as they traverse the microcirculation[17]. Sickled erythrocytes may 'sludge' in capillary beds, leading to chronic hemolysis, anemia and vaso-occlusion. However, other factors involved in vaso-occlusion may include abnormal adhesion, hypercoagulability, inflammation and endothelial activation[18–20]. Vaso-occlusion explains one of the most common clinical manifestations of SCD – the pain crisis – but the role of this well studied sickle cell phenomenon in organ infarction, such as stroke, is not clear.

EPIDEMIOLOGY OF STROKE AND INTRACRANIAL HEMORRHAGE IN SCD

Previous reports suggested that the prevalence of stroke in SCD ranges from 5% to 17% for patients 15 years of age and under[14,21–25]. More recent data on the prevalence and incidence of this disease have been obtained from the Cooperative Study of Sickle Cell Disease (CSSCD), a natural history study of 4082 homozygous HbSS and compound heterozygous patients, observed in 23 US clinical centers from 1978 to 1988. The investigators in this study reported an overall age-specific incidence of a first stroke in HbSS patients of 0.13% at an age of less than 24 months, increasing to a peak of over 1% at ages 2–5 years, with only a slight decrease to 0.79% at ages 6–9 years. Thereafter, the risk of brain infarction declines until a second peak that occurs at over age 50 years,

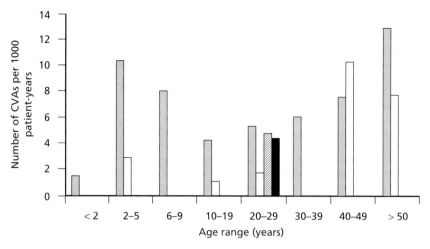

Figure 2   Incidence of stroke by age group from the Cooperative Study in Sickle Cell Disease (CSSCD). CVA, cerebrovascular accidents; ■, sickle cell disease; □, sickle/C hemoglobin disease; ▨, sickle/β^+-thalassemia; ■, sickle/β^0-thalassemia

when the incidence again increases to nearly 1.3% (Figure 2). In contrast, the subgroup of hemorrhagic stroke peaks sharply in the 20–29 years age range[26].

Compared to this homozygous HbSS population, the incidence of first stroke was lower for compound heterozygous groups (HbSC, HbS/β-thalassemia) studied at all ages, except for HbSC disease patients, whose risk was slightly higher for stroke only in the 40–49 years age range. Stroke incidence for HbS/β-thalassemia patients was lower than for the HbSC patients at all ages except for the 20–29 years age range, that showed a higher incidence in HbS/β-thalassemics, possibly indicating a propensity for hemorrhagic events in this age group. The incidence rate of having a first stroke by 20 years of age was calculated to be 11% in HbSS patients versus 2% in HbSC patients and essentially 0% for HbS/β-thalassemia patients, confirming the higher risk of stroke in HbSS, particularly in childhood[26].

The CSSCD study further divided the stroke into transient ischemic attack (TIA), cerebral infarction and cerebral hemorrhage. Among

the HbSS patients with strokes, 53.9% were infarctions, 34.2% were hemorrhages, and 10.5% were TIAs[26]. In a different study, intracranial hemorrhage (ICH) was reported to be as high as 20% of all stroke in SCD, followed by subarachnoid hemorrhage (SAH), that accounted for only 1–2%[23,27]. With 75% of the intracranial hemorrhages occurring in patients older than 14 years of age, SAH and ICH are more common in older children and adults. In addition, cerebral hemorrhage was more frequent in patients with prior infarction[23,28].

Sickle cell disease patients seem to be at a higher risk for SAH than the general population, and aneurysms, usually of smaller size if present, tend to bleed at a younger age[29]. However, 30% of children with SAH have angiograms showing no aneurysms, but instead have multiple distal branch occlusions and leptomeningeal collateralization. On computed tomography (CT) examination of these patients, evidence of blood within the superficial cortical sulci may be seen. SCD adults with SAH, in contrast, typically have aneurysms, often multiple in number, with blood in the basal cisterns on CT [28,30]. A case report[31] adds credence to earlier observations[32] that in SCD patients there is a heightened incidence of multiple aneurysms that have an unusual predilection for the posterior circulation when compared to the general population. There are several factors that may be responsible for the development of aneurysms in SCD disease: large vessel vasculopathy with stenosis that increases local and alternative path hemodynamic stress, greater cerebral blood flow and velocities secondary to a low hematocrit, and abnormal HbS erythrocyte interactions with endothelial surfaces that induce vessel wall damage. With life expectancies of SCD patients in developed countries dramatically increasing from less than 20 years to 40 to 50 years, it is possible that aneurysm and SAH will be seen with increased frequency in this population[33].

In the CSSCD study by Ohene-Frempong and colleagues[26] the incidence of stroke showed no significant gender difference. However, the Baltimore–Washington Cooperative Young Stroke Study, a retrospective investigation of stroke frequency in the Baltimore–Washington, DC area, showed a male preponderance of stroke in SCD[34]. Another study conducted at the Children's Hospital of Philadelphia reported that 57% of all SCD patients with stroke were male[35]. Balkaran et al. reported that males comprised 73.3% of the Jamaican SCD population that suffered stroke[36]. However, these clinical series, although suggestive, are not as convincing as the CSSCD, which did not find a male predominance in stroke. The question of gender difference in the stroke frequency of SCD sufferers remains unresolved.

The above stroke frequency data were based on patients who manifested overt clinical signs and symptoms of stroke. However, magnetic resonance imaging (MRI) has allowed the estimation of the prevalence and incidence of subclinical ischemic events, which may more often be associated with impaired performance on standardized psychometric testing[37]. Moser et al. showed that lesions of cerebral infarction or ischemia, in the absence of a history suggestive of stroke, are a common finding in SCD children. This group of investigators sought to define the spectrum of MRI abnormalities in 312 SCD children from the CSSCD, prospectively evaluating a cohort of newborns followed over the first two decades of life. Their data showed that 17% of HbSS patients had silent lesions, as compared to 3% of HbSC patients. The overall prevalence of silent stroke lesions was 13% in this patient population[38].

For patients with SCD and a history of stroke, cerebral infarction or ischemic lesions typically involve both the cortex and deep white matter, while silent lesions are usually confined to the deep white matter. A multivariate model for silent infarction in the CSSCD group proposed by Kinney et al. identified the following as risk factors for such events: low pain event rate, history of seizure, leukocyte count $\geq 11.8 \times 10^9/l$, and HbS/SEN β gene haplotype. A risk factor analysis for this group showed that silent infarcts were present in 18.3% of 230 subjects selected with HbSS[37]. The frequency of these lesions did not increase significantly between the ages of 6 and 14 years, suggesting that they were already present by age 6 years. However, older patients tended to have a greater number of lesions than their juniors, consistent with a progression of brain injury with age[38].

PATHOPHYSIOLOGY OF STROKE IN SCD

The mechanism of stroke in SCD has been better defined at the vascular level with advances in the understanding of this disease. Vaso-occlusion in the microcirculation is, at most, only part of the story. The majority of strokes in SCD do not result from vaso-occlusion in the microcirculation, but rather

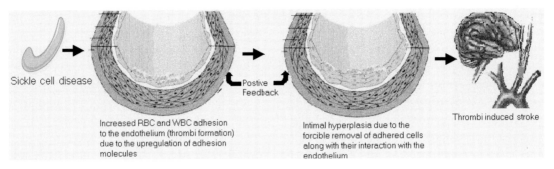

Figure 3 Possible mechanism of large vessel occlusion in sickle cell disease

from large-vessel vasculopathy primarily at three locations: the distal supraclinoid portion of the internal carotid artery (ICA), the proximal middle cerebral artery (MCA), and the proximal anterior cerebral artery (ACA). Such lesions have been demonstrated in about 80% of angiograms of SCD patients with stroke[39–43]. Also consistent with large-vessel etiology, MRI and CT studies of patients with SCD and stroke have shown that 80% have major distal-vessel occlusion or distal vessel insufficiency patterns[44]. In the later stages of vasculopathy there may be a striking similarity to the angiographic picture of 'moyamoya', with its abnormal network of subcortical vessels. The 'puff of smoke' appears in as many as 30% of SCD patients with vasculopathy[39–45]. Moyamoya and SCD show parallels in the risk of early infarction coupled with a later risk of hemorrhage, possibly due to the rupture of dilated, weakened collateral vessels[46].

Pathological examination of large vasculopathic segments reveals striking intimal proliferation with discontinuity of the internal elastic lamina. The cause of intimal hyperplasia and why it occurs at specific proximal sites in the anterior circulation are not fully known. However, there is evidence from pathologic sections that this intimal hyperplasia is mediated by endothelial damage. It has been postulated that adherent sickled red blood cells (RBCs) and or mini-thrombi are being forcibly removed, causing intimal denudation injury with the deposition of platelets and the release of platelet granules[47]. These granules release mitogens such as platelet-derived growth factor or endothelin-1 (ET-1), that have effects on vascular smooth muscle and fibroblast proliferation[48]. The concomitant thrombus formation in areas of endothelial damage may not only perpetuate the vicious cycle of intimal changes but also serve as the proximal source of artery-to-artery emboli responsible for some distal vessel occlusions (Figure 3)[49,50].

One area of research currently attracting much interest is the role of vascular endothelium in the process of intimal hyperplasia. SCD patients have been shown to have molecular abnormalities in the expression of adhesion molecules, that is intercellular adhesion molecule (ICAM), vascular cell adhesion molecule (VCAM) and E-selectin, that cause RBCs and white blood cells to adhere to the endothelium[18]. Vascular endothelium can be damaged by several mechanisms: (1) abnormal RBC adhesion[18], (2) reaction to endotoxin during infection[20], or (3) activated monocytes that express cytokines that upregulate adhesion molecules in endothelial cells[19]. A combination of all these processes may result in increased vascular damage and thrombus formation. Discussion of these mechanisms may be found in excellent reviews[50–53] as well as in reports by Hebbel and his colleagues[47,54–56].

Another area of investigation pertains to the role of an underlying hypercoagulable state in causing stroke in SCD. A recent study compared coagulation in 20 HbSS patients and 17 HbSC patients. In the HbSS group, antiphospholipid antibodies (particularly IgGs to phosphatidylserine that are exposed by red cell membrane damage) were elevated. The presence of such antibodies is known to lead to a hypercoagulable state. In addition, this study revealed that protein C and S activities were lower in HbSS patients compared to those with HbSC. Other measures of coagulation activation were also abnormal only in the HbSS group. The significant differences in coagulation indices were consistent with observed differences in the clinical severity between the two diseases[57].

RISK FACTORS FOR STROKE IN SCD

A number of risk factors have been implicated in SCD patients who had a stroke, but the strength of the data varies considerably among the studies. That a previous stroke was the single greatest risk factor for stroke in SCD is shown in the CSSCD, in which the patients were particularly at increased risk for intracranial hemorrhage[58]. Recalling the above epidemiologic data on stroke in SCD, patients aged 2–5 years old had the highest incidence of infarction, while young adults (aged 20–29 years) had a higher incidence of hemorrhagic stroke[26]. Hematologic characteristics have also been shown to correlate with stroke risk. SCD patients with lower average hemoglobin concentrations, increased steady state HbA_2 values, and decreased reticulocyte count were at increased risk for stroke[1,36]. A compensatory increase in cerebral blood flow due to severe anemia may cause flow disturbances that may lead to cerebrovascular damage[15]. Also, the proportion of HbF is inversely correlated with the incidence of stroke, owing to the mitigating

effects of HbF on sickling in SCD[59]. In addition, because SCD patients are more prone to infection, other systemic illnesses and pain crises[60], they have a higher incidence of increased leukocyte count, which has also been implicated as a risk factor for stroke in SCD[61].

Hyperhomocysteinemia is a known predisposing condition for ischemic complications in non-SCD patients. Whether elevated homocysteine adds to the complications of SCD is unclear. Houston and colleagues showed that homocysteine may be a risk factor for the development of stroke in SCD, and the increased homocysteine levels were correlated with low folate levels[62]. But more recent studies have shown that patients with SCD have elevated plasma concentrations of homocysteine, even when elevated plasma folate levels and vitamin B_{12} concentrations were similar to those in controls[63]. This may be the result of a higher folate requirement in SCD patients. Kennedy *et al.* showed that 15% of SCD subjects showed low folate levels, despite folate supplementation[64]. SCD patients with a homozygous mutation of C677T in the gene encoding for the enzyme responsible for metabolizing homocysteine, methylenetetrahydrofolate reductase (MTHFR), showed that hyperhomocysteinemia was not a significant factor in the pathogenesis of stroke in children with SCD. This casts doubt on the significance of elevated homocysteine in SCD[65,66].

Compared to patients with HbS/α-thalassemia, patients with HbSS disease and HbSC are at increased risk for stroke overall[26]. In addition, the HbS/α-thalassemia state may even protect against strokes because of a decrease in the number of HbS molecules in this condition[1,10,11]. On the other hand, certain haplotypes in SCD may be associated with a greater stroke risk. For example, the haplotype of the HbS/SEN β globin gene has been shown to increase silent infarcts, although the overall risk for clinical signs of stroke is lower than with other haplotypes[37]. The human leukocyte antigen (HLA) system may also influence

Table 1 Stroke incidence in the transfusion arm and standard care arm in the Stroke Prevention Trial in Sickle Cell Anemia (STOP)

Variable	Total number (n = 130)	Transfusion arm (n = 63)	Standard care arm (n = 67)
Follow-up (months)			
Total	2550	1321	1229
Median	21.1	22.2	18.3
Mean ± SD	19.6 ± 6.5	21.0 ± 5.7	18.3 ± 7.0
Intracerebral hematoma	1	0	1
Cerebral infarction	11	1	10
Number of strokes	12	1	11

stroke risk in SCD. Styles and colleagues studied 53 SCD patients, of whom 22 had MRI-documented evidence of cerebral infarction; the remaining 31 had a negative MRI. The HLA-DRB1*0301 and *0302 alleles were associated with increased risk of stroke, while protective associations were found with the DR2 group and the DRB1*1501 allele[67].

IMAGING IN SCD

Historically, imaging of the central nervous system in the SCD population was only prompted by symptoms such as stroke, seizure and altered mental status. The most commonly used techniques in these clinical situations were angiography, radionucleotide scanning, and cranial CT[1]. SCD patients who had imaging abnormalities showed more extensive involvement than anticipated from their clinical signs and symptoms. These early imaging observations prompted studies to define the types of lesions and their frequency. As a result of such studies, screening SCD children at risk for neurologic complications, such as stroke, was initiated and deemed worthwhile.

The Stroke Prevention Trial in Sickle Cell Anemia (STOP), a randomized clinical trial, established that chronic transfusion therapy can reduce the risk of first stroke by 92% in high-risk children 2–16 years old who are selected by screening with transcranial Doppler (TCD)

ultrasonography. Therefore, TCD screening of patients with SCD was considered useful. The children in this study, none of whom had a history of stroke at entry, were identified by TCD as having time-averaged maximal mean (as opposed to peak systolic) velocities ≥ 200 cm/sec in the ICA or MCA (normal adult velocities are 62 ± 12 cm/sec). Children with SCD generally have TCD velocities in the range of 130 to 140 cm/sec. Thus, the 200 cm/sec cut-off is about two standard deviations above the median for children of this age with SCD, taking the degree of anemia into account. Children in the untreated arm had a stroke risk of 10% per year, which is about 10–20 times the baseline risk in children with SCD in the same age group not selected by TCD criteria. Eleven strokes occurred in the untreated group, versus only one in the transfused group ($p < 0.0001$) (Table 1). An interim analysis showing these impressive results led to the early termination of the trial. The report was published as a *Clinical Alert* by the National Heart, Lung, and Blood Institute. TCD screening and consideration of transfusion in high-risk cases was encouraged based on the STOP study results[68,69].

MRI has also been used to determine the spectrum of brain abnormalities in SCD. In the CSSCD cranial MRI was performed on 312 patients and showed that 17% of patients without a history of stroke had MRI lesions consistent with ischemia; the ischemic lesions were usually small[38] and typically in the border zone region. Steen and colleagues showed that gray matter is selectively vulnerable in SCD patients during childhood and that white matter damage occurs later in the course of the disease[70]. In addition, the CSSCD performed neuropsychological testing along with MRI imaging of the brain on 135 children aged 6–12 years. Nine (6.7%) had a history of stroke in addition to abnormal MRI and neuropsychological testing results. Twenty-one others (15.6%) had no stroke history but did have MRI lesions indicative of infarction, while the remaining 105 (77.8%) had normal MRI findings. An abnormal MRI was associated with one or more cognitive deficits. 'Silent' MRI lesions were not uncommon and were also associated with abnormalities on cognitive testing. However, it was not clear at the time of these reports whether such lesions predisposed to subsequent clinical strokes[71].

To better understand the relationship between the anatomical lesions seen on MRI and the functional study of TCD, a multicenter comparison was conducted on a subset of 78 children with SCD, who had participated in both the CSSCD and STOP. Patients who had suffered an overt stroke were excluded. MRI findings in the 78 patients were classified as normal or 'silent stroke'. TCD results were classified as normal, conditional, or abnormal, based on the time-averaged maximal mean flow velocity in the proximal middle cerebral and distal internal carotid arteries. In the 61 patients with a normal MRI examination, 11 (18%) had either conditional (five) or abnormal (six) TCD results. Among 17 patients in whom silent infarction was seen on MRI, only five (29%) had a conditional (one) or abnormal (four) TCD velocity. Discordant results were seen in 23 cases. In 12 of these 23 patients, the TCD result was normal while the MRI was abnormal; and in 11 patients, the TCD velocity was elevated while the MRI was normal. From these results, it was concluded that abnormal TCD and MRI examinations reveal different aspects of the pathophysiology of CNS injury in SCD and may be discordant. Although TCD abnormality is predictive of overt stroke, the discordance between TCD and MRI findings in some patients suggests a need to develop more sensitive and specific indicators of early CNS pathology in SCD[72].

Newer MRI techniques, such as diffusion and perfusion imaging, may help decrease the discordance between MRI and TCD. Gadian and co-workers have shown that diffusion-weighted imaging (DWI) can be very sensitive in detecting early cerebral ischemia[73]. When DWI is combined with T_2-weighted imaging, the time at which the stroke occurred can be estimated more accurately. In addition, perfusion imaging, a technique that assesses cerebral perfusion, has shown promise in revealing deficits that are not seen on standardized MRI. The investigators in this study cited the case of an 11-year-old boy with SCD who had abnormal TCD results of the ICA and MCA, with velocities of 203 cm/sec and 185 cm/sec in the right and left side, respectively. T_2 and diffusion imaging showed no abnormalities. However, perfusion imaging showed abnormalities in the anterior and posterior border zone in the left hemisphere. Based on these results, this child was considered at high risk for stroke and placed on transfusion therapy[73].

Magnetic resonance angiography (MRA) is another non-invasive technique for evaluating the brain vascular anatomy in SCD patients. Currently, the sensitivity and specificity of a routine MRA are not well known and may vary from site to site. Kandeel and colleagues suggest that MRA may be 85% as accurate as conventional angiography. In this study, long segments (≥ 6 mm) of abnormal signal with reduced blood flow correlated with sub-clinical infarcts[74]. Seibert and colleagues have shown that an abnormal MRA, in combination with abnormal TCD, may be the best way to identify SCD patients at greatest risk for stroke[75].

Moreover, the use of MRA can be justified even in young SCD patients, because stenotic lesions can occur early in life in this population[76].

Positron emission tomography (PET) using fluorodeoxyglucose F18, a tracer analogue of glucose, has been used to evaluate local metabolic abnormalities in SCD. Initial studies have shown decreased frontal lobe activity, even when CT imaging is normal[77]. Reed *et al.* showed that PET may enhance the detection of impaired metabolism in the areas surrounding a major vessel infarct; however, this technique does not appear to be generally useful in characterizing small watershed lesions or deep white matter infarcts[78]. Powars *et al.* believe that PET may be useful, in conjunction with MRI, in identifying a greater number of SCD patients with neuroimaging abnormalities who do not yet have overt clinical signs. PET may also serve to monitor metabolic improvement after therapeutic intervention[79].

Recently computer-assisted intravital microscopy (CAIM) has been used to evaluate small-vessel abnormalities, as reflected by abnormal bulbar conjunctival vessel velocities. These measurements have been compared to TCD velocities in large-vessel vasculopathies. In one investigation, 18 children with SCD were examined with both TCD and CAIM. The MCA velocities were found to correlate significantly with bulbar conjunctival flow velocities ($p \leq 0.008$). Three patients (one with immeasurable MCA flow and two with normal MCA velocity) had abnormal conjunctival velocities on CAIM. Thus, CAIM may detect a sub-group at high risk for stroke even though MCA velocities on TCD are not increased[80].

PREVENTION OF STROKE IN SCD

Transfusion

Considerable evidence has accrued indicating that transfusion therapy helps prevent stroke in children with SCD. Following a first stroke, as many as two-thirds of untreated children experience a subsequent stroke, with the majority of these occurring within 36 months[23]. Although not tested in a clinical trial, chronic transfusion therapy with a goal of HbS reduction to < 30% has been reported to reduce stroke recurrence to as low as 10%[39,81]. Moreover, the STOP trial established that chronic transfusion therapy can reduce the risk of a first stroke by 92% in high-risk children aged 2 to 16 years old who were selected by screening with TCD[68]. A transfusion program should be developed in consultation with a pediatric hematologist. Exchange or simple transfusions are options. In the acute setting, using exchange transfusions avoids the potential adverse effect of raising hemoglobin toward a higher level, thereby raising blood viscosity. Over time, exchange transfusion, when compared to chronic transfusion, reduces iron loading, but requires more blood and thus exposes the patient to more transfusion hazards. With increased surveillance over the blood supply, this hazard has been reduced. For example, in the STOP study, there were no reports of HIV or hepatitis C transmission in over 1500 transfusions. Wayne *et al.* have provided further details on transfusion management in SCD[82].

While effective in carefully selected cases, transfusion is not a panacea. Although used in the acute setting immediately following stabilization after a stroke in children with SCD, there are no controlled data on the effect of the transfusion. Furthermore, there are no data supporting its use in adults, either for stroke prevention or treatment of acute stroke. It is also unclear whether transfusion is helpful in preventing recurrent intracranial brain hemorrhage, although it is frequently given in this setting in preparation for cerebral angiography to exclude aneurysms and vascular malformation. It may be of some benefit in reducing hemodynamic stress, that in turn may lower the risk of cerebral aneurysm rupture, but studies are needed to test this.

Chronic transfusion has many drawbacks, including alloimmunization[83] and iron overload. After only a few years of transfusion, treatment with chelation is needed to reduce iron overload. Untreated transfusion siderosis leads to organ damage, most prominently cardiomyopathy and hepatic dysfunction. Desferoxamine is the only FDA-approved chelation therapy available in the United States and is usually recommended when serum ferritin reaches 2500 ng/ml. The initial dose of desferoxamine is 50 mg/kg, administered by subcutaneous infusion over an eight-hour period daily for several days a week. The treatment is arduous and painful. It may cause hearing loss and, in rare cases, acute respiratory distress syndrome (ARDS)[84]. Long-term compliance with chelation becomes a problem, as no oral chelator is approved by the FDA. However, ICL 670A (4-(3,5-bis-(hydroxyphenyl)-[1,2,4] triazol-1-yl]-benzoic acid), an oral chelator, is in Phase I dose-finding clinical trials. This drug has great promise and has shown a good safety profile[85]. Deferiprone, another oral chelator, has shown promise but is not approved in the United States[86]. A modified transfusion protocol, not yet widely used, which allows HbS levels of 50%, may also be effective in preventing recurrent stroke[87,88].

It has not yet been established when the discontinuation of chronic transfusion following stroke is safe. As SCD children on chronic transfusion mature into adulthood, hematologists often discontinue transfusion therapy. Some patients choose to discontinue regular transfusions. The rate of stroke after discontinuation has not been adequately reported. Studies by Wilimas *et al.* have shown that discontinuation of transfusion after a stroke was followed by recurrent stroke within one year in 7 out of 10 patients[40]. However, another group observed no recurrences in seven children who had received transfusion for an average of two years prior to cessation[25]. More recently, Rana *et al.* reported that nine patients of various ages who had transfusions for an average of six years (minimum three years), had no strokes over an observation period ranging from 3 to 18.5 years. At the time of cessation of transfusions, two patients were approximately ten years of age and others were 17–25 years of age[89]. Wang *et al.* followed ten patients after an average duration of 9.5 years of transfusions were stopped and five recurrent cerebrovascular events ensued in a 12-month period. In addition, one death of unknown cause occurred. Ages at the time of discontinuation in patients with a stroke were 10, 13, 15, 16 and 17 years; the four without stroke were aged 7, 17, 20 and 21 years[90]. Existing guidelines recommend transfusion after infarction for at least five years or until the age of 18[91].

Hydroxyurea

Research has shown that an increased percent of HbF correlates with reduced disease severity in SCD[92]. After decades of unsuccessful efforts to find agents capable of elevating the percent HbF, therapy with hydroxyurea (HU) was developed. HU is the only chemotherapeutic agent approved for the treatment of SCD in the USA. A double-blind, placebo-controlled study of HU in 299 adults with SCD that investigated the reduction of painful episodes was terminated early when significant reductions became evident in the frequencies of pain episodes, acute chest syndrome, hospitalization and the need for blood transfusions[93]. However, in this study there were too few patients with strokes to determine any effect of the drug on the risk of stroke. No controlled study has since specifically addressed the question of whether HU is effective in stroke prevention. Ware and colleagues reported the outcomes of secondary stroke treatment with HU and phlebotomy in 16 young patients, in whom transfusion was no longer an option[94]. They reported a

19% reduction in recurrent events, but comparison with an appropriate control is needed[23,90]. In addition, the sample size was small, and randomization was not performed.

On theoretical grounds, HU offers promise for stroke prevention. In addition to elevating percent HbF, HU reduces many of the markers of severe SCD. HU results in an improvement of RBC deformability, a reduction in cellular dehydration and potassium content, a decrease in the irreversible sickled cell fraction and improvements in rheology and RBC survival[95]. Abnormal adhesion of blood cells may also be modified[96–98]. Increased levels of granulocytes, reticulocytes and platelets, that are putative markers of an increased risk for cerebral vasculopathy, are also ameliorated with HU treatment[84]. HU therapy is initiated at 15 mg/kg/day and is typically raised by 5 mg/kg/day. Every 8 to 12 weeks platelets, reticulocytes and neutrophils are monitored, and treatment is interrupted temporarily or permanently if toxicity is evident. Few patients can tolerate over 30 mg/kg/day. It is not clear how important it is to reach the maximal tolerated dose, as opposed to maintaining a lower dose for the control of pain crises[93,94].

In pilot studies over an average of 137 weeks, HU used in SCD has been shown to be safe and effective[99]. Negative effects on growth and development cannot yet be excluded, and questions regarding a predisposition to malignancy remain to be answered. These concerns have arisen because of observations of DNA mutations occurring at very low frequency in *in vivo* studies of HU therapy[100]. Other side-effects of HU are cutaneous lesions such as leg ulcers, and it may also exacerbate the ulcers that can occur in SCD even without HU[101].

Bone marrow transplant

Bone marrow transplant (BMT) may cure SCD and is potentially an option for stroke prevention. Data are available showing that HLA-identical sibling stem cell allografts can successfully replace sickle cells with normal donor-derived RBCs[102,103]. Such a stable mixed chimerism, even with a relatively low proportion of donor cells, can ameliorate many of the symptoms and complications of SCD, although an effect specifically on stroke is not clear. The survival of BMT patients has been in the 90% range, and event-free survival about 85%[102]. The cumulative incidence of graft rejection or return of SCD is 11%. Although most transplanted patients have survived free of SCD, approximately 8% have died, and about half of these deaths have occurred in the setting of graft-versus-host disease (GVHD)[103]. In addition to acute and chronic GVHD, seizures and intracerebral hemorrhage have been reported in stroke patients who received BMT, in addition to other transient but benign complications of the procedure.

The study by Walters *et al.* examined 22 patients with stable donor engraftment over two years for the impact of BMT on CNS disease[102]. Ten patients had a history of stroke, four had silent infarcts revealed by MRI, one had a TIA and one had positive TCD screening prior to BMT. Based on clinical and MRI follow-up, it was concluded that no significant CNS events had occurred and that most had shown a 'stabilization' of underlying cerebral vasculopathy. Bernaudin states that a history of stroke has become the main indication for BMT in SCD and recommended that it be considered in patients with silent cerebral infarcts associated with cognitive impairment or TCD evidence of increased stroke risk[104]. However, the paucity of available HLA-identical sibling donors is a major obstacle to BMT in SCD, but it remains an option for some patients, particularly those at highest risk of significant adverse events, such as stroke[103].

Other treatments

Gene therapy offers hope as a future intervention in SCD. However, it will probably be several years before it can be applied clinically.

Obstacles include the expected problems of efficient gene transfer into hematopoietic cells and regulation of gene expression. Successful gene therapy in SCD must not only increase production of a normal hemoglobin chain, but also ameliorate the effects of abnormal HbS. Since patients with an increased percent of HbF are known to have a milder disease course, efforts are currently being directed toward gene therapy that would increase the production of HbF. Preliminary findings in mice suggest the possibility of a hemoglobin chain regulatory mechanism that increases the gene production of HbF, while decreasing that of HbS[105,106]. Such a switching mechanism, if identified and manipulated, could be of potential benefit in the treatment of SCD.

Warfarin is another unproven alternative for children who cannot be transfused over the long term, and also for reducing the recurrence of stroke in adult SCD patients. It may serve as a reasonable therapy if there is evidence of intracranial arterial stenosis. No systematic studies have been conducted on either anticoagulation or antiplatelet agents in this setting, but, given the support for the use of these agents in adults generally, it is reasonable to use them in adults with SCD when no other specific stroke prevention strategy is available.

In cases of treatment failure and recurrent strokes despite medical therapy, and also in the setting of severe vascular disease, vascular surgery is an option. There are a few reports of the successful establishment of collateral blood supply using an operation called encephaloduroarteriosynangiosis, in which a superficial scalp artery and its adjacent galea are mobilized, passed through the dura, and placed onto the arachnoid surface of the brain[107].

CONCLUSION

SCD disease, a prototypical hemoglobinopathy, has throughout its history been a disease that has had many neurologic sequelae, including stroke. Through the efforts of the scientific community, immense strides in the prevention and treatment of stroke in the SCD patient have been made, and a practicable primary prevention strategy is now available. With the implementation of widespread screening combined with intervention, the frequency of severe cerebrovascular disease in these patients may be reduced.

References

1. Pavlakis SG, Prohovnic I, Piomelli S, *et al.* Neurologic complications of sickle cell disease. *Adv Pediatr* 1989;36:247–76

2. Syndenstricker VP, Mulherin WA, Houseal RW. Sickle cell anemia. *Am J Dis Child* 1923;26:132–54

3. Herrick JB. Peculiar elongated and sickle-shaped red corpuscles in a case of severe anemia. *Arch Intern Med* 1910;6:517–24

4. Cook JE, Myers J. Severe anemia with remarkable elongated and sickle-shaped red blood cells and chronic leg ulcers. *Arch Intern Med* 1915;16:644–51

5. Mason VR. Sickle cell anemia. *J Am Med Assoc* 1922;79:1318–20

6. Leikin SL, Gallagher D, Kinney TR, *et al.* Mortality in children and adolescents with sickle cell disease. *Pediatrics* 1989;84:500–8

7. Platt OS, Brambilla DJ, Rosse WF, *et al.* Mortality in sickle cell disease. *N Engl J Med* 1994;330:1639–44

8. Steinberg MH. Management of sickle cell disease. *N Engl J Med* 1999;340:1021–30

9. Steinberg M, Embury S. Natural history: Overview. In Embury SH, Hebbel RP, Mohandas N, Steinberg M, eds. *Sickle Cell Disease: Basic Principles and Practice.* New York: Raven, 1994:349–52

10. Sergeant GR. Sickle-cell disease. *Lancet* 1997;350:725–30

11. Adams RJ, Kutlaer A, Mckie V, *et al.* Alpha thalassemia and stroke risk in sickle cell anemia. *Am J Hematol* 1994;45:279–82

12. Ingram VM. Gene mutation in human hemoglobin: the chemical difference between normal and sickle cell hemoglobin. *Nature* 1957; 180:326–9

13. Alavi JB. Sickle cell anemia: Pathophysiology and treatment. *Med Clin N Am* 1984;68: 545–55

14. Sergeant G. The nervous system. In Seargent G, ed. *Sickle Cell Disease*. Oxford: Oxford University Press, 1985:233–46

15. Adams RJ. Neurologic complications. In Embury SH, Hebbel RP, Mohandas N, Steinberg M, eds. *Sickle Cell Disease: Basic Principles and Practice*. New York: Raven, 1994:599–621

16. Schechter AN, Noguchi CT. Sickle hemoglobin polymer: structure-function correlates. In Embury SH, Hebbel RP, Mohandas N, Steinberg M, eds. *Sickle Cell Disease: Basic Principles and Practice*. New York: Raven, 1994:33–51

17. Mozzarelli A, Holrichter J, Eaton WA. Delay time of HbS polymerization prevents most cells from sickling *in vivo*. *Science* 1987;237:500–6

18. Kaul DK, Fabry ME, Costantini F, *et al. In vivo* demonstration of red cell–endothelial interaction, sickling and altered microvascular response to oxygen in the sickle transgenic mouse. *J Clin Invest* 1995;96:2845–53

19. Belcher JD, Marker PH, Weber JP, *et al.* Activated monocytes in sickle cell disease: potential role in the activation of vascular endothelium and vaso-occlusion. *Blood* 2000; 96:2451–9

20. Sultana C, Shen Y, Ratten V, *et al.* Interaction of sickle erythrocytes with endothelial cells in the presence of endothelial cell conditioned medium induces oxidant stress leading to transendothelial migration of monocytes. *Blood* 1998;92:3924–35

21. Portnoy BA, Herion JC. Neurologic manifestations in sickle cell disease: with a review of the literature and emphasis on the prevalence of hemiplegia. *Ann Intern Med* 1972;76:643–52

22. Greer M, Schotland D. Abnormal hemoglobin as a cause of neurological disease. *Neurology* 1962;12:114–20

23. Powers D, Wilson B, Imbus C, *et al.* The natural history of stroke in sickle cell disease. *Am J Med* 1978;65:461–71

24. Sarniak SA, Lusher JM. Neurological complications of sickle cell anemia. *J Pediatr Hematol Oncol* 1982;4:386–94

25. Moohr JW, Wilson H, Pang E. Strokes and their management in sickle cell disease. In Fried W, ed. *Comparative Clinical Aspects of Sickle Cell Disease*. New York: Elsevier North Holland, 1982:101–11

26. Ohene-Frempong K, Weiner SJ, Sleeper LA, *et al.* Cerebrovascular accidents: rates and risk factors. *Blood* 1998;91:288–94

27. Wood DH. Cerebrovascular complications of sickle cell anemia. *Stroke* 1978;9:73–5

28. Van Hoff J, Ritchey AK, Shaywitz BA. Intracranial hemorrhage in children with sickle cell disease. *Am J Dis Child* 1985;139:1120–2

29. Anson JA, Koshy M, Ferguson L, *et al.* Subarachnoid hemorrhage in sickle cell disease. *Hematology* 1991;75:552–8

30. Love LC, Mickle JP, Sypert GW. Ruptured intracranial aneurysms in cases of sickle cell anemia. *Neurosurgery* 1985;16:808–12

31. Preul MC, Cendes F, Just N, Mohr G. Intracranial aneurysms and sickle cell anemia: multiplicity and propensity for vertebrobasilar territory. *Neurosurgery* 1998;42:971–7

32. Oyesiku NM, Barrow DL, Eckman JR, *et al.* Intracranial aneurysms in sickle cell anemia: clinical features and pathogenesis. *J Neurosurg* 1991;75:356–63

33. Diggs LW, Brookoff D. Multiple cerebral aneurysms in patients with sickle cell disease. *South Med J* 1993;86:377–9

34. Earley CJ, Kitter SJ, Feeser BR, *et al.* Stroke in children and sickle-cell disease: Baltimore–Washington cooperative young stroke study. *Am Acad Neurol* 1998;51:169–76

35. Ohene-Frempong K. Stroke in sickle cell disease: demographic, clinical, and therapeutic considerations. *Semin Hematol* 1991;28:213–19

36. Balkaran B, Char G, Morris JS, *et al.* Stroke in a cohort of patients with homozygous sickle cell disease. *J Pediatr* 1992;120:360–6

37. Kinney TR, Sleeper LA, Wang WC, *et al.* Silent cerebral infarcts in sickle cell anemia: a risk factor analysis. *Pediatrics* 1999;103:640–5

38. Moser FG, Miller ST, Bello JA, *et al.* The spectrum of brain MR abnormalities in sickle cell disease: a report from the cooperative study of sickle cell disease. *Am J Neuroradiol* 1996; 17:965–72

39. Russell MO, Goldgerg HI, Hodson A, *et al.* Effect of transfusion therapy on arteriographic

abnormalities and on recurrence of stroke in sickle cell disease. *Blood* 1984;63:162–9

40. Wilimas J, Goff JR, Anderson HR, *et al.* Efficacy of transfusion for one to two years in patients with sickle cell disease and cerebrovascular accidents. *J Pediatr* 1980;96: 205–8

41. Jeffries BF, Lipper MH, Kishore PRF. Major intracerebral involvement in sickle cell disease. *Surg Neurol* 1980;14:291–5

42. Gerald B, Sebes JI, Langston JW. Cerebral infarction secondary to sickle cell disease: arteriographic findings. *Am J Radiol* 1980;134: 1209–12

43. Baird RL, Weiss DL, Ferguson AD, *et al.* Studies in sickle cell anemia: XII. Clinico-pathological aspects of neurological manifesta-tions. *Pediatrics* 1964;34:92–100

44. Adams RJ, Nichols FT, McKie V, *et al.* Cerebral infarction in sickle cell anemia: mech-anism based on CT and MRI. *Neurology* 1988; 38:1012–17

45. Seeler RA, Royal JE, Powe L, *et al.* Moya moya in children with sickle cell anemia and cere-brovascular occlusion. *J Pediatr* 1978;93: 808–10

46. Suzuki J, Takaku A. Cerebrovascular moya moya disease: disease showing abnormal net-like vessels in the base of the brain. *Arch Neurol* 1969;20:288–99

47. Hebbel RP. Adhesive interactions of sickle erythrocytes with endothelium. *J Clin Invest* 1997;99:2561–4

48. Francis RB. Large vessel occlusion in sickle cell disease: pathogenesis, clinical consequences, and therapeutic implications. *Med Hypotheses* 1991;35:88–95

49. Merkel KHH, Ginsberg PL, Parker JC, *et al.* Cerebrovascular disease in sickle cell anemia: a clinical pathological and radiological correla-tion. *Stroke* 1978;9:45–52

50. Rothman SM, Fulling KH, Nelson JS. Sickle cell anemia and central nervous system infarc-tion: a neuropathological study. *Ann Neurol* 1986;20:684–90

51. Hess DC, Adams RJ, Nichols FT. Sickle cell anemia and other hemoglobinopathies. *Semin Neurol* 1991;11:314–28

52. Stehbens WE. Localization of atherosclerotic lesions in relation to hemodynamics. In Olson AG, ed. *Atherosclerosis: Biology and Clinical Science.* New York: Churchhill Livingstone, 1987:175–82

53. Kaul DK, Fabry ME, Nagel RL. The patho-physiology of vascular obstruction. *Blood Rev* 1996;10:29–44

54. Solovey A, Gui L, Key NS, Hebbel RP. Tissue factor expression by endothelial cells in sickle cell anemia. *J Clin Invest* 1998;101:1899–904

55. Solovey A, Lin Y, Browne P, *et al.* Circulating activated endothelial cells in sickle cell anemia. *N Engl J Med* 1997;337:1584–90

56. Barabino GA, Wise RJ, Woodbury VA, *et al.* Inhibition of sickle erythrocyte adhesion to immobilized thrombospondin by von Willebrand factor under dynamic flow condi-tions. *Blood* 1997;89:2560–7

57. Westerman MP, Green D, Gilman-Sacks A, *et al.* Antiphospholipid antibodies, proteins C and S and coagulation changes in sickle cell disease. *J Clin Invest* 1999;134:352–62

58. Powars DR, Schroeder WA, Weiss JN, *et al.* Lack of influence of fetal hemoglobin levels of erythrocyte indices on the severity of sickle cell anemia. *J Clin Invest* 1980;65:732–40

59. Franco RS, Yasin Z, Lohmann JM, *et al.* The survival characteristics of dense sickle cells. *Blood* 2000;96:3610–17

60. Osuntokun BO. Undernutrition and infectious disorders as risk factors for stroke. *Adv Neurol* 1979;25:161–74

61. Miller ST, Sleeper LA, Pegelow CH. Prediction of adverse outcomes in children with sickle cell disease. *N Engl J Med* 2000;342:83–9

62. Houston PE, Rana S, Sekhsaria S, *et al.* Homocysteine in sickle cell disease: relation-ship with stroke. *Am J Med* 1997;103:192–6

63. Lowentthal EA, Mayo MS, Cornwell PE, *et al.* Homocysteine elevation in sickle cell disease. *J Am Coll Nutr* 2000;19:608–12

64. Kennedy TS, Fung EB, Kawchak DA, *et al.* Red blood cell folate and serum vitamin B12 status in children with sickle cell disease. *J Pediatr Hematol Oncol* 2001;23:165–9

65. Balasa VV, Gruppo RA, Gartside PS, *et al.* Correlation of C677T MTHFR genotype with homocysteine levels in children with sickle cell disease. *J Pediatr Hematol Oncol* 1999;21: 397–400

66. Cumming AM, Olujohungbe A, Keeny S, *et al.* The methylenetetrahydrofolate reductase gene C677T polymorphism in patients with sickle cell disease and stroke. *Br J Haematol* 1999; 107:569–71

67. Styles LA, Hoppe C, Klitz W, *et al.* Evidence for HLA-related susceptibility for stroke in

children with sickle cell disease. *Blood* 2000;95:3562–7

68. Adams RJ, Mckie VC, Hsu L, *et al.* Prevention of first stroke by transfusions in children with sickle sell anemia and abnormal results on transcranial ultrasonography. *N Engl J Med* 1998;339:5–11

69. Clinical Alert from the National Heart, Lung, and Blood Institute, Dept of Health and Human Services. 18 Sept 1997

70. Steen RG, Langston JW, Ogg RJ, *et al.* Diffuse T_1 reduction in gray matter of sickle cell disease patients: evidence of selective vulnerability to damage? *Mag Res Imag* 1999;17:503–15

71. Armstrong FD, Thompson RJ, Wang W, *et al.* Cognitive functioning and brain magnetic resonance in children with sickle cell disease. *Pediatrics* 1996;97:864–70

72. Wang WC, Gallagher DM, Pegelow CH, *et al.* Multicenter comparison of magnetic resonance imaging and transcranial Doppler ultrasonography in the evaluation of the central nervous system in children with sickle cell disease. *J Pediatr Haematol Oncol* 2000;22:335–9

73. Gadian DG, Calamante F, Kirkham F, *et al.* Diffusion and perfusion magnetic resonance imaging in childhood stroke. *J Child Neurol* 2000;15:279–83

74. Kandeel AY, Zimmerman RA, Ohene-Frempong K. Comparison of magnetic resonance angiography and conventional angiography in sickle cell disease: clinical significance and reliability. *Neuroradiology* 1996;38:409–16

75. Seibert JJ. Transcranial Doppler, MRA, and MRI as a screening examination for cerebrovascular disease in patients with sickle cell anemia: an 8-year study. [published erratum appears in *Pediatr Radiol* 1998;28:546.] *Pediatr Radiol* 1998;28:138–42

76. Gilliams AR, McMahon L, Weinber G, *et al.* MRA of the intracranial circulation in asymtomatic patients with sickle cell disease. *Pediatr Radiol* 1998;28:283–7

77. Rodgers GP, Clark CM, Larson SM, *et al.* Brain glucose metabolism in neurologically normal patients with sickle cell disease. *Arch Neurol* 1998;45:78–82

78. Reed W, Jagust W, Al-Mateen M, *et al.* Role of positron emission tomography in determining the extent of CNS ischemia in patients with sickle cell disease. *Am J Hematol* 1999;60:268–72

79. Powars DR, Conti PS, Wong WY, *et al.* Cerebral vasculopathy in sickle cell anemia: diagnostic contribution of positron emission tomography. *Blood* 1999;93:71–9

80. Cheung AT, Harmatz P, Wun T, *et al.* Correlation of abnormal intracranial vessel velocity, measured by transcranial Doppler ultrasonography, with abnormal conjunctival vessel velocity, measured by computer-assisted intravital microscopy, in sickle cell disease. *Blood* 2001;97(11):3401–4

81. Pegelow CH, Adams RJ, Mckie V, *et al.* Risk of recurrent stroke in patients with sickle cell disease treated with erythrocyte transfusions. *J Pediatr* 1995;126:896–9

82. Wayne AS, Kevy SV, Nathan DG. Transfusion management of sickle cell disease. *Blood* 1993;81:1109–23

83. Rosse WR, Gallagher D, Kinney TR, *et al.* Transfusion and alloimunization in sickle cell disease. *Blood* 1990;76:1431–7

84. Powars DR. Management of cerebral vasculopathy in children with sickle cell anemia. *Br J Haematol* 2000;108:666–78

85. Galanello R. Iron chelation: new therapies. *Semin Hematol* 2001;38:73–6

86. Rombos Y, Tzanetea R, Konstanopoulos K, *et al.* Chelation therapy in patients with thalassemia using the orally active iron chelator deferipone. *Hematologica* 2000;85:115–17

87. Cohen AR, Martin MB, Silber JH, *et al.* A modified transfusion program for prevention of stroke in sickle cell disease. *Blood* 1992;79:1657–61

88. Miller ST, Jensen D, Rao SP. Less intensive long-term transfusion therapy for sickle cell anemia and cerebrovascular accident. *J Pediatr* 1992;120:54–7

89. Rana S, Houston PE, Surana N, *et al.* Discontinuation of long term transfusion therapy in patients with sickle cell disease and stroke. *J Pediatr* 1997;131:757–60

90. Wang WC, Kovnar EH, Tonkin IL, *et al.* High risk of recurrent stroke after discontinuation of five to twelve years of transfusion therapy in patients with sickle cell disease. *J Pediatr* 1991;118:377–82

91. Charache S, Lubin B, Reid CD. Management and therapy of sickle cell disease. Washington, DC, US Dept of Health and Human Services Public Health Service, National Institutes of Health, 1992: Publication No. 92-2117:22

92. Platt OS, Thorington BD, Brambilla DJ, *et al.* Pain in sickle cell disease: rates and risk factors. *N Engl J Med* 1991;325:11–16

93. Charache S, Terrin ML, Moore RD, *et al.* Effect of hydroxyurea on the frequency of painful crisis in sickle cell anemia. *N Engl J Med* 1995;332:1317–22

94. Ware WE, Zimmerman SA, Schultz WH. Hydroxyurea as an alternative to blood transfusions for the prevention of recurrent stroke in children with sickle cell disease. *Blood* 1999;94:3022–6

95. Ballas SK, Marcolina MJ, Dover GJ, *et al.* Erythropoietic activity in patients with sickle cell anaemia before and after treatment with hydroxyurea. *Br J Haematol* 1999;105:491–6

96. Bridges KR, Barabino GD, Brugnara C, *et al.* A multiparameter analysis of sickle erythrocytes in patients undergoing hydroxyurea therapy. *Blood* 1996;88:4701–10

97. Saleh AW, Hillen HF, Duits AJ. Levels of endothelial, neutrophil and platelet-specific factors in sickle cell anemia patients during hydroxyurea therapy. *Acta Haematol* 1999;102:31–7

98. Styles LA, Lubin B, Vichinsky E, *et al.* Decrease of very late activation of antigen-4 and CD-36 on reticulocytes in sickle cell patients treated with hydroxyurea. *Blood* 1997;89:2554–9

99. Hoppe C, Vinchinsky E, Quirolo K, *et al.* Use of hydroxyurea in children aged 2 to 5 years with sickle cell disease. *J Pediatr Hematol Oncol* 2000;22:330–4

100. Hanft VN, Fruchtman ST, Picken CV, *et al.* Acquired DNA mutations associated with *in vivo* hydroxyurea exposure. *Blood* 2000;95:3589–93

101. Chaine B, Neonato MG, Girot R, *et al.* Cutaneous adverse reactions to hydroxyurea in patients with sickle cell disease. *Arch Dermatol* 2001;137:467–70

102. Walters MC, Storb R, Patience M, *et al.* Impact of bone marrow transplantation for symptomatic sickle cell disease: an interim report. *Blood* 2000;95:1918–24

103. Walters MC. Bone marrow transplantation for sickle cell disease: where do we go from here? *J Pediatr Haematol Oncol* 1999;21:467–74

104. Bernaudin F. Results and current indications of bone marrow allograft in sickle cell disease. *Pathol Biol* 1999;47:59–64

105. Karsson S. The first steps on the gene therapy pathway to anti-sickling process. *Nat Med* 2000;6:139–40

106. Blouin MJ, Beauchemin H, Wright A, *et al.* Genetic correction of sickle cell disease: insights using transgenic models. *Nat Med* 2000;6:177–82

107. Vernet O, Montes JL, O'Gorman AM, *et al.* Encephaloduroarteriosynangiosis in a child with sickle cell disease and moyamoya disease. *Pediatr Neurol* 1996;14:226–30

Chapter 7

Oral contraception and postmenopausal estrogen replacement therapy

Gretchen E. Tietjen, MD, and Robin L. Brey, MD

INTRODUCTION

Stroke prevention necessitates an understanding of stroke risk. This chapter examines the risk of stroke related to the use of oral contraceptive pills and estrogen replacement therapy. The focus of stroke risk is hence restricted to the adult female population. Overall, adult females have a lower frequency of stroke than adult males. However, among individuals younger than 45 years and older than 80 years, women have more strokes than men. Among younger women, those in their reproductive years, use of estrogen-containing pharmaceuticals is most prevalent. An estimated 65 million women worldwide, corresponding to 6% of all women of reproductive age, use the oral contraceptive pill (OCP)[1]. Developed to prevent pregnancy, OCP are also widely used to treat menorrhagia, irregular menstrual periods, peri-menopausal symptoms and even menstrual migraine. Estrogen replacement therapy (ERT), used by an estimated 38% of postmenopausal women in the United States[2], is commonly prescribed to prevent osteoporosis and alleviate symptoms of menopause, including hot flashes, night sweats, insomnia and mood swings.

With hormonal contraceptives as well as with hormone replacement therapy (ERT), there are also potential effects of estrogen that may be harmful. The increased risk of thrombosis, predominantly in the systemic venous circulation, has long been acknowledged as a risk of OCP use. Reports of the magnitude of the risk of OCP-related stroke have varied, depending on pill type, population and methodology of the study. The increased risk for endometrial and breast cancer due to supplemental ERT is well recognized[3] but the impact of a theoretical risk for heart disease and stroke due to adverse effects on coagulation is unclear. With widespread use of OCP and ERT, effects on hemostasis and their impact on stroke is germane to the discussion of stroke prevention.

MECHANISMS OF STROKE WITH OCP AND ERT

Beneficial effects of OCP and estrogen replacement therapy (ERT) include improved endothelial vascular function, reduction of Lp(a) lipoprotein, reduction of plasma levels of low-density lipoprotein (LDL), and increase of plasma levels of high-density lipoprotein (HDL)[4]. These effects decrease the risk of atherosclerosis. However, an adverse effect of ERT and OCP that increases stroke risk, both in the arterial and venous circulations, is most probably related to the effects on hemostasis, the equilibrium of coagulation and fibrinolysis[5].

In women taking synthetic ethinylestradiol containing OCP, hypercoagulability is related to elevated levels of fibrinogen and coagulation factors (VII, VIII and X), as well as to decreased levels of physiologic anticoagulants (antithrombin III, protein S) and acquired activated protein C (APC) resistance. These effects are balanced by increased fibrinolysis related to increased plasminogen and a decrease in its physiologic inhibitor, plasminogen activating inhibitor 1 (PAI-1). In total, these changes are more likely to affect the venous than the arterial system. Observational studies have suggested that the tendency toward thrombosis rises with the ethinylestradiol dose. Progesterone, the other component in the combined OCP, adversely affects lipids and lipid metabolism, possibly increasing atherogenic potential. Evidence of the variability of stroke risk based on the type of progesterone is conflicting[6–8]. Studies suggest that when combined with synthetic estrogen, the less androgenic third generation progestogens (desogestrel, gestodene and norgestimate) predispose to venous thrombosis through decreased antithrombin, protein C activation and increased coagulation factors[9–11]. Progestogen-only contraception does not affect coagulation or fibrinolysis, and there are no data suggesting that it predisposes to thromboembolism[12].

In similar fashion to synthetic estrogen-containing OCP, ERT using oral conjugated equine estrogens and oral 17-β-estradiol predisposes to thrombosis by decreasing antithrombin III, protein S, and abnormal APC resistance. Profibrinolytic effects of ERT include a decrease in PAI-1 and decrease in fibrinogen[5]. A shift from hemostasis toward hypercoagulability appears to increase with an increasing dose of conjugated estrogen[13]. Favorable alterations of LDL and HDL levels with oral estrogens at doses of 0.625 and 1.25 mg/day have been reported[14]. The decrease in LDL levels resulted from accelerated LDL catabolism, and an increase in triglycerides resulted from an increased production of large, triglyceride-rich very-low-density lipoprotein (VLDL). This large VLDL fraction is cleared directly from the circulation and not converted into small VLDL or LDL. Postmenopausal estrogens may also lower the risk of vascular disease by beneficial effects on serum glucose and insulin levels as well as on blood pressure[15,16]. Transdermal 17-β-estradiol preparations may lack deleterious effects on hemostasis[17], but their benefits are also less certain.

ORAL CONTRACEPTIVE PILLS AND STROKE

Assessment of the risk of stroke associated with combined OCP is difficult because their composition has changed substantially over the forty years since they were introduced. The estrogen content has decreased at least fivefold (from 150 micrograms to 20–35 micrograms). With decreasing estrogen content, the risk of stroke decreases significantly. A causal relationship with this reduction has been assumed but not proven. The type of progestogen (first, second and third generation) with which estrogen is combined has changed as well.

Cerebral ischemic infarction (arterial)

The safety of lower dose estrogen with respect to stroke risk is illustrated by a number of studies. The World Health Organization (WHO) study of OCP was a multi-center hospital-based, case–control study with centers throughout Europe, and in developing countries in Asia, Africa and Latin America. Although in the developing countries the risk of stroke was increased regardless of the pill dosage, in the European countries the risk of stroke was elevated five-fold for women using OCP preparations with estrogen levels higher than 50 µg, but was negligible (OR, 1.53; 95% CI, 0.71–3.31) with formulations containing less than 50 µg[7]. Similarly, a Danish case–control study reported an increased risk of thrombotic stroke with formulations containing 50 µg estrogen (OR, 2.9) and 30–40 µg estrogen (OR, 1.8) but not with those containing 20 µg[18]. The Royal College of General Practitioners' (RCGP) study showed that for normotensive, non-smoking women, the sub-50 µg estrogen OCP was not associated with increased risk of stroke (OR, 0.6; 95% CI, 0.1–2.9). In this study, the risk was significantly higher with 50 µg (OR, 2.9; 95% CI, 1.7–5.0) and preparations containing more than 50 µg (OR, 5.8; 95% CI, 1.5–22.8)[19]. In the Oxford Family Planning Association study, no thrombotic strokes occurred in women using OCP with less than 50 µg estrogen[20]. A California HMO-based case–control study of sub-50 µg estrogen OCP and stroke showed a non-significant, adjusted OR of 1.18; 95% CI, 0.54–2.59[21]. When these data were pooled with a similar US population-based case–control study[22], analysis suggested that the risk of ischemic stroke (adjusted pOR, 0.66; 95% CI, 0.20–1.47) in low-dose OCP users was not greater than for the cohort that had never used OCP, even in those who smoked cigarettes (pOR, 0.72; 95% CI, 0.17–3.02), were obese (pOR, 0.59; 95% CI, 0.16–2.12) or were older than 35 years (pOR, 0.61; 95% CI, 0.13–2.08). Although the estrogen content of the OCP was not specified, in the US Health and Nutrition Survey of 12 000 people there was no increased risk of ischemic stroke in OCP users[23].

In contrast to the data on the effect of estrogen dose on stroke risk, data on the effect of progestogen type is less uniform. The Danish study showed an increased ischemic stroke risk with second generation OCP[8], whereas in the Transnational study the greatest risk was with the use of first generation OCP[24]. There is no evidence that progesterone-only OCP predisposes to arterial or venous thrombosis.

Cerebral venous thrombosis (CVT)

CVT is rarer than arterial stroke, but two studies suggest that CVT is strongly and independently associated with the use of OCP (OR, 13[25]; OR, 22.1; 95% CI, 5.9–84.2[26] respectively). OCP users with congenital thrombophilia, including factor V Leiden and the prothrombin gene mutation, are at even higher risk. For example, in a recent report, the risk of CVT for women with the prothrombin gene mutation was increased dramatically in OCP users compared with those without these factors (OR, 10.2; 95% CI, 2.3–31.0) and OR, 149.3; 95% CI, 31.0–711 respectively)[26]. However, since factor V Leiden and the prothrombin gene mutation are present in less than 5% of the population, and the incidence of CVT is probably less than 1 per 1000 persons per year, screening for these mutations prior to prescribing OCP is arguably not cost effective[26].

Subarachnoid and intracerebral hemorrhage (SAH)

The effects of OCP on the vasculature and coagulation system do not appear to predispose to an increased risk of primary hemorrhage, but studies examining the risk of SAH in users of combined OCP have yielded conflicting results. A recent meta-analysis of 11 observational studies suggests that even when controlling for smoking and hypertension, there is an increase in the risk of SAH in current users of OCP (RR, 1.57; 95% CI, 1.25–1.99), with no significant difference based on estrogen content[27]. In the WHO study an increased risk of hemorrhagic stroke with current use of combined OCP was significant in developing countries, but not in Europe, in women over 35 years old[28].

ADDITIONAL RISK FACTORS FOR STROKE IN OCP USERS

While the use of combined OCP may increase the overall risk of stroke, the risk varies with estrogen dose and, for reasons that are not entirely clear, the risk also varies in different parts of the world; the risk declines with discontinuation of the OCP. Two studies have suggested that prior use of OCP may even have a protective effect[21,24]. While the risk of stroke in OCP users increases only slightly with advancing age, it rises quite dramatically in the presence of other vascular risk factors, particularly hypertension and cigarette smoking.

Hypertension

Elevated blood pressure substantially increases the risk of stroke in OCP users. The increase of ischemic stroke risk in such individuals doubled in the RCGP study[19] and rose seven-fold in the European arm of the WHO study[7]. The effect of hypertension on ICH risk was similar[28]. The impact of hypertension in developing countries, where the overall risk with the OCP is higher, was also substantial (OR 14)[28]. The mechanism by which the interaction of OCP use and hypertension increases stroke risk is unclear and confounded by the fact that OCP use may lead to elevation in blood pressure.

Cigarette smoking

Overall, in women of childbearing age, smoking increases the risk of both cerebral ischemia (OR 2.5) and cerebral hemorrhage (OR 5). Studies have also consistently shown a substantial increase in stroke risk with OCP use in women smokers over 35 years of age[7,28].

Migraine

The first suggestion that migraine was an independent risk factor for stroke came in 1975 from the collaborative group for the study of stroke in young women (Table 1)[29]. Migraine was associated with a significant relative risk (RR 2.0) for thrombotic stroke using neighbor controls but, while also increased in hospital controls (RR 1.2), the increase was not significant. In this study the relative stroke risk for women with migraine using OCP was 5.9 compared to women without migraine who did not use OCP. A French case–control study found that migraine was only related to ischemic stroke in women less than 45 years of age[30]. A follow-up case–control study restricted to women under 45 years of age showed an odds ratio of 3.5; 95% CI, (1.8–6.4) for women with migraine and 13.9 for women with migraine using OCP[31]. The WHO sub-study also suggests that migraine is an independent risk factor for stroke in women of childbearing age. Migraineurs who used OCP were at increased risk of stroke (OR 16.9), although the risk was lower (OR 6.6) with low dose estrogen (< 50 μg) formulations[32]. With the additional risk from cigarette smoking, the OR for ischemic stroke was 34.4. A retrospective case–control study in Denmark involving 497 women with stroke and 1370 controls found that migraine is associated with a three-fold independent risk of stroke, but there was no increase in stroke with OCP use[33].

Although there was no difference between the risk of stroke for the different subtypes of migraine in the WHO study, migraine with aura had a stronger association with stroke than migraine without aura in three other case–control studies[31,34,35], including the one limited to women less than 45 years of age. All were inadequately powered for a definitive result in stroke risk based on the migraine subtype.

The mechanisms of stroke, both associated with and remote from the migraine attack, are

Table 1 Studies of migraine as a risk factor for stroke

Study	Population	Cases, controls	Risk ratio (RR)/Odds ratio (OR)
Collaborative Group for the Study of Stroke in Young Women[29]	Women, 15–44 years old	430, 429	RR = 2.0 (neighbor) RR = 1.2 (hospital) RR = 5.9 (+OCP)
National Health and Nutrition Examination Survey, Merikangas *et al.*[23],	Men and women, 25–74 years old	423, 11 777	OR = 2.1
Tzourio *et al.*[30]	Men and women 18–80 years old	212, 212	OR = 1.3 OR = 4.3 (women < 45)
Tzourio *et al.*[31]	Women, < 45 years old	72, 173	OR = 3.0 without aura OR = 6.2 with aura OR = 10.9 (+ smoking) OR = 13.9 (+OCP)
Lidegaard[33]	Women, 15–44 years old	497, 1370	OR = 2.8
Carolei *et al.*[35]	Men and women, < 45 years old	308, 591	OR = 1.0 without aura OR = 8.6 with aura OR = 3.7 (women < 35)
Chang *et al.*[32]	Women, 20–44 years old	291, 736	OR = 3.0 without aura OR = 3.8 with aura OR = 17 (+OCP) OR = 34 (OCP, smoking)

uncertain and probably multifactorial. Serotonin function in platelets has been widely studied as playing a potential role. Platelet aggregation studies have yielded conflicting results, and drugs that inhibit platelet function are not consistently effective in migraine prophylaxis[36]. Recent findings implicate the endothelial glycoprotein von Willebrand factor. It is elevated in migraineurs, both during[37] and between attacks[38], suggesting that migraine-induced endothelial changes may activate platelets and predispose to thrombosis. Migraineurs with OCP-induced elevated fibrinogen levels may have an increased risk of stroke. Antiplatelet agents would be expected to decrease the risk of migraine-related stroke but not necessarily prevent or alleviate migraine. In primary and secondary antiphospholipid (aPL) syndromes there is an increased frequency of migraine-like headache and transient focal neurological events. Two small studies of aPL in migraine-induced infarction[39,40] were conflicting in their conclusions,

and a large study of migraine, both with and without aura[41], failed to substantiate an independent association of migraine with aPL. The precise mechanism by which aPL leads to thrombosis is uncertain, as is the interaction of this risk factor with OCP. There has also been some work on the prevalence of familial thrombophilia in migraineurs[42–45]. Most of the factors studied to date in migraineurs cause venous thrombosis and, thus, are unlikely to be involved in migraine-related stroke.

POSTMENOPAUSAL ESTROGEN REPLACEMENT THERAPY AND STROKE

Postmenopausal estrogen replacement therapy is used by over 3 million women in the United States to treat the symptoms associated with menopause and to prevent osteoporosis after menopause. Postmenopausal ERT is not without risk. Therefore, information about cardiovascular risk associated with ERT is essential for decisions regarding ERT for treating menopausal symptoms or preventing osteoporosis. Observational studies have not provided clear information about the effect of ERT on stroke risk. Recent case–control and cohort studies have concluded that ERT increases[46], decreases[47–51] or has no effect on stroke risk[52–58]. It is also not clear whether there may be a difference in efficacy or risk associated with ERT in primary as compared to secondary stroke prevention.

The Heart and Estrogen Replacement Study (HERS) was a randomized trial of estrogen plus progestin for secondary prevention of coronary artery disease in 2763 postmenopausal women with an average follow-up of 4.1 years. It did not show a significant difference in the main outcome of non-fatal myocardial infarction (MI) or coronary heart disease and death although there was a beneficial effect on lipid levels[59]. This trial admitted women with a prior history of coronary artery disease. The highest risk for non-fatal MI was within the first year of treatment in women who had not received estrogen plus progestin before. This suggested that an early adverse effect on coagulation may increase the MI risk before longer-term beneficial effects of ERT on lipid levels or atherogenesis could be realized. Data from the Nurses' Health Study support this interpretation[60]. In the latter study, postmenopausal ERT use and secondary prevention of coronary events were studied in 2489 women with a previous MI or documented atherosclerosis followed for 20 years. A trend of decreasing risk for recurrent major coronary heart disease events with increasing duration of ERT use was observed (*p* for trend = 0.002). The risk for short-term use, comparable to the first year of follow-up in HERS, was increased compared to never-users. However, after longer term use the rate was lower than in never-users. No differences were seen between users of estrogen alone compared with

estrogen plus progestin. Overall, the relative risk for a second event among current users of ERT was 0.65; (95% CI, 0.45–0.95) compared to never-users. Thus, HERS may have failed to find a benefit from ERT owing to insufficient length of follow-up. In contrast, the Nurses' Health Study may have a selection bias, with healthier women making up the group who comply with long-term treatment with ERT.

The Women's Estrogen Stroke Trial (WEST) was a prospective, randomized controlled trial of 17-β-estradiol with placebo in women who had experienced a transient ischemic attack or non-disabling stroke[61]. In the WEST trial estrogen alone was compared with placebo. This trial did not show a reduction in recurrent stroke or in all-cause mortality in ERT users during a mean follow-up of 2.7 years. In a post-hoc analysis, fatal and non-fatal strokes, as well as severity of subsequent neurologic impairment, might actually have been increased by treatment with the human estrogen 17-β-estradiol. There was an increase in events in the first year as compared to the second and third years of follow-up. These results are similar to those reported from the HERS primary results. Both studies used ERT in a secondary prevention trial, both found no benefit for cardiovascular disease prevention and both suggest an early increased risk in the first year of treatment. The HERS investigators have recently published the results of their pre-specified secondary endpoints, transient ischemic attacks and ischemic and hemorrhagic strokes[62]. The main finding was the absence of any significant beneficial or detrimental effect of ERT on the risk of cerebrovascular disease events with coronary disease over four years of follow-up. Unlike the pattern observed for non-fatal MI and death in the initial report and the pattern reported in the WEST, there was neither an early increased risk of stroke in the ERT group nor a later decrease. There was no adverse interaction between ERT and stroke among smokers as was described in the Framingham Heart Study[46]. The Women's Health Study, when completed, may provide strong evidence regarding the effect of a combined estrogen–progesterone regimen on the risk of first stroke.

Animal studies have found that estrogen may be neuroprotective in an acute stroke setting[63]. However, WEST found no difference in stroke severity between women randomized to ERT and placebo. Another group evaluated stroke severity associated with ERT in women with acute stroke using a case–control design and also failed to find a benefit[64]. Why neuroprotective effects in models of experimental stroke are so much better than in human studies are unclear, but could relate to dose or formulation of ERT and species differences in vascular endothelial responsiveness to estrogen or estrogen/progesterone combinations.

SUMMARY

The risk of thrombotic stroke with the current formulations of estrogen-containing OCP and ERT is negligible, in the absence of other risk factors. The risk of stroke rises substantially in those who smoke or who have hypertension or migraine. When evaluating the studies concerning risks of stroke with OCP, it must be kept in mind that for all non-smoking women the risk of serious morbidity and death is still greater with pregnancy than with OC use[65]. Estrogen replacement therapy, which has some beneficial effects in atherogenesis, has shown no benefit in secondary prevention trials of stroke or of MI. Concerns have been raised over possible increased thrombosis early in the course of therapy. The effect of OCP and ERT on first stroke remains uncertain.

References

1. Lidegaard O, Milsom I. The pill. The controversy continues. *Acta Obstet Gynecol Scand* 1996;75:93–7

2. Keating NL, Cleary PD, Rossi AS, *et al.* Use of hormone replacement therapy by postmenopausal women in the United States. *Ann Intern Med* 1999;130:545–53

3. Notelovitz M. Estrogen replacement therapy: indications, contraindications, and agent selection. *Am J Obstet Gynecol* 1989;161:1832–41

4. Herrington DM, Rebousin DM, Brosnihan KB, *et al.* Effects of estrogen replacement on the progression of coronary artery atherosclerosis. *N Engl J Med* 2000;343:522–9

5. Conrad J, Samama MM. Oral contraceptives, hormone replacement therapy and haemostasis. *Cephalagia* 2000;20:175–82

6. Schwartz SM, Petitti DB, Siscovick DS, *et al.* Stroke and use of low-dose oral contraceptives in young women. A pooled analysis of two US studies. *Stroke* 1998;29:2277–84

7. WHO Collaborative Study. Cardiovascular disease and steroid hormone contraception. Ischemic stroke and combined oral contraceptives: results of an international, multicentre, case-control study. *Lancet* 1996;348:498–505

8. Lidegaard O, Kreiner S. Cerebral thrombosis and oral contraceptives: a case control study. *Contraception* 1998;57:303–14

9. Cohen H, Mackie IJ, Walshe K, *et al.* A comparison of the effects of two triphasic oral contraceptives on haemostasis. *Br J Haematol* 1988;69:259–63

10. Rosing J, Tans G, Nicolaes GAD, *et al.* Oral contraceptives and venous thrombosis: different sensitivities to activated protein C in women using second and third generation oral contraceptives. *Br J Haematol* 1997;97:233–8

11. Rakoczi I, Gero G, Demeter J, *et al.* Comparative metabolic effects of oral contraceptive preparations containing different progestogens. Effects of desogestrel and ethinylestradiol on the haemostatic balance. *Drug Res* 1985;35:630–3

12. Kuhl H. Effects of progestogens on haemostasis. *Maturitas* 1996;24:1–19

13. Caine YG, Bauer KA, Barzegar S, *et al.* Coagulation activation following estrogen administration to postmenopausal women. *Thromb Haemost* 1992;4:392–5

14. Walsh BW, Schiff I, Rosner B, *et al.* Effects of postmenopausal estrogen replacement on the

concentrations and metabolism of plasma lipoproteins. *N Engl J Med* 1991;325: 1196–204

15. Barrett-Connor E. Putative complications of estrogen replacement therapy: hypertension, diabetes, thrombophlebitis, and gallstones. In Korenman SG, ed. *The Menopause; Biological and Clinical Consequence of Ovarian Failure; Evolution and Management.* Norwel, MA: Serono Symposi 1990;199–209

16. Lobo RA. Estrogen replacement therapy and hypertension. *Postgrad Med* 1987;September 14:48–54

17. Conrad J, Samama M, Basdevant A, *et al.* Differential AT III response to oral and parenteral administration of 17beta estradiol. *Thromb Haemost* 1983;49:245

18. Lidegaard O. Oral contraception and risk of a cerebral thromboembolic attack: results of a case control study. *Br Med J* 1993;306:956–63

19. Hannaford PC, Croft PR, Kay CR. Oral contraception and stroke: evidence from the Royal College of General Practitioners' oral contraception study. *Stroke* 1994;25:935–42

20. Vessey MP, Lawless M, Yeates D. Oral contraceptives and stroke: findings in a large prospective study. *Br Med J* 1984;289:530–1

21. Pettiti DB, Sidney S, Bernstein A, *et al.* Stroke in users of low-dose oral contraceptives. *N Engl J Med* 1996;335:8–15

22. Schwartz S, Siscovick D, Longstreth WT, *et al.* Use of low-dose oral contraceptives and stroke in young women. *Ann Intern Med* 1997;127: 596–603

23. Merikangas KR, Fenton BT, Cheng SH, *et al.* Association between migraine and stroke in a large-scale epidemiological study of the United States. *Arch Neurol* 1997;54:362–8

24. Heineman LAJ, Lewis MA, Thorogood M, *et al.* The Transnational Research Group on Oral Contraceptives and the Health of Young Women. *Br Med J* 1997;315:1502–4

25. De Bruijn SFTM, Stam J, Koopman MM, *et al.* Case-control study of risk of cerebral sinus thrombosis in oral contraceptive users and in carriers of hereditary prothrombotic condition. The Cerebral Venous Sinus Thrombosis Study Group. *Br Med J* 1998;316:589–92

26. Martinelli I, Sacchi E, Landi G, *et al.* High risk of cerebral-vein thrombosis in carriers of a prothrombin-gene mutation and in users of oral contraceptives. *N Engl J Med* 1998;338:1793–7

27. Johnston SC, Colford JM, Gress DR. Oral contraceptives and the risk of subarachnoid hemorrhage. A meta-analysis. *Neurology* 1998; 51:411–18

28. WHO Collaborative Study of cardiovascular disease and steroid hormone contraception. Haemorrhagic stroke, overall stroke risk, and combined oral contraceptives: results of an international, multicentre, case-control study. *Lancet* 1996;348:505–10

29. Collaborative Group for the Study of Stroke in Young Women. Oral contraceptives and stroke in young women. *J Am Med Assoc* 1975;231: 718–22

30. Tzourio C, Iglesias S, Hubert JB, *et al.* Migraine and risk of ischemic stroke: a case-control study. *Br Med J* 1993;308:289–92

31. Tzourio C, Tehindrazanarivelo A, Iglesias S, *et al.* Case-control study of migraine and risk of ischemic stroke in young women. *Br Med J* 1995;310:830–3

32. Chang CL, Donaghy M, Poulter N. Migraine and stroke in young women: the World Health Organisation Collaborative Study of Cardiovascular Disease and Steroid Hormone Contraception. *Br Med J* 1999;318:13–18

33. Lidegaard O. Oral contraceptives, pregnancy and the risk of cerebral thromboembolism: the influence of diabetes, hypertension, migraine and previous thrombotic disease. *Br J Obstet Gynaecol* 1995;102:153–9

34. Henrich JB, Horowitz RI. A controlled study of ischemic stroke risk in migraine patients. *J Clin Epidemiol* 1989;42:773–80

35. Carolei A, Marini C, De Matteis G. History of migraine and risk of cerebral ischaemia in young adults. *Lancet* 1996;347:1503–6

36. Crassard I, Conrad J, Bousser M-G. Migraine and haemostasis. *Cephalagia* 2001;21:630–6

37. Cesar JM, Garcia-Avello A, Vecino AM, *et al.* Increased levels of plasma von Willebrand factor in migraine crisis. *Acta Neurol Scand* 1995;91:412–13

38. Tietjen GE, Al-Qasmi MM, Athanas K, *et al.* Increased von Willebrand factor in migraine. *Neurology* 2001;57:334–6

39. Montalban J, Titus F, Ordi J, *et al.* Anti-cardiolipin antibodies and migraine-related strokes (letter). *Arch Neurol* 1988;45:603

40. Silvestrini M, Matteis M, Troisi E, *et al.* Migrainous stroke and antiphospholipid antibodies. *Eur Neurol* 1994;34:316–19

41. Tietjen GE, Day M, Norris L, *et al.* Role of anticardiolipin antibodies in young persons with migraine and transient focal neurological events. *Neurology* 1998;50:1433–40

42. Haan J, Kapelle LJ, de Ronde H, *et al*. The factor V Leiden is not a major risk factor for migrainous cerebral infarction. *Cephalalgia* 1997;17:605–7

43. Soriani S, Borgna-Pignatti C, Trabetti E, *et al*. Frequency of Factor V Leiden in juvenile migraine with aura. *Headache* 1998;38:779–81

44. Corral J, Iniesta JA, Gonzales-Conejero R, *et al*. Migraine and prothrombotic risk factors. *Cephalalgia* 1998;18:27–60

45. D'Amico F, Moschiano F, Leone M, *et al*. Genetic abnormalities of the protein C system: shared risk factors in young adults with migraine with aura and with ischemic stroke? *Cephalalgia* 1998;18:618–21

46. Wilson PW, Garrison RJ, Castelli WP. Postmenopausal estrogen use, cigarette smoking and cardiovascular morbidity in women over 50: the Framingham Study. *N Engl J Med* 1985;313:1038–43

47. Falkeborn M, Persson I, Terent A, *et al*. Hormone replacement therapy and the risk of stroke: follow-up of a population-based cohort in Sweden. *Arch Intern Med* 1993;153:1201–9

48. Finucane FF, Madans JH, Bush TL, *et al*. Decreased risk of stroke among postmenopausal hormone users: results from a national cohort. *Arch Intern Med* 1993;153:73–9

49. Henderson BE, Paganini-Hill A, Ross RK. Decreased mortality in users of estrogen replacement therapy. *Arch Intern Med* 1991;151:75–8

50. Hunt K, Vessey M, McPherson K. Mortality in a cohort of long-term users of hormone replacement therapy: an updated analysis. *Br J Obstet Gynaecol* 1990;97:1080–6

51. Schairer C, Adami H-O, Hoover R, *et al*. Cause-specific mortality in women receiving hormone replacement therapy. *Epidemiology* 1997;8:59–65

52. Stampfer MJ, Coldwitz GA, Willett WC, *et al*. Postmenopausal estrogen therapy and cardiovascular disease. Ten-year follow-up from the nurses' health study. *N Engl J Med* 1991;325:756–62

53. Lindenstrom E, Boysen G, Nyboe J. Lifestyle factors and risk of cerebrovascular disease in women: the Copenhagen City Heart Study. *Stroke* 1993;24:1468–72

54. Folsom AR, Mink PJ, Sellers TA, *et al*. Hormonal replacement therapy and morbidity and mortality in a prospective study of postmenopausal women. *Am J Pub Health* 1995;85:1128–32

55. Grodstein F, Stampfer MJ, Manson JE, *et al*. Postmenopausal estrogen and progestin use and the risk of cardiovascular disease. *N Engl J Med* 1996;335:453–61

56. Pedersen AT, Lidegaard O, Kreiner S, *et al*. Hormone replacement therapy and risk of non-fatal stroke. *Lancet* 1997;350:1277–83

57. Petitti DB, Sidney S, Quesenberry CP, *et al*. Ischemic stroke and use of estrogen and estrogen/progestogen as hormone replacement therapy. *Stroke* 1998;29:23–8

58. Grodstein F, Stampfer MJ, Falkeborn M, *et al*. Postmenopausal hormone therapy and risk of cardiovascular disease and hip fracture in a cohort of Swedish women. *Epidemiology* 1999; 5:476–80

59. Hulley S, Grady D, Bush T, *et al*. Randomized trial of estrogen plus progestin for secondary prevention of coronary heart disease in postmenopausal women. *J Am Med Assoc* 1998; 280:605–13

60. Grodstein F, Manson JE, Stampfer MJ. Postmenopausal hormone use and secondary prevention of coronary events in the Nurses' Health Study: a prospective, observational study. *Ann Intern Med* 2001;135(1):1–9

61. Kernan WN, Brass LM, Viscoli CM, *et al*. Estrogen after ischemic stroke: clinical basis and design of the women's estrogen for stroke trial. *J Stroke Cerebrovas Dis* 1998;7:85–95

62. Simon JA, Hsia J, Cauley JA, *et al*., for the HERS Research Group. Postmenopausal hormone therapy and risk of stroke: the Heart and Estrogen-progestin Replacement Study (HERS). *Circulation* 2001;103:638–42

63. Lee SJ, McEwen BS. Neurotropic and neuroprotective actions of estrogens and their therapeutic implications. *Ann Rev Pharmacol Toxicol* 2001;41:569–91

64. Bushnell CD, Samsa GP, Goldstein LB. Hormone replacement therapy and ischemic stroke severity in women: a case-control study. *Neurology* 2001;56:1304–7

65. Harlap S, Kost K, Forrest JD. *Preventing Pregnancy, Protecting Health: a New Look at Birth Control Choices in the United States*. New York: Alan Guttmacher Institute, 1991

Chapter 8

Genetics and stroke

John W. Cole, MD, and Steven J. Kittner, MD, MPH

INTRODUCTION

The completion of the human genome project[1] should now enhance our ability to understand the interplay between genetics and environment in the pathogenesis of many common chronic diseases, including stroke, and to develop new approaches to disease prevention. There are four principal lines of evidence supporting a genetic contribution to stroke risk. First, there are numerous monogenetic disorders associated with stroke, including the recently described disorder cerebral autosomal dominant arteriopathy with subcortical infarcts and leukoencephalopathy (CADASIL)[2]. These conditions are considered simple Mendelian traits because they exhibit a dominant or recessive inheritance pattern attributable to a single gene[3]. Second, studies of human populations have shown strong evidence for the familial aggregation of stroke[4]. Since it is common for stroke to run in families but dominant or recessive modes of inheritance are uncommon, these studies have supported a complex (unknown) mode of inheritance or a role for a shared environment. Third, twin studies have shown concordance rates of 3.6% for dizygotic twins and 17.7% for monozygotic twins[5], suggesting a genetic basis for the familial aggregation. Fourth, candidate gene studies have been increasingly productive. For example, studies of the stroke-prone spontaneously hypertensive

rat have shown the existence of a blood pressure-independent single gene locus predisposing to stroke[6]; the same locus has been demonstrated to be associated with ischemic stroke in human populations[7].

This chapter will discuss clues to genetic disease from the history and physical examination, including important monogenetic disorders; stroke as a polygenetic or complex genetic disorder; and responsible genetic testing. We will focus on clinically relevant information and secondarily discuss concepts important for interpreting the evolving literature on stroke genetics.

DEFINITION OF TERMS

Several terms used throughout this chapter require definition:

(1) Allele – Alternative form of a gene or marker locus due to changes at the level of DNA;

(2) Complex trait – A trait with a genetic component that is not strictly Mendelian (dominant, recessive, sex-linked). Complex traits may involve the interaction of two or more genes to produce a phenotype or may involve gene–environment interactions;

(3) Genotype – The observed alleles at a genetic locus for an individual. For an autosomal locus, a genotype is composed of two alleles, one transmitted maternally and the other transmitted paternally;

(4) Linkage – Two loci which are physically connected to one another on the same chromosome and are so close that they usually fail to be transmitted to offspring independently from one another;

(5) Phenotype – The observed manifestations of a genotype. The phenotype may be an observed trait, a particular type of clinical event, or may be expressed physiologically;

(6) Polymorphism – Genetic loci at which there are two or more alleles that are each present at a frequency of at least 1% in the population; and

(7) Recombination – The formation of new arrangements of genes on chromosomes by the crossing over of the two partners of a chromosome pair during meiosis.

MONOGENETIC OR MENDELIAN DISORDERS

Rare Mendelian disorders arising from single-gene defects have been described in which stroke is a prominent presenting feature. It should be emphasized that these are not 'stroke genes' but rather mutations that may have stroke as an accompanying manifestation. There are several reasons to recognize monogenetic conditions associated with stroke[3]. There may be specific treatments that can alter the course of the disease. Natural history or prognostic information may be available, including the possibility of anticipating problems in other organ systems. Finally, diagnosis and counseling may be of benefit to family members of the affected patient, potentially leading to the prevention of disease.

The search for monogenetic stroke etiologies begins with the history and physical examination. We have chosen to illustrate several monogenetic disorders categorized by general descriptive categories. Table 1[8-13] highlights clues to these disorders from the history and examination respectively. Table 2[8-13] describes other features of these disorders including associated laboratory findings, mode of inheritance, resulting pathophysiologic defects, and diagnostic testing. More comprehensive listings can be found in Natowicz and Kelley[3] and Hademenos et al.[14], and The National Library of Medicine database, Online Mendelian Inheritance in Man (*http://www.ncbi.nlm.nih.gov/entrez/query.fcgi?db=OMIM*). This database is particularly useful because it can be searched for any combination of specific clinical features. Another federally funded online database, Gene Test-Gene Clinics (*http://www.genetests.org/*), provides an international directory of genetic testing laboratories and genetics clinics.

A genetic cause should be considered in any young stroke patient who lacks established vascular risk factors. To maximize the likelihood of detecting a familial condition, a structured approach to the family history is needed. This should include recording the family pedigree in detail, including, at a minimum, all first-degree relatives. The major medical conditions of all members should be recorded as well as age at onset for relevant medical conditions and age at death. Depending on the context, this information from the pedigree should be included for second and third degree relatives.

STROKE AS A POLYGENIC OR COMPLEX GENETIC DISORDER

Compelling evidence from epidemiologic and animal studies[7] shows that stroke is a complex genetic disorder, determined by multiple genes and environmental influences, but there is still limited understanding of its genetic basis. There is evidence that the genetic contribution

Table 1 Mendelian disorders: history and findings

	History				System based findings		
Disease type	Patient and family history	Age of onset, predilection	General appearance	HEENT	CVS/respiratory/abdomen	Extremities/skin	Nervous system
Large artery disease							
Homocystinuria[8,10-13] OMIM: 236200	Seizures Arterial and venous thrombotic events Osteoporosis PVD Psychiatric disorders	Occasional failure to thrive in infancy High risk of thrombotic events in childhood	Marfanoid habitus – tall, thin body habitus Kyphoscoliosis Pectus excavatum	Sparse brittle hair Crowded teeth Myopia Glaucoma Ectopia lentis Elevated palate	MVP MI Inguinal hernia	Genu valgum Livedo reticularis Foot deformities – high arched feet Arachnodactyly Biconcave 'codfish' vertebrae	Cognitive impairment – mental retardation Seizures Myelopathy and neuropathy are less common
Familial hypercholesterolemia (Type II-a)[10,12,13] OMIM: 143890	Early MI PVD Hereditary dyslipidemia	CAD after 30 years in heterozygotes, childhood in homozygotes	At birth – web xanthomas between first and second digits	Corneal arcus (by 3rd decade) Xanthelasma Bruit – atherosclerosis	CAD	Tendon xanthomas – Achilles common Decreased peripheral pulses	
Tangier disease[8,10-12] (Familial HDL deficiency, Type I) OMIM: 205400	Extremity pain Asymmetric sensory deficits or abnormalities Hereditary dyslipidemia Early MI	Infancy or childhood with pharyngeal findings	Adenopathy	Orange tonsils – cholesterol laden	Hepatosplenomegaly Intestinal lipid storage		Facial diplegia Weak intrinsic hand muscles Asymmetric polyneuropathy – motor and sensory, deficit of pain/temp.
Small vessel disease							
CADASIL – Cerebral autosomal dominant arteriopathy with subcortical infarcts and leukoencephalopathy[8,10,12] OMIM: 125310	Migraines – with prolonged aura Familial hemiplegic migraine Early onset dementia Manic episodes Depression Seizures	Early adulthood Migraines by age 30 First stroke by age 45	Lumbar spondylosis				Cognitive impairment Pseudobulbar palsy and dementia Progressive motor disability
Fabry disease[8,10-13] OMIM: 301500	Anhidrosis Periodic fever Lancinating pain in hands and feet – often initial symptom, heat or exercise may induce Cardiomegaly with MI Arthritis	Children and young adults with paresthesias Stroke occurs in adults	Retarded growth Delayed puberty	Corneal opacity Tortuous retinal conjunctive vessels Crystalline deposits in conjunctiva Oral, conjunctival lesions (vascular)	Cardiomegaly MI Mild obstructive lung disease Episodic GI disturbances Renal disease	Telangiectasias Angiokeratomas with primary locations on lower abdomen, scrotum, upper thigh Arthritic changes Hypohidrosis	Neuropathy – limb paresthesias Autonomic dysfunction Pain episodes induced by exercise Seizures

(Continued)

Table 1   (Continued)

Disease type	History			System based findings			
	Patient and family history	Age of onset, predilection	General appearance	HEENT	CVS/respiratory/abdomen	Extremities/skin	Nervous system
Hematologic diseases							
Sickle cell disease[8–13] OMIM: 603903	Acute pain crisis with physical exertion; Unexplained fevers; Abdominal, bone and chest pain; Large or small vessel occlusive disease; Intracerebral epidural or subdural hemorrhages; Subarachnoid hemorrhages	Black children	Slow growth; Jaundice	Proliferative retinopathy	Acute chest syndrome; Asplenia – autosplenectomy; Cor pulmonale; Painless hematuria; Cholelithiasis	Hand foot syndrome with swollen joints, short middle finger, short 2nd toe, non-healing ulcers; Cyanosis	
Protein C deficiency[8,10–12] OMIM: 176860 Protein S deficiency[8,10–12] OMIM: 176880	DVT; Recurrent thrombotic events; Warfarin induced skin necrosis; Purpura fulminalis neonatalis	Young adults; Occasional late onset with homozygosity with protein C deficiency		Neonatal vitreous hemorrhages	Pulmonary embolism; Intra-abdominal venous thrombosis	Superficial thrombophlebitis	Cerebral arterial and venous thrombosis
Factor V Leiden mutation[8,10,12] OMIM: 227400	Cerebral venous thrombosis; DVT	Young adults					Cerebral venous thrombosis
Mitochondria based disease							
MELAS – Mitochondrial encephalopathy lactic acidosis and stroke[8–12] OMIM: 540000	Seizures – grand mal; Episodic vomiting; Visual disturbances; Episodic migraines; Deafness; Maternally inherited diabetes	Infancy – failure to thrive; Children or young adults – stroke	Short stature, children	Ophthalmoplegia; Pigmentary retinal degeneration; Bilateral cataracts	Cardiomyopathy; Cardiac conduction defects; Progressive renal dysfunction	Myalgias	Seizures; Myoclonus; Dementia; Weakness – reduced muscle mass; Deafness

(Continued)

Table 1 (Continued)

Disease type	History		General appearance	HEENT	System based findings		Nervous system
	Patient and family history	Age of onset, predilection			CVS/respiratory/abdomen	Extremities/skin	
Connective tissue disorders							
Ehlers-Danlos syndrome (type IV)[8,10–13] OMIM: 130050	Cerebral aneurysms, Arterial dissections, Easy bruising – vascular fragility, Excessive scarring s/p surgery	Typically death by age 40–50 years secondary to dissecting aneurysms	Short stature, Alopecia of scalp, Gingival recession	Pinched thin nose, Thin lips, Lobeless ears, Keratoconus, Peridontal disease, Early loss of teeth, Horner's syndrome with carotid dissection	MVP, ASD/VSD, Aortic insufficiency, Spontaneous pneumothorax, Colon rupture, Bladder prolapse, Uterine prolapse	Hyper-mobile joints, Hyper-extensible skin, Acrogeria (skin over hands and feet thin and finely wrinkled), Prominent veins	Cerebral hemorrhage
Marfan syndrome[8,10–13] OMIM: 154700	Cerebral aneurysms, Internal carotid artery dissection, Premature arthritis	Typically death by age 40–50 years secondary to dissecting aneurysms	Tall, thin body habitus, Pectus exacutum, Bossing of frontal eminences, Prominent supra-orbital ridge	Ectopia lentis, Retinal detachment, Early cataracts and glaucoma, Lens subluxation, Micrognathia, Horner's syndrome with carotid dissection	Aortic dissection, MVP, Aortic valve insufficiency, CHF, Recurrent incisional hernias	Excessive joint laxity, Kyphoscoliosis, Striae distensae	Cerebral hemorrhage
Fibromuscular dysplasia[8,10,12,13] OMIM: 135580	Headaches, Myocardial infarction, Tinnitus and/or vertigo, Transient retinal or cerebral ischemia, Dissection – carotid aneurysms, SAH, HTN	Female > Male, Typically middle aged females, White > Blacks	Neck pain, carotidynia	Carotid bruits, Transient retinal ischemia, Carotidynia, Horner's syndrome with carotid dissection	Renal FMD – leading to hypertension	Claudication	Cerebral hemorrhage
Pseudoxanthoma elasticum AD form[8,10,12] OMIM: 177850 AR form[8,10,12] OMIM: 264800	Angina – CAD, MI, Gradual vision loss, Epistaxis, Hematuria, Arterial dissections, GI hemorrhages, PVD		Pectus deformities	Angiod retinal streaks, Macular degeneration, Retinal hemorrhages, High arched palate, Yellowish lip mucosal nodules, Horner's syndrome with carotid dissection	MVP, Gastric microaneurysms	Loose skin; Small, raised orange-yellow papules – 'plucked chicken skin' located on neck, axilla, abdomen, inguinally	Cerebral hemorrhage

AD, autosomal dominant; AR, autosomal recessive; ASD, atrial septal defect; CAD, coronary artery disease; CHF, congestive heart failure; CVS, cardiovascular systems; DVT, deep venous thrombosis; FMD, fibromuscular dysplasia; GI, gastrointestinal; HEENT, heart, eyes, ears, nose, throat; HDL, high density lipoprotein; HTN, hypertension; MI, myocardial infarction; MVP, mitral valve prolapse; OMIM, Online mendelian inheritance in man; PVD, peripheral vascular disease; SAH, subarachnoid hemorrhage; VSD, ventricular septal defect

Table 2 Mendelian disorders: other features and diagnostic tests

Disease type/ OMIM number	Associated abnormal findings and laboratory tests	Inheritance and chromosomal location	Resulting defect/ basis for disease	Availability of genetic test	Ancillary diagnostic tests
Large artery disease					
Homocystinuria[8,10–13] OMIM: 236200	Homocystine is elevated in blood, CSF and urine Methionine elevated in blood and urine	AR, 21q22.3	Deficiency of cystathione beta-synthase	Yes, DNA	Urine/serum homocystine Urine/serum methionine
Familial hyper-cholesterolemia (Type II-a)[10,12,13] OMIM: 143890	Serum: elevated LDL, elevated cholesterol	AD, 19p13.2	Abnormal LDL receptor	Yes, DNA	Fasting lipid panel
Tangier disease (familial HDL deficiency, type I)[8,10–12] OMIM: 205400	Serum: low HDL, low LDL, low cholesterol, elevated triglycerides, low phospholipids, abnormal chylomicron remnants	AR, 9q22–q31	HDL – Apo-Gln-I very low Severe atherosclerosis Thymus and reticuloendothelial cells filled with cholesterol esters	No	Fasting lipid panel Denervation apparent on EMG
Small vessel disease					
CADASIL – Cerebral autosomal dominant arteriopathy with subcortical infarcts and leukoencephalopathy[8,10,12] OMIM: 125310	MRI with multiple subcortical infarcts, both clinically evident and silent	AD, 19p13.2–p13.1 Notch 3 gene	Non-amyloid eosinophilic material in small vessel walls and reduplicated internal elastic lamella	Yes, DNA	MRI
Fabry disease[8,10–13] OMIM: 301500	Proteinuria Lipid laden macrophages in bone marrow	X-linked, Xq21.33–q22 Complete form in males Incomplete form in female carriers	Alpha-galactosidase A deficiency Leads to accumulation of ceramide trihexidose in peripheral nerves and blood vessels	Under development Prenatal diagnosis available	

(Continued)

Table 2 (Continued)

Disease type/ OMIM number	Associated abnormal findings and laboratory tests	Inheritance and chromosomal location	Resulting defect/ basis for disease	Availability of genetic test	Ancillary diagnostic tests
Hematologic diseases					
Sickle cell disease[8–13] OMIM: 603903	Aplastic crisis induced with parvo B-19 virus	AR, 11p15.5 Missense mutation, valine for glutamate in position 6 of beta hemoglobin chain	Defective beta-chain hemoglobin molecule	Yes, DNA Can also screen using electrophoresis or chromatography tests	Follow-up with transcranial Doppler studies recommended
Protein C deficiency[8,10–12] OMIM: 176860 Protein S deficiency[8,10–12] OMIM: 176880	Vitamin K antagonists may worsen Acquired deficiencies may occur with pregnancy, liver disease, DIC, oral contraceptive use, warfarin use, and following surgery	Protein C – AD, 2q13–q14 Protein S – AD, 3p11.1–q11.2	Deficiency of functional proteins	Yes, DNA	Protein function test No heparin for more than 72 hours
Factor V Leiden mutation[8,10,12] OMIM: 227400	Prolonged bleeding time Prolonged clotting time Prolonged one-stage prothrombin time, corrected by rabbit plasma	AR, 1q23 Point mutation G to A nucleotide 1691R506Q protein mutation, glutamine for arginine at residue 506	Abnormal factor V molecule	Yes, DNA	Protein function test No heparin for more than 72 hours Preferably off warfarin
Mitochondria based disease					
MELAS – Mitochondrial encephalopathy lactic acidosis and stroke[8–12] OMIM: 540000	Elevated serum lactic acid and pyruvic acid; Ragged red fibers on muscle biopsy; Progressive renal dysfunction MRI – multifocal infarcts in non vascular distribution	Mitochondrial Defect in transfer RNA for leucine	Abnormal leucine processing	Yes, mitochondria DNA	Serum lactic and pyruvic acid levels elevated at rest, markedly increase with exercise Muscle biopsy

(Continued)

Table 2 (Continued)

Disease type/ OMIM number	Associated abnormal findings and laboratory tests	Inheritance and chromosomal location	Resulting defect/ basis for disease	Availability of genetic test	Ancillary diagnostic tests
Connective tissue disorders					
Ehlers–Danlos syndrome (type IV)[8,10–13] OMIM: 130050	Premature delivery because of cervical insufficiency or membrane fragility	AD, 2q31 Collagen III, alpha-1 gene – COL3A1	Type III collagen abnormal	Yes, DNA	Echocardiogram
Marfan syndrome[8,10–13] OMIM: 154700	Dilated aortic root Coarctation of aorta	AD, 15q21.1 Fibrillin 1 gene	Defective fibrillin 1	Yes, DNA – linkage and mutation based tests available	Protein based – immunohistochemistry Echocardiogram
Fibromuscular dysplasia[8–13] OMIM: 135580	MRA – 'String of beads' in carotid arteries @ cervical levels C1and C2	AD, location unknown	Degradation of elastic tissue of vessel wall	No	Carotid Doppler ultrasound
Pseudoxanthoma elasticum AD form[8,10,12] OMIM: 177850 AR form[8,10,12] OMIM: 264800	Females – estrogen, pregnacy, puberty may increase skin lesions	AD and AR forms, 16p13.1	Defective transmembrane protein ABCC6 (ATP-binding casette subfamily C, member 6 gene), substrate and function unknown	Research only, DNA	Skin biopsy – fragmented elastic fibers

AD, autosomal dominant; AR, autosomal recessive; ATP, adenosine triphosphate; CSF, cerebrospinal fluid; DIC, disseminated intravascular coagulation; DNA, deoxyribonucleic acid; EMG, electromyogram; HDL, high density lipoprotein; LDL, low density lipoprotein; MRI, magnetic resonance imaging; OMIM, online mendelian inheritance in man; RNA, ribonucleic acid to stroke risk is particularly strong in early-onset cases[15,16]. How should new knowledge accrue and how should new research findings be evaluated? Several recent papers have reviewed the methods for generating new knowledge pertaining to the genetic basis for complex diseases, including stroke[4,15,16]. These methods, quantitative trait locus mapping using experimental crosses, linkage analysis, allele sharing methods, and association studies, will be briefly discussed.

Quantitative trait locus mapping using experimental crosses is based on the very close homology of man's genetic code with that of experimental animals such as mice and rats, and the simplification which occurs when studying large numbers of offspring from a single set of parents. The power of this approach has been elegantly demonstrated by a genotype/phenotype co-segregation analysis of stroke-prone spontaneously hypertensive rats and stroke-resistant spontaneously hypertensive rats in which three quantitative trait loci were found to account for stroke susceptibility independently of blood pressure levels[6]. The region with the highest association with stroke susceptibility coincided with the atrial natriuretic peptide and brain natriuretic peptide gene locus on rat chromosome 5. Subsequently, in an epidemiologic association study in the Physician's Health Study, the same investigators found that two polymorphisms in the atrial natriuretic peptide gene were significantly associated with stroke risk[7].

Linkage analysis involves specifying a model to explain the transmission pattern of a trait within families. In this approach one calculates the probability of the transmission pattern assuming linkage to a specific genetic region under a given model and compares it to the probability of the transmission data assuming no linkage. This approach has been hugely successful for simple Mendelian traits because there are only a small number of easily tested models. The method has had more limited success with complex traits because the large number of possible models introduces a multiple testing problem, requiring the use of a higher significance level and a resultant lower power to associate a locus with a trait. In addition, if the model is not specified correctly one may accept false linkages and miss true linkages.

Allele sharing methods also examine the transmission pattern of a trait within families in order to identify genetic loci associated with disease. However, in contrast to linkage analysis, they do not require specifying a model of inheritance. Allele sharing is based on showing that affected relatives inherit certain regions of the genome more often than expected by chance under random segregation. The advantage of this approach is that it will provide evidence for or against the association of a particular genetic region with disease, regardless of the genetic mode of transmission. Neither linkage analysis nor allele sharing methods can provide information on the frequency in the population of the genetic variant associated with disease or how often the variant is associated with disease (penetrance). Although finding linkage in a set of families may provide clues to the biological mechanisms of the disease, the genetic basis for the disease in that set of families may differ from that of the general population. Association studies can address these limitations.

Association studies are not based on the transmission pattern of a trait within families; rather, the analysis is performed across families. Association is established by comparing the prevalence of an allele or the genotype in affected as compared with unaffected individuals within a population. There are many candidate genes that have shown an association with stroke risk[15] and the list is increasing at a rapid rate. As in all epidemiologic association studies, it is important to recognize that association between an allele and disease does not necessarily imply causation. A positive association will also occur if the allele does not cause the trait but is in linkage disequilibrium with the allele that does cause the trait. Linkage disequilibrium occurs in a population when two conditions are met[17]: (1) most cases of the disease are due to only a few ancestral mutations at the trait-causing locus and (2) the marker allele was close enough on one of these ancestral chromosomes that an association between these two alleles has not yet been removed by recombination during the evolution of that population. Thus, an association between the marker allele and disease may occur in one population, but not in another population that has evolved differently. Despite inconsistent findings between studies, this type of indirect association can be a clue to the genetic site of a disease-causing locus.

Association studies are also prone to another and more problematic type of indirect association due to population admixture. An allele may be associated with disease if it is more common in a particular ethnic group and that ethnic group is more likely to develop the disease. This is a particularly important problem in ethnically mixed populations like American Caucasians and African-Americans. Fortunately, this type of confounding can be controlled by performing association studies using parental or other within-family controls. Such studies are based on the idea that transmission of alleles from parents to offspring should be random, with each allele having an equal probability of transmission. If a particular allele is transmitted to affected individuals more often than expected, then this is evidence for an association between that allele and disease.

Regardless of whether the study methodology is quantitative trait locus mapping, linkage analysis, allele sharing, or association studies, it is necessary to be cautious in deriving clinical implications from genetic studies. There are a number of conditions that must be met before genetic testing is indicated, even if multiple studies demonstrate with confidence that a particular allele has a causal association with stroke risk. These are alluded to in the section on monogenetic disorders and discussed in detail in the next section.

RESPONSIBLE GENETIC TESTING

This section will address the questions of when genetic testing is indicated and what is the appropriate context of genetic testing. Genetic tests include analyses not only of DNA or RNA for the purpose of detecting a genetic condition, but also analyses of proteins and certain metabolites for the same purpose. Unlike other types of laboratory tests, genetic tests provide information not only about the tested person, but also about his or her relatives or descendants. The most appropriate criteria to be used to evaluate the risks and benefits of genetic tests and how these criteria should apply to different categories of genetic tests have been the subject of much societal scrutiny and a recent federal task force report[18]. It has been proposed that the decision to use a particular genetic test in a particular individual should include consideration of analytical validity, clinical validity and clinical utility, including social consequences.

Analytical validity refers to whether the test is reliable and valid in measuring what it purports to measure. Clinical validity refers to the accuracy of the test in diagnosing or predicting the risk of disease and is measured by sensitivity and specificity, which are test characteristics, and predictive value, which is a function of the prevalence of the disease in the population. Clinical utility refers to outcomes associated with a positive or negative test result. It is important to emphasize that genetic testing may have unintended social consequences. While the need for federal legislation to limit this risk is widely recognized, there is at present no protection from discrimination in employment or health insurance based on genetic information. Other family members may be inadvertently affected by this type of discrimination, or by unwanted dissemination of knowledge about the existence of a genetic condition. Genetic testing may also provide unintended information about paternity.

Consideration of the above factors implies the need to individualize the decision for genetic testing. It should be apparent that the clinical validity, clinical utility and social consequences of a test could vary greatly depending on whether it is performed for diagnostic or prognostic purposes, individual testing or population screening, whether a treatment is available for the condition, and whether the genotype has a high or low probability of being associated with the disease phenotype. While there is currently no legal mandate, there is an evolving consensus[18] that genetic education and counseling, as well as written informed consent, should accompany certain types of 'high scrutiny' genetic testing. 'High scrutiny' tests include those that have a relatively low clinical validity and utility and a high risk of adverse social consequence. For example, a test whose purpose is predictive, which detects a variant with a low probability of being associated with disease, and for which there is no proven intervention would fall into this category. It follows from this line of reasoning that the obligation to ensure that the patient is well informed and participates in the decision to proceed with genetic testing depends on where the test falls on the spectrum from low to high scrutiny.

Several examples serve to illustrate these considerations in the case of genetic screening in stroke prevention. The value of screening young African-American stroke patients for sickle cell disease is widely accepted because this information directly influences treatment of the initial stroke and strategies for preventing recurrent stroke. The issues relating to factor V Leiden mutation testing are more complex. A recent consensus statement by the American College of Medical Genetics

recommends that factor V Leiden mutation testing be performed in any person with venous thrombosis in an unusual site, including cerebral vein thrombosis[19]. Although the finding of heterozygosity for this mutation (lifetime risk of venous thrombosis approximately 10%) does not currently change the management or prophylaxis for most patients, the finding of homozygosity (lifetime risk of venous thrombosis > 80%) would dictate the consideration of lifelong antithrombotic prophylaxis. While more controversial[20], another benefit of testing for factor V Leiden mutation in cerebral venous thrombosis is that relatives of those possessing one or more of the mutant alleles could choose to be screened. Knowledge of factor V Leiden status in asymptomatic relatives could influence a woman's decision to use oral contraceptives or could lead to antithrombotic prophylaxis during periods of increased risk, such as the postpartum period. Routine testing is not currently recommended for young patients with arterial stroke, even those with a family history[19], although testing could play a role in the evaluation of persons with suspected paradoxical embolism. In contrast to stroke attributable to a Mendelian trait, most candidate genes for stroke have a low probability of being associated with disease and do not have proven interventions. For these reasons, testing for such candidate stroke genes would fall into the category of high scrutiny genetic tests at this time.

ACKNOWLEDGEMENT AND DISCLAIMER

Dr Kittner's effort on this project was supported by the Baltimore Veterans Administration (VA) Geriatrics Research, Education, and Clinical Center and through a cooperative agreement between the Centers for Disease Control and Prevention (CDC) and the

Association of Teachers of Preventive Medicine (ATPM) award number TS499-16/16; its contents are the responsibility of the authors and do not necessarily reflect the official views of the CDC, ATPM or VA. Dr Cole's effort on this project was supported by an American Academy of Neurology clinical research fellowship and by the National Institutes of Health Research Training in the Epidemiology of Aging (Grant T32-AG00262-04).

References

1. Venter JC, Adams MD, Myers EW, *et al*. The sequence of the human genome. *Science* 2001; 291(5507):1304–51

2. Joutel A, Corpechot C, Ducros A, *et al*. E notch 3 mutations in CADASIL, a hereditary adult-onset condition causing stroke and dementia. *Nature* 1996;383:707–10

3. Natowicz M, Kelley RI. Mendelian etiologies of stroke. *Ann Neurol* 1987;22:175–92

4. Elbaz A, Amarenco P. Genetic susceptibility and ischaemic stroke. *Curr Opin Neurol* 1999; 12:47–55

5. Brass LM, Isaacson JL, Mericangas KR, Robinnette CD. A study of twin and stroke. *Stroke* 1992;3:221–3

6. Rubattu S, Volpe M, Kreutz R, *et al*. Chromosomal mapping of quantitative trait loci contributing to stroke in a rat model of complex human disease. *Nat Genet* 1996;13:429–34

7. Rubattu S, Ridker P, Stampfer MJ, *et al*. The gene encoding atrial natriuretic peptide and the risk of human stroke. *Circulation* 1999; 100(16):1722–6

8. Bradley WG, Daroff RB, *et al. Neurology in Clinical Practice*, vols. 1 and 2, 3rd edn. Woburn, MA: Butterworth-Heinmann, 2000

9. Fenichel GM. *Clinical Pediatric Neurology*, 3rd edn. Philadelphia, PA: W.B. Saunders, 1998

10. McKusick VA. *Menedelian Inheritance in Man*, 12th edn. Baltimore, MD: Johns Hopkins Press, 1997

11. Menkes JH, Sarnat HB. *Child Neurology*, 6th edn. Philadelphia, PA: Lippincott Williams and Wilkins, 2000

12. Online Mendelian Inheritance in Man (OMIM). www.ncbi.nlm.nih.gov/entrez/query. fcgi?db=OMIM

13. Robbins SL, Cotran RZ, Kumar V. *Robbin's Pathologic Basis of Disease*, 6th edn. Philadelphia, PA: W.B. Saunders, 1998

14. Hademenos GJ, Alberts MJ, Awad I, *et al*. Advances in the genetics of cerebrovascular disease and stroke. *Neurology* 2001;56: 997–1008

15. Hassan A, Markus HS. Genetics and ischaemic stroke. *Brain* 2000;123:1784–812

16. Hassan A, Sham P, Markus H. Modeling feasibility of genetic approaches to human stroke. Abstracts of the international stroke conference. *Stroke* 2001;32:322

17. Lander ES, Schork NJ. Genetic dissection of complex traits. *Science* 1994;265:2037–48

18. Secretary's Advisory Committee on Genetic Testing. Enhancing the oversight of genetic tests: recommendations of the SACGT. 19 January 2001. http://www4.od.nih.gov/oba/ sacgt.htm

19. Grody WW, Griffin JH, Taylor AK, *et al*., for the ACMG factor V Leiden working group. American College of Medical Genetics consensus statement on factor V Leiden mutation testing. *Gen Med* 2001;3:139–48

20. Vandenbroucke JP, van der Meer FJ, Helmerhorst FM, Rosendaal FR. Factor V Leiden: should we screen oral contraceptive users and pregnant women?

Chapter 9

Markers of subclinical vascular disease and stroke

Monika Hollander, MD, and Monique M.B. Breteler, MD, PhD

INTRODUCTION

It is estimated that 70% of all strokes are related to vascular disease caused by atherosclerosis. Nowadays, a large arsenal of techniques is available to measure subclinical vascular pathology in various arterial segments. To the extent that subclinical vascular pathology predicts stroke risk, it can be used to identify persons who are at increased risk of stroke and, hence, may benefit most from preventive interventions. In this chapter, we review the relation between markers of subclinical vascular disease and their relation with stroke, focusing, when possible, on population-based evidence. Some measures of vascular disease are relatively new and their relation with stroke in the population still has to be explored. In those cases, we discuss results from hospital-based studies. First, we focus on measures of generalized atherosclerosis. Then, we discuss some structural and functional properties of vascular disease. Finally, possible expressions of vascular disease as detected by brain magnetic resonance imaging (MRI) are discussed.

MEASURES OF GENERALIZED ATHEROSCLEROSIS

Ankle–brachial index

The ankle–brachial index is a relatively simple and non-invasive measure that is used to assess peripheral arterial disease and atherosclerosis[1,2]. The ankle–brachial index is the ratio of systolic blood pressure measured at the ankle to systolic blood pressure at the arm. An ankle–brachial index below 0.90 is considered to reflect the presence of peripheral arterial disease[3]. Peripheral arterial disease is common in elderly persons without overt symptoms of claudication, and its prevalence in subjects over 65 years of age is estimated to be 10%[4]. Several studies have consistently shown that a low ankle–brachial index is a predictor of stroke (Table 1)[5–9].

It has been suggested that a low ankle–brachial – or ankle–arm – index can be used as a screening tool to identify subjects at high risk for disease, although a high ankle–brachial index does not rule out the presence of atherosclerosis. The Atherosclerosis Risk in Communities Study has shown that the risk associated with a low ankle–arm index diminished after adjustment for cardiovascular risk factors including systolic blood pressure, antihypertensive medication, diabetes, smoking, pack-years smoking, LDL cholesterol, HDL cholesterol and prevalent coronary heart disease. Therefore, it is doubtful whether assessment of the ankle–arm index has prognostic ability beyond traditional risk factors in the prediction of stroke.

Table 1 Prospective population-based cohort studies on ankle–arm index and risk of stroke

Study	Study population (age, years)	Follow up	No of strokes	Relative risk (95% CI) of stroke in low (< 0.9) vs high (> 0.9) ankle–arm index
Edinburgh Artery Study[5]	1592 subjects (55–74)	5 years	50	1.9 (1.0–3.5)* 1.9 (1.0–3.4)¶
Cardiovascular Health Study[6]	5714 subjects (≥ 65)	6 years	67	1.4 (0.9–2.2)*§ 1.4 (0.9–2.3)¶§ 1.6 (1.1–2.4)*‡ 1.1 (0.7–1.7)¶‡
Atherosclerosis Risk in Communities Study[7]	14 839 subjects (45–64 years)	7 years	206	5.7 (2.8–11.7)*† 1.4 (0.7–2.6)¶†
Rotterdam Study[8]	6450 subjects (≥ 55)	3.7 years	135	2.3 (1.5–3.3)*
Honolulu Heart Program[9]	2767 men (71–93)	3.6 years	91	2.0 (1.1–3.5)¶

*, Adjusted for age and gender; ¶, adjusted for age, gender and cardiovascular risk factors; ‡, in participants without previous cardiovascular disease; †, relative risk in ankle–arm index < 0.8 vs > 1.2; §, in participants with previous cardio-vascular disease

Carotid artery intima-media thickness

Atherosclerosis is accompanied by thickening of the intimal layer of the artery. B-mode ultrasonography allows non-invasive visualization of intima-media thickness. Although no distinction is made between the intimal and medial arterial layer, intima-media thickness has been shown to be related to cardiovascular risk factors and other measures of atherosclerosis. Therefore, an increased intima-media thickness is considered to reflect generalized atherosclerosis[10]. Carotid intima-media thickness can be measured in different carotid arterial segments (common carotid artery, bifurcation or internal carotid artery). Several studies have shown that the carotid intima-media thickness is positively related to the risk of stroke[11,12] and cerebral infarction[13], irrespective of its location in the carotid artery[12]. Table 2 gives an overview of these studies. In summary, carotid intima-media thickness is related to all subtypes of stroke and cerebral infarction.

Carotid plaques

Plaques represent more advanced stages of atherosclerosis and are predominantly present in arterial segments with a turbulent blood flow like the carotid bifurcation. The presence of carotid plaques and plaque characteristics like echolucency, ulceration, intraplaque hemorrhage and surface regularity can be assessed through ultrasonography or angiography. Carotid plaques are frequently found in stroke patients and are related to the risk of stroke in the population[14–17]. It is still a matter of debate as to what the underlying mechanism is that relates carotid plaques and stroke. One proposed mechanism is rupture and intraplaque hemorrhage, leading to superimposed emboli. The finding that plaques with characteristics like echolucency, ulceration, intraplaque bleeding and irregularity of the plaque surface are associated with symptoms supports this[14–19]. Furthermore, it has been reported that hypoechoic, but not hyperechoic, plaques were related to an increased risk of non-cardioembolic ischemic stroke in the population[17]. Another explanation is that carotid plaques simply reflect generalized atherosclerosis. The finding in the Rotterdam Study that total plaque score is related to the risk of stroke, cerebral infarction and lacunar infarction confirms that carotid plaques are markers of generalized atherosclerosis. Table 3 gives an

Table 2 Studies on intima-media thickness (IMT) and risk of stroke

Study	Study design	Population	Determinant	Unit of IMT	Outcome	Relative risk (95% CI) of stroke per SD increase in CCA-IMT
Cardiovascular Health Study[12]	Population-based cohort	4476 subjects aged > 65 years	Maximal IMT in CCA and ICA	Per SD increase and in quartiles	Stroke	1.4 (1.3–1.5)*
Atherosclerosis Risk in Communities Study[13]	Population-based cohort	14 214 subjects aged 45–64 years	Mean IMT in CCA, BIF and ICA	Per SD increase and in tertiles and quintiles	Ischemic stroke caused by thrombosis or embolism	Women: 1.7 (1.5–2.0)¶ Men: 1.5 (1.3–1.8)¶
Génétique de l'Infarctus Cerebral Study[60]	Hospital-based case–control	470 stroke cases and 463 controls	Mean far wall IMT in CCA	Per SD increase	Cerebral infarction and subtypes	1.8 (1.5–2.2)¶
Rotterdam Study	Population-based cohort	5679 subjects aged > 55 years	Mean, maximal IMT and mean far wall IMT in CCA	Per SD increase and in quartiles	Stroke, hemorrhagic stroke and subtypes of infarction	1.5 (1.4–1.6)* 1.4 (1.2–1.6)¶

CCA, common carotid artery; BIF, carotid bifurcation; ICA, internal carotid artery; *, per SD increase in maximal IMT; ¶per SD increase in mean IMT.

Table 3 Prospective studies on carotid plaques and stroke

Study	Study design	Population	Determinant	Outcome	Results[§]
Cardiovascular Health Study[17]	Population-based cohort	4886 asymptomatic subjects aged > 65 years	Echogenicity of dominant plaque in internal carotid artery	Non-cardioembolic ischemic strokes	Hypoechoic plaques increase the risk of stroke in asymptomatic adults (2.5 (10.4–4.5))*[†]
Rotterdam Study	Population-based cohort	4217 neurologically asymptomatic subjects aged > 55 years	Plaques in six locations in the carotid artery	Stroke and subtypes of cerebral infarction	Plaques increase risk of stroke (2.4 (1.4–4.2)) lacunar (10.8 (1.70–69.7)) and non-lacunar infarction in anterior (3.2 (1.1–2.6)), but not in posterior circulation (0.6 (0.1–4.9))*[†‡]
Tromsø Study[18]	Population-based follow-up study	223 subjects with and 215 without carotid stenosis	Echogenicity of plaque	Stroke, cerebral infarction and TIA	Subjects with both stenosis and echolucent plaques have increased risk of stroke compared to subjects without carotid stenosis (2.8 (4.4–37.2))*
Grønholdt et al.[19]	Hospital-based follow-up study	111 asymptomatic and 135 symptomatic patients with > 50% carotid stenosis	Echogenicity of plaque	Ischemic stroke in ipsilateral hemisphere	Echolucent plaques compared to echorich plaques increase risk of stroke in symptomatic (2.9 (1.2–7.0)), but not in asymptomatic subjects (1.0 (0.3–3.3))[¶]

* Adjusted for age and gender; [¶]adjusted for age, gender and cardiovascular risk factors; [†]subjects without plaques as reference; [‡]relative risk in subjects with 5 to 6 plaques in the carotid arteries; [§]figures represent relative risk (95% CI)

overview of prospective studies that have been carried out on carotid plaques and stroke.

Aortic arch atherosclerosis

Atherosclerosis in the aortic arch, and in particular disrupted and protruding plaques as assessed by transesophageal echocardiography, is frequently observed in stroke patients[20]. Follow-up studies have shown that aortic plaque morphology (ulceration, calcification, hypoechoic plaques, irregularities and mobile thrombus[21,22] and thickness[23]) is related to the risk of recurrent stroke. Several mechanisms have been proposed to explain the relationship between aortic plaques and stroke[24]. First, aortic plaques are potential sources of thromboemboli, as indicated by patient series in which a relationship between aortic arch atheroma and cerebral micro-emboli was found[25]. Second, obstruction of the origin of the carotid and vertebral arteries could lead to hemodynamic obstruction of the cerebral blood flow. Third, aortic plaques are considered to be markers of generalized atherosclerosis. However, thus far the relationship between plaques in the aortic arch and stroke has not yet been investigated in a population-based setting.

STRUCTURAL AND FUNCTIONAL PROPERTIES OF SUBCLINICAL VASCULAR DISEASE

Calcifications in the vessel wall

Calcium deposits in the coronary and extra-coronary vessels are considered to indicate the extent of atherosclerotic lesions. Therefore, they are putative markers of subclinical vascular disease. Calcifications in the coronary arteries can be visualized very sensitively by electron-beam tomography. Quantitative measures of coronary calcification are closely related to the amount of atherosclerotic plaques in histopathologic investigation[26]. Several population-based studies have explored the relation between calcifications and stroke. Iribarren and colleagues investigated the relation between calcification of the aortic arch, detected by X-ray, and risk of stroke in a population of 139 849 subjects aged 30 to 89 years[22]. They found that aortic arch calcification increased the risk of ischemic stroke in women (RR, 1.46; 95% CI, 1.28–1.67), but not significantly in men (RR, 1.17; 95% CI, 0.97–1.42). The Rotterdam Study investigated the relation between coronary calcification and the presence of stroke in 2013 men and women in whom 34 men and 16 women had experienced a stroke[27]. Coronary calcifications in the epicardial arteries were assessed on electron-beam tomography and the calcium score was obtained. Participants with a higher calcium score were more likely to have experienced a stroke than subjects in the reference category (RR, 5.2; 95% CI, 1.5–17.8 in men and 2.4; 95% CI, 0.7–7.8 in women). These results indicate that electron-beam tomography is promising for the selection of subjects at high risk for cerebrovascular events, but prospective studies are needed to confirm these findings.

Arterial stiffness

An important risk factor for stroke is hypertension; the prevalence of isolated systolic hypertension increases with age[28,29]. Stiffening of the arterial tree is seen as the main cause of an elevated systolic blood pressure and a decreased diastolic blood pressure, and thus an elevated pulse pressure in the arterial system. Recently, accurate methods to non-invasively measure arterial stiffness have become available. One of these methods is the measurement of arterial distensibility, that is the change in arterial diameter due to the change in arterial pressure over the cardiac cycle[30,31]. The relationship between carotid distensibility and risk of stroke has been scarcely addressed, though the Rotterdam Study investigated the relation between carotid distensibility and history of stroke[32]. The study was performed in 3818 subjects, of whom 78 had experienced a previous stroke. Participants in the lowest quartile of carotid distensibility were more than 12 times more likely to have experienced a stroke (OR, 12.6; 95% CI, 2.7–58.1), compared to those in the highest quartile. This relationship remained significant after adjustment for carotid plaques and ankle–brachial index. The most likely underlying mechanism of this association is an elevation of pulse pressure, induced by increased arterial stiffness. In addition, it has been suggested that the risk of embolism due to rupture of plaques is increased in stiff arteries[33]. Additional prospective studies are needed to confirm the result from this cross-sectional study.

Another measurement of arterial stiffness is the pulse-wave velocity, which is the ratio between the transit time for the foot of the pulse wave to travel along the arterial tree and the distance of the arterial segment. A higher pulse-wave velocity reflects a stiff artery. The pulse-wave velocity can be measured in the thoraco-abdominal aorta. One case–control study investigated the relationship between pulse-wave velocity and stroke in 20 stroke patients and 20 controls without cardiovascular disease[34]. The pulse-wave velocity was significantly higher in stroke patients compared to controls, independently of blood pressure level. These findings, however, were not confirmed by researchers from the Rotterdam Study, who failed to find a clear relationship with a history of stroke[32]. More studies are needed to elucidate the relationship between arterial stiffness and stroke.

Indices of cerebral circulation, measured by transcranial Doppler ultrasonography

Transcranial Doppler ultrasonography allows the detection of micro-embolic signals and the evaluation of cerebral hemodynamics such as cerebral blood flow and vasomotor reactivity. Various hospital-based studies have shown that the presence of micro-emboli as assessed by transcranial Doppler has diagnostic and prognostic value for stroke[35–37], as the presence of micro-embolic signals was related to cardio-embolic strokes[38], severe carotid stenosis[39], poorer outcome[37] and a higher recurrence rate of stroke[36,40]. Transcranial Doppler can also be used to assess cerebral hemodynamic parameters such as the blood flow velocity, pulsatility index and reactivity to CO_2, all of which have been shown to be related to cardiovascular risk factors[41,42]. However, the prognostic value of these hemodynamic measurements themselves still needs to be investigated.

CONSEQUENCES OF VASCULAR DISEASE

Silent brain infarctions and white matter lesions are frequently observed in elderly subjects. It is estimated that 20 to 33% of the healthy elderly have silent brain infarctions[43–45] and that, depending on the scoring method, 5 to 90% have white matter lesions[46], the prevalence of which substantially increases with age[43,44,47–49]. These lesions are associated with cardiovascular risk factors[43,50–52] and are considered to reflect small vessel pathology.

Silent brain infarctions as a risk factor for stroke

One hospital-based study investigated the relationship between the presence of silent brain infarctions and the risk of vascular events in stroke patients with non-rheumatic atrial fibrillation[53]. The investigators observed that the presence of silent brain infarctions is associated with an increased risk of vascular events, and stroke in particular. Kobayashi and colleagues followed 933 healthy subjects aged 30 to 81 years for 1 to 7 years[47] and reported that the presence of silent brain infarctions was related to a more than 10-fold increased risk of stroke. The Cardiovascular Health Study followed 3324 participants aged 65 years or over for 4 years[45]. The presence of silent brain infarctions almost doubled the risk of stroke (RR, 1.9; 95% CI, 1.2–2.8).

White matter lesions as a risk factor for stroke

It has been observed that white matter lesions are related to all kinds of stroke subtypes, but especially lacunar infarctions and deep cerebral hemorrhages[54]. These findings suggest that lacunes and white matter lesions share a common type of vasculopathy located either in the deep perforator vessels or deep medullary arterioles. Little data exist on the relationship between white matter lesions and the risk of future stroke or other cardiovascular events. The studies that have been performed were based on patient series and have shown that the presence of white matter lesions in elderly neurological patients is related to an increased risk of cardiovascular death[55,56]. In addition higher recurrence rates of stroke in patients with white matter lesions have been reported[57–59]. These studies, however, were based on selected patient groups, and prospective population-based studies are awaited.

SUMMARY

Various measures of subclinical vascular disease are related to stroke and its subtypes. Ankle–arm index, carotid intima-media thickness and plaques are markers of generalized atherosclerosis and are related to the risk of stroke in the general population. Plaque characteristics like echodensity and surface regularity may provide additional information. It is still debated whether these measures have prognostic value beyond traditional risk factors. Less well established measures are aortic arch atherosclerosis, calcifications in the vessel wall and arterial stiffness and indices of cerebral circulation measured by transcranial Doppler. They have been shown to be related to stroke, but quantification of this relationship in prospective population-based studies is needed. Finally, the consequences of vascular disease – like silent brain infarctions – have recently been confirmed as risk factors for stroke.

References

1. Yao ST, Hobbs JT, Irvine WT. Ankle systolic pressure measurements in arterial disease affecting the lower extremities. *Br J Surg* 1969;56:676–9
2. Fowkes FG, Housley E, Macintyre CC, *et al.* Variability of ankle and brachial systolic pressures in the measurement of atherosclerotic peripheral arterial disease. *J Epidemiol Commun Health* 1988;42:128–33
3. Fowkes FG, Housley E, Cawood EH, *et al.* Edinburgh Artery Study: prevalence of asymptomatic and symptomatic peripheral arterial disease in the general population. *Int J Epidemiol* 1991;20:384–92
4. Newman AB, Siscovick DS, Manolio TA, *et al.* Ankle-arm index as a marker of atherosclerosis in the Cardiovascular Health Study. Cardiovascular Health Study (CHS) Collaborative Research Group. *Circulation* 1993;88:837–45
5. Leng GC, Fowkes FG, Lee AJ, *et al.* Use of ankle brachial pressure index to predict cardiovascular events and death: a cohort study. *Br Med J* 1996;313:1440–4
6. Newman AB, Shemanski L, Manolio TA, *et al.* Ankle-arm index as a predictor of cardiovascular disease and mortality in the cardiovascular Health Study. The Cardiovascular Health Study Group. *Arterioscler Thromb Vasc Biol* 1999;19:538–45

7. Tsai AW, Folsom AR, Rosamond WD, Jones DW. Ankle-brachial index and 7-year ischemic stroke incidence: the ARIC study. *Stroke* 2001;32:1721–4

8. Meijer WT. *Peripheral Arterial Disease in the Elderly*. (Thesis) Epidemiology & Biostatistics. Erasmus Medical Centre, Rotterdam, 1999

9. Abbott RD, Rodriguez BL, Petrovitch H, *et al*. Ankle-brachial blood pressure in elderly men and the risk of stroke: the Honolulu Heart Program. *J Clin Epidemiol* 2001;54:973–8

10. Bots ML, Hofman A, de Bruyn AM, *et al*. Isolated systolic hypertension and vessel wall thickness of the carotid artery. The Rotterdam Elderly Study. *Arterioscler Thromb* 1993;13:64–9

11. Bots ML, Hoes AW, Koudstaal PJ, *et al*. Common carotid intima-media thickness and risk of stroke and myocardial infarction: the Rotterdam Study. *Circulation* 1997;96:1432–7

12. O'Leary DH, Polak JF, Kronmal RA, *et al*. Carotid-artery intima and media thickness as a risk factor for myocardial infarction and stroke in older adults. Cardiovascular Health Study Collaborative Research Group. *N Engl J Med* 1999;340:14–22

13. Chambless LE, Folsom AR, Clegg LX, *et al*. Carotid wall thickness is predictive of incident clinical stroke: the Atherosclerosis Risk in Communities (ARIC) Study. *Am J Epidemiol* 2000;151:478–87

14. Sabetai MM, Tegos TJ, Nicolaides AN, *et al*. Hemispheric symptoms and carotid plaque echomorphology. *J Vasc Surg* 2000;31:39–49

15. Golledge J, Cuming R, Ellis M, *et al*. Carotid plaque characteristics and presenting symptoms. *Br J Surg* 1997;84:1697–701

16. Gomez RG. Carotid plaque morphology and risk for stroke. *Stroke* 1990;21:148–51

17. Polak JF, Shemanski L, O'Leary DH, *et al*. Hypoechoic plaque at US of the carotid artery: an independent risk factor for incident stroke in adults aged 65 years or older. Cardiovascular Health Study. *Radiology* 1998;208:649–54

18. Mathiesen EB, Bonaa KH, Joakimsen O. Echolucent plaques are associated with high risk of ischemic cerebrovascular events in carotid stenosis: The Tromsø study. *Circulation* 2001;103:2171–5

19. Grønholdt ML, Nordestgaard BG, Schroeder TV, *et al*. Ultrasonic echolucent carotid plaques predict future strokes. *Circulation* 2001;104:68–73

20. Tenenbaum A, Fisman EZ, Schneiderman J, *et al*. Disrupted mobile aortic plaques are a major risk factor for systemic embolism in the elderly. *Cardiology* 1998;89:246–51

21. Cohen A, Tzourio C, Bertrand B, *et al*. Aortic plaque morphology and vascular events: a follow-up study in patients with ischemic stroke. FAPS investigators. French Study of Aortic Plaques in Stroke. *Circulation* 1997;96:3838–41

22. Iribarren C, Sidney S, Sternfeld B, Browner WS. Calcification of the aortic arch: risk factors and association with coronary heart disease, stroke, and peripheral vascular disease. *J Am Med Assoc* 2000;283:2810–5

23. Mitusch R, Doherty C, Wucherpfennig H, *et al*. Vascular events during follow-up in patients with aortic arch atherosclerosis. *Stroke* 1997;28:36–9

24. Sen S, Wu K, McNamara R, *et al*. Distribution, severity and risk factors for aortic atherosclerosis in cerebral ischemia. *Cerebrovasc Dis* 2000;10:102–9

25. Rundek T, Di Tullio MR, Sciacca RR, *et al*. Association between large aortic arch atheromas and high-intensity transient signals in elderly stroke patients. *Stroke* 1999;30:2683–6

26. Rumberger JA, Simons DB, Fitzpatrick LA, *et al*. Coronary artery calcium area by electron-beam computed tomography and coronary atherosclerotic plaque area. A histopathologic correlative study. *Circulation* 1995;92:2157–62

27. Vliegenthart R, Hollander M, Breteler MMB, *et al*. Stroke is associated with coronary calcification as detected on electron-beam computed tomography: The Rotterdam Coronary Calcification Study. *Stroke* 2002;33:4625

28. Ekpo EB, Ashworth IN, Fernando MU, *et al*. Prevalence of mixed hypertension, isolated systolic hypertension and isolated diastolic hypertension in the elderly population in the community. *J Hum Hypertens* 1994;8:39–43

29. Aguero Torres H, Fratiglioni L, Lindberg J, Winblad B. Hypertension in the elderly population: prevalence data from an urban area in Sweden. *Aging (Milano)* 1994;6:249–55

30. Reneman RS, van Merode T, Hick P, *et al*. Age-related changes in carotid artery wall properties in men. *Ultrasound Med Biol* 1986;12:465–71

31. Lehmann ED. Terminology for the definition of arterial elastic properties. *Pathol Biol (Paris)* 1999;47:656–64

32. Popele van N. *Causes and Consequences of Arterial Stiffness. An Epidemiological Approach.* (Thesis) Epidemiology & Biostatistics. Erasmus Medical Center, Rotterdam, 2000

33. Lee RT, Kamm RD. Vascular mechanics for the cardiologist. *J Am Coll Cardiol* 1994;23: 1289–95

34. Lehmann ED, Hopkins KD, Jones RL, *et al.* Aortic distensibility in patients with cerebrovascular disease. *Clin Sci (Colch)* 1995;89: 247–53

35. Valton L, Larrue V, le Traon AP, *et al.* Microembolic signals and risk of early recurrence in patients with stroke or transient ischemic attack. *Stroke* 1998;29:2125–8

36. Valton L, Larrue V, Le Traon AP, Geraud G. Cerebral microembolism in patients with stroke or transient ischaemic attack as a risk factor for early recurrence. *J Neurol Neurosurg Psychiatry* 1997;63:784–7

37. Serena J, Segura T, Castellanos M, Davalos A. Microembolic signal monitoring in hemispheric acute ischaemic stroke: a prospective study. *Cerebrovasc Dis* 2000;10:278–82

38. Lund C, Rygh J, *et al.* Cerebral microembolus detection in an unselected acute ischemi stroke population. *Cerebrovasc Dis* 2000;10: 403–8

39. Eicke BM, von Lorentz J, Paulus W. Embolus detection in different degrees of carotid disease. *Neurol Res* 1995;17:181–4

40. Baracchini C, Manara R, Ermani M, Meneghetti G. The quest for early predictors of stroke evolution: can TCD be a guiding light? *Stroke* 2000;31:2942–7

41. Bakker SL, de Leeuw FE, Koudstaal PJ, *et al.* Cerebral CO_2 reactivity, cholesterol, and high-density lipoprotein cholesterol in the elderly. *Neurology* 2000;54:987–9

42. Bakker SL, de Leeuw FE, de Groot JC, *et al.* Cerebral vasomotor reactivity and cerebral white matter lesions in the elderly. *Neurology* 1999;52:578–83

43. Vermeer SE, Koudstaal PJ, Oudkerk M, *et al.* Prevalence and risk factors of silent brain infarcts in the population-based Rotterdam Scan Study. *Stroke* 2002;33:21–5

44. Longstreth WT Jr, Manolio TA, Arnold A, *et al.* Clinical correlates of white matter findings on cranial magnetic resonance imaging of 3301 elderly people. The Cardiovascular Health Study. *Stroke* 1996;27:1274–82

45. Bernick C, Kuller L, Dulberg C, *et al.* Silent MRI infarcts and the risk of future stroke: the cardiovascular health study. *Neurology* 2001;57:1222–9

46. de Leeuw FE, De Groot JC, Breteler MMB. White matter changes: frequency and risk factors. In Pantoni L, Inzitari D, Wallin A, eds. *The Matter of White Matter. Clinical and Pathophysiological Aspects of White Matter Disease Related to Cognitive Decline and Vascular Dementia,* 1998

47. Kobayashi S, Okada K, Koide H, *et al.* Subcortical silent brain infarction as a risk factor for clinical stroke. *Stroke* 1997;28:1932–9

48. Liao D, Cooper L, Cai J, *et al.* Presence and severity of cerebral white matter lesions and hypertension, its treatment, and its control. The Atherosclerosis Risk in Communities (ARIC) Study. *Stroke* 1996;27:2262–70

49. de Leeuw FE, de Groot JC, Achten E, *et al.* Prevalence of cerebral white matter lesions in elderly people: a population based magnetic resonance imaging study. The Rotterdam Scan Study. *J Neurol Neurosurg Psychiatry* 2001;70:9–14

50. Kobayashi S, Okada K, Yamashita K. Incidence of silent lacunar lesion in normal adults and its relation to cerebral blood flow and risk factors. *Stroke* 1991;22:1379–83

51. Bots ML, van Swieten JC, Breteler MM, *et al.* Cerebral white matter lesions and atherosclerosis in the Rotterdam Study. *Lancet* 1993;341: 1232–7

52. de Leeuw FE, De Groot JC, Oudkerk M, *et al.* Aortic atherosclerosis at middle age predicts cerebral white matter lesions in the elderly. *Stroke* 2000;31:425–9

53. The EAFT study group. Silent brain infarction in nonrheumatic atrial fibrillation. European Atrial Fibrillation Trial. *Neurology* 1996;46: 159–65

54. Leys D, Englund E, Del Ser T, *et al.* White matter changes in stroke patients. Relationship with stroke subtype and outcome. *Eur Neurol* 1999;42:67–75

55. Tarvonen-Schroder S, Kurki T, Raiha I, Sourander L. Leukoaraiosis and cause of death: a five year follow up. *J Neurol Neurosurg Psychiatry* 1995;58:586–9

56. Inzitari D, Cadelo M, Marranci ML, *et al.* Vascular deaths in elderly neurological patients with leukoaraiosis. *J Neurol Neurosurg Psychiatry* 1997;62:177–81

57. van Swieten JC, Kappelle LJ, Algra A, *et al.* Hypodensity of the cerebral white matter in patients with transient ischemic attack or minor stroke: influence on the rate of subsequent

stroke. Dutch TIA trial study group. *Ann Neurol* 1992;32:177–83

58. Miyao S, Takano A, Teramoto J, Takahashi A. Leukoaraiosis in relation to prognosis for patients with lacunar infarction. *Stroke* 1992; 23:1434–8

59. Inzitari D, Di Carlo A, Mascalchi M, *et al*. The cardiovascular outcome of patients with motor impairment and extensive leukoaraiosis. *Arch Neurol* 1995;52:687–91

60. Touboul PJ, Elbaz A, Koller C, *et al*. Common carotid artery intima-media thickness and brain infarction: the Étude du Profil Génétique de l'Infarctus Cerebral (GENIC) case-control study. The GENIC investigators. *Circulation* 2000;102:313–18

Chapter 10

Community mass and high risk strategies

Philip B. Gorelick, MD, MPH, FACP

INTRODUCTION

Stroke is the second most common cause of death worldwide and is responsible for about 5.1 million or 9.5% of all deaths[1]. In Asian countries such as Japan and China stroke is the most common cause of mortality, whereas in most developed countries it is the third leading cause of death. Although stroke takes a substantial personal and financial toll, it is well suited for prevention as it has a high prevalence of disease, burden of illness and economic cost, and there are effective prevention measures[2-7]. However, there are gaps between actual physician prevention practices and implementation of stroke clinical preventative services[8,9]. These gaps must be bridged if we are to reduce the risk of stroke and attain national goals for stroke prevention. In this chapter we review approaches to stroke prevention in the community.

RATIONALE FOR PREVENTION

The goal to prevent disease by reducing its risk factors has become well ingrained in the cultures of developed countries. Yet physicians are trained primarily to care for the sick and may be less familiar with prevention guidelines and measures for the community at large[10,11]. Rose has summarized the rationale for preventive services

and programs[12]. As prosperity has risen over time and people live longer, we have witnessed a growth of interest in healthy living, and thus, a growing interest in preventive services. Many continue to search for the 'fountain of youth' and hope to add 'life to years' rather than merely 'years to life'. Our quest for healthy living inspires preventive measures. In addition there are economic arguments whereby a decline in the incidence of a disease brings about savings, as well as the humanitarian argument that being healthy is better than being ill.

Screening for disease

Screening is a public health prevention tool whereby persons with higher probabilities of getting a disease are identified from among the general population[13]. Those who are at higher risk can then be referred for a definitive diagnosis. For screening to be useful the following guides must be considered[13]: (1) Is the disease sufficiently prevalent in the community to warrant screening? (2) Is there an effective screening test? (3) Will the screening program reach those at risk? (4) Are there effective treatment or prevention measures for the disease? (5) Is the program cost-effective for the public health system? (6) Will those who screen positive be able to adhere to advice and apply the prevention measure(s)?

Screening and early intervention are thought to be most effective when the risk factor is common amongst the target population; screening procedures and therapy are safe, valid and cost-effective; and therapy for the risk factor is associated with favorable effects. Therefore, screening programs are aimed primarily at the 'susceptibility' and 'presymptomatic' stages of disease as prevention is possible during these stages[2].

Diagnostic technology is employed in the screening process to determine who screens positive or negative for the disease or risk marker of interest. For a diagnostic technology to be considered useful it must be safe and effective, have the technical capacity to detect disease when present and exclude it when not present (diagnostic accuracy), and add significant information regarding diagnosis or patient management (diagnostic and therapeutic impact)[14–17]. The reader is referred to a review by Nuwer for a discussion of the process for evaluating a new diagnostic technology[18].

Measures of the diagnostic accuracy of a proposed test should be scrutinized[16]. For example, is the test valid (does it measure what it is intended to) and is there reliability of the measure (reproducibility)? Evidence-based measures such as sensitivity (true-positive rate), specificity (true-negative rate), positive predictive value (probability of disease if a test is positive) and negative predictive value (probability of absence of disease if a test is negative) may be applied. As sensitivity and specificity measures may have limitations, a more powerful measure, the likelihood ratio, which takes into account multiple test level results, sensitivity and specificity, and pretest probabilities to generate post-test probabilities, may be used[16]. Thus, the likelihood ratio measures the probability of a test result among persons with a target disorder in relation to the probability of the same result among those free of the disorder.

Strategies for prevention

In discussing strategies for stroke prevention in the community, we will focus on means to reduce the risk of a first stroke in the community at large[5]; means to reduce the risk of a recurrent stroke or cerebral ischemia are discussed in Chapters 19–21 of this book.

Surprisingly, acute treatment of stroke appears to have little impact on the overall stroke burden[19]. For example, it is estimated that acute thrombolysis if given to as many as 10% of appropriate stroke patients (a figure far greater than the 1% cited in the United States as actually given) would reduce stroke mortality by only 0.5%. Aspirin in acute stroke patients is estimated to reduce mortality by only 1.5%, whereas treatment in a stroke unit might reduce overall mortality by 3%. Thus, a weak treatment (for example aspirin) or one that is applied to only a small proportion of acute stroke patients (for example thrombolysis) is unlikely to substantially reduce stroke mortality. Furthermore, the ability of acute stroke treatments to reduce even post-stroke dependency, let alone overall stroke burden, is limited, given the modest absolute risk reduction of available treatments such as administration of intravenous tissue plasminogen activator within three hours of the onset of ischemic stroke. Despite these limitations, community strategies to reduce the risk of a first stroke merit substantial consideration, because only when evaluating the overall effect of preventive measures in the population can the benefits be perceived in proper perspective.

THE HIGH-RISK STRATEGY

The strategy of chronic disease prevention that targets individuals at high risk of stroke (for example smokers, hypertensives, diabetics and those with atrial fibrillation or severe carotid stenosis) is widely accepted[19]. However, the process whereby one identifies or screens for those with high blood pressure or cholesterol levels, heavy alcohol consumption or cigarette use, or high degrees of carotid stenosis is generally an expensive and labor intensive activity. The 'high-risk' approach becomes even more challenging when one attempts to identify and treat those at lower risk. Not surprisingly, in lower risk persons the strategy becomes less cost-effective because the number needed to be treated to prevent one stroke is higher than in higher risk persons for any given risk factor[19]. Furthermore, by identifying and treating only individuals at highest risk, those with moderate risk – among whom most strokes arise – may be missed. This is an example of the prevention paradox in that what is best for the individual may not necessarily be best for the community.

The approach that targets those at high risk usually requires pharmacologic intervention to achieve reduction of the risk factor with drug therapy. However, it is difficult to conclude that published reports of non-randomized studies using drug therapy in high-risk individuals have conclusively shown a reduction of stroke or coronary events[20,21]. Thus, the high-risk strategy is by no means ideal as it may be an expensive strategy, may distract one from those at moderate risk (in whom a higher absolute number of stroke events occur), and treatment may be too risky or impracticable in those at highest risk[19]. Furthermore, for example, physicians in community practice may not be able to achieve blood pressure reductions as great as those reported in clinical trials[19].

MASS STRATEGY

The mass strategy for community prevention focuses on achieving a modest or small downward shift in risk factors among an entire population[2,4,6,19]. This may be accomplished by lifestyle changes and through health education, legislation and economic measures to discourage harmful behavior or exposure to harmful factors. By reducing levels of risk factors in an entire population, a greater number of strokes may be eliminated because a greater number of events will be avoided in a larger number of persons[19]. An example of the mass strategy is the reduction of mean daily salt intake in the population by health education and legislative measures which can lead to a reduction in the prevalence of hypertension and subsequent stroke rates[22]. It is estimated that a 1–2% reduction in the population mean systolic blood pressure could result in a 10% reduction in the incidence of stroke[19].

In theory, the success of the mass strategy is based on lowering blood pressure at least slightly in a large number of hypertensives in the population, reducing the number of cigarettes smoked and an overall reduction in the number of smokers in the population, and encouraging other healthy behaviors such as exercise, moderate rather than heavy alcohol consumption for drinkers, and healthy diets for all[19]. Although this approach could have a high impact on stroke reduction, it may be challenging to obtain individual compliance, as individuals may not find immediate reward from lifestyle changes, have difficulty sustaining these changes, and as individuals may not benefit as they are already at lower risk for stroke. Furthermore, the mass strategy has its detractors who claim it would be impractical to treat an entire community, and there could be risks (for example injuries related to exercise, potential danger of low blood pressure, and the potential risk of low cholesterol on cancer and hemorrhagic stroke risk). Moreover, the societal need for quick or short-term results may not be met[19]. Even with these potential drawbacks, the mass approach to prevention has persuasive advantages, at least in theory.

PREVENTION PROGRAMS AND PUBLIC HEALTH POLICY

Stroke is a disease with high financial costs. For example, in the United States the aggregate cost per year is estimated to be at least

Table 1 Key results of stroke and cardiovascular disease community intervention studies[6]

Study location	Focus	Results
Stroke		
Rural north–eastern Japan[36]	Hypertension control (pharmacologic and lifestyle modification)	Decline in stroke incidence for men in full intervention group but no sustained difference for women through 1987
Urban China[37]	Intervention for hypertension, heart disease, and diabetes mellitus (pharmacologic, traditional and lifestyle modification)	Decline in incidence of stroke, more favorable blood pressure profile, but no change in the prevalence of heart disease and diabetes
Coronary heart disease		
Northern California[38–40]	Community organization and health education on cardiovascular risk factors	Improvements in blood pressure, coronary heart disease and all-cause mortality risk scores
Minnesota[41–43]	Hypertension prevention/control, diet, smoking cessation, physical activity to improve risk factors, health behavior and morbidity/mortality	Modest effects on risk factors within chance variation, coronary rates ↓ but no major trends for stroke
Rhode Island[44]	Target cardiovascular risk factors, behavior change and community activation to ↓ population risk factors and cardiovascular disease risk	Risk reduction feasible but there was no maintenance of significant trends
Finland[20,45–47]	Systematic and comprehensive cardiovascular disease risk modification	Intervention feasible but inconclusive if decrease in cardiovascular mortality related to program alone

$30–40 billion, with an average cost of $50 000/case[23]. However, public health policy barriers appear to exist that inhibit the development of prevention programs[24,25]. Essential components of successful preventive action include a better knowledge base, political support, and a sophisticated social strategy designed to accomplish change[26]. Prevention policy could be enhanced by informing key decision makers about such aspects of prevention as effectiveness of the strategy, cost, risks, and the multiplicity of preventatives[27,28]. It is estimated that less than 5% of healthcare dollars are spent on health promotion and disease prevention, and essential public health services have averaged less than a dime/day/capita in the United States[24,29]. Despite this low support, favorable cardiovascular risk profiles are already discernible and may be predictive of lower average medical charges in the elderly[28,30]. Gains in life expectancy through preventive interventions are estimated to be highest for those at high risk[31], and may occur quickly after the institution of the preventive measure, although the cost may be high[32]. Cost-effective interventions and detection of new risk factors that can be modified in a cost-effective manner are needed. With this type of evidence in hand, it will be easier to approach policy makers who allocate health care expenditure and who have competing financial demands.

Most screening activities for stroke and cardiovascular disease risk in the United States occur in the physician's office or local health clinics. Community-based stroke and cardiovascular disease prevention programs that have focused on detection, reduction and maintenance of reduction of risk factors, and surveillance of stroke and cardiovascular disease morbidity and mortality, have achieved only modest benefits[6]. This has been attributed to the educational message aimed at the intervention communities having influenced the control communities, insufficient sample size or inconsistent and insensitive outcome measures, and favorable secular trends in general risk factor awareness, knowledge and behavior that may be propagated via national mass media campaigns[33–35].

Table 1 lists key findings from selected stroke and cardiovascular disease community intervention studies[36–47]. Two stroke studies are featured, one from rural Japan and one from urban China. Four cardiovascular disease studies are featured (three from the United States [Stanford Five-City Project, Minnesota Heart Health Program, and Pawtucket Heart Health Program] and one from Europe [North Karelia]). Overall, the studies suggest that the interventions were feasible and effective. In general, at least modest reductions in risk factors were achieved, but it is still uncertain whether a reduction in key disease outcomes has occurred.

CONCLUSION

Secular trends in cardiovascular risk factors portend higher stroke rates in the United States

and other places in the world[4,48]. As developing countries modernize, smoking, obesity, unhealthy diet and hypertension become more prevalent. In the United States, an epidemic of obesity and overweight is alleged and trends toward reduced awareness, lower treatment and less adequate control of hypertension are suspected. The earliest signals of cardiovascular disease or its precursors may be observed in children, adolescents and young adults[49–52]. Stroke and cardiovascular disease risk factors may cluster early in life and provide an opportunity for intervention by lifestyle modification. New low-cost, high-yield population prevention strategies to control disease risk early as well as later in life need to be explored[53]. Cardiovascular risk factors earlier in life predict illness, disability and cognitive impairment later in life[54,55]. The strategies targeting high risk individuals as well as the general population offer an opportunity to delay and diminish the risk of stroke and its damaging consequences.

ACKNOWLEDGEMENT

Supported in part by NIH/NINDS grant # R01NS33430.

References

1. Bonita R. Stroke Prevention: A Global Perspective. In Norris J, Hachinski V, eds. *Stroke Prevention*. New York: Oxford University Press, 2001:259–74
2. Gorelick PB. Stroke prevention. An opportunity for efficient utilization of health care resources during the coming decade. *Stroke* 1994;25:220–4
3. Gorelick PB. Stroke prevention. *Arch Neurol* 1995;52:347–55
4. Gorelick PB. Stroke prevention: windows of opportunity and failed expectations? A discussion of modifiable cardiovascular risk factors and a prevention proposal. *Neuroepidemiology* 1997;16:163–73
5. Gorelick PB, Sacco RL, Smith DB, *et al*. Prevention of a first stroke. A review of guidelines and a multidisciplinary consensus statement from the National Stroke Association. *J Am Med Assoc* 1999;281:1112–20
6. Gorelick PB. Prevention and screening programs. In Norris J, Hachinski V, eds. *Stroke Prevention*. New York: Oxford University Press, 2001: 117–36
7. Goldstein LB, Adams R, Becker K, *et al*. Primary prevention of ischemic stroke. A statement for healthcare professionals from the Stroke Council of the American Heart Association. *Stroke* 2001;32:280–99

8. Goldstein LB. Evidence-based medicine and stroke. *Neuroepidemiology* 1999;18:120–4

9. Ferguson JH. Curative and population medicine: bridging the great divide. *Neuroepidemiology* 1999;18:111–19

10. Kottke TE, Brekke ML, Solberg LI. Making time for preventive services. *Mayo Clin Proc* 1993;68:785–91

11. Kottke TE, Solberg LI, Brekke ML, *et al.* Delivery rates for preventive services in 44 Midwestern clinics. *Mayo Clin Proc* 1997;72: 515–23

12. Rose G. *The Strategy of Preventive Medicine.* Oxford: Oxford University Press, 1994 (reprinted):1–138

13. Sackett DL, Haynes RB, Tugwell P. *Clinical Epidemiology. A Basic Science for Clinical Medicine.* Boston: Little, Brown Company, 1985:139, 302–10

14. Sox H, Stern S, Owens D, Abrams HL. *Assessment of Diagnostic Technology in Health Care. Rationale, Methods, Problems and Directions.* Washington, DC: Institute of Medicine, National Academy Press, 1989:8–54

15. Silverman WA. Doing more good than harm. In Warren KS, Mosteller F, eds. *Doing More Good than Harm. The Evaluation of Health Care Interventions.* Annals of the New York Academy of Sciences, 1993, vol. 703:5–11

16. Sackett DL, Straus S. On some clinically useful measures of the accuracy of diagnostic tests. *ACP Journal Club* 1998;Sept/Oct:A17–A19

17. Ahlbom A, Norell S. *Introduction to Modern Epidemiology.* Chestnut Hills, MA: Epidemiology Resources, Inc., 1990:24–7, 57–60

18. Nuwer M. On the process for evaluating proposed new diagnostic EEG tests. *Brain Topography* 1992;4(4):243–7

19. Reducing the burden of stroke and improving the public health. In Warlow CP, Dennis MS, van Gijn J, *et al.*, eds. Oxford: Blackwell Science, 2001:762–84

20. Salonen JT. Did the North Karelia project reduce coronary mortality (letter)? *Lancet* 1987;2:269

21. Iso H, Shimamoto T, Naito Y, *et al.* Effects of a long-term hypertension control program on stroke incidence and prevalence in a rural community in Northeastern Japan. *Stroke* 1998;29:1510–18

22. Hankey GJ. Stroke. How large a public health problem, and how can the neurologist help? *Arch Neurol* 1999;56:748–54

23. Matchar DB. The value of stroke prevention and treatment. *Neurology* 1998;51(Suppl 3): S31–S35

24. Atwood K, Colditz GA, Kawachi I. From public health science to prevention policy: placing science in its social and political contexts. *Am J Pub Health* 1997;87:1603–6

25. Brownson RC, Newschaffer CJ, Ali-Abarghoui F. Policy research for disease prevention: challenges and practical recommendations. *Am J Pub Health* 1997;87:735–9

26. Richmond JB, Kotelchuck M. Co-ordinating and development of strategies and policy for public health promotion in the United States. In Holland WW, Detels L, Knox G, eds. *Oxford Textbook of Public Health.* Oxford, England: Oxford Medical Publications, 1991

27. Russell LB. The knowledge base for public health strategies (annotation). *Am J Pub Health* 1997;87:1597–8

28. Russell LB. Prevention and Medicare costs. *N Engl J Med* 1998;339:1158–60

29. Gordon RL, Gerzoff RB, Richards TB. Determinants of US local health department expenditures, 1992 through 1993. *Am J Pub Health* 1997;87:91–5

30. Daviglus ML, Greenland P, Dyer AR, *et al.* Benefit of a favorable cardiovascular risk-factor profile in middle age with respect to Medicare costs. *N Engl J Med* 1998;339: 1122–9

31. Wright JC, Weinstein MC. Gains in life expectancy from medical interventions – standardizing data on outcome. *N Engl J Med* 1998;339:380–6

32. Detsky AS, Redelmeier DA. Measuring health outcomes – putting gains into perspective. *N Engl J Med* 1998;339:402–4

33. Feinlieb M. New directions for community intervention studies (editorial). *Am J Pub Health* 1996;86:1696–8

34. Fishbein M. Great expectations, or do we ask too much from community-level interventions (editorial)? *Am J Pub Health* 1996;86:1075–6

35. Niknian M, Lefebvre C, Carleton RA. Are people more health conscious? A longitudinal study of one community. *Am J Pub Health* 1991;81:203–5

36. Iso H, Shimamoto T, Naito Y, *et al.* Effects of a long-term hypertension control program on stroke incidence and prevalence in a rural community in northeastern Japan. *Stroke* 1998;29:1510–18

37. Fang Y-H, Kronmal RA, Li S-C, *et al.* Prevention of stroke in urban China. A community-based intervention trial. *Stroke* 1999;30:495–506

38. Farquhar JW, Fortmann SP, Flora JA, *et al.* Effects of community-wide education on cardiovascular disease risk factors. The Stanford Five-City Project. *J Am Med Assoc* 1990;264:359–65

39. Frank E, Winkleby M, Fortmann SP, Farquhar JW. Cardiovascular disease risk factors: improvements in knowledge and behavior in the 1980s. *Am J Pub Health* 1993;83:590–3

40. Winkleby MA, Taylor LB, Jatulis D, Fortmann SP. The long-term effects of a cardiovascular disease prevention trial: the Stanford Five-City Project. *Am J Pub Health* 1996;86:1773–9

41. Murray DM. Design and analysis of community trials: lessons from the Minnesota Heart Health Program. *Am J Epidemiol* 1995;142:569–75

42. Luepker RV, Murray DM, Jacobs DR, *et al.* Community education for cardiovascular disease prevention: Risk factor changes in the Minnesota Heart Health Program. *Am J Pub Health* 1994;84:1383–93

43. Luepker RV, Rastam L, Hannan PJ, *et al.* Community education for cardiovascular disease prevention. Morbidity and mortality results from the Minnesota Heart Health Program. *Am J Epidemiol* 1996;144:351–62

44. Carleton RA, Lasater TM, Assaf AR, *et al.*, and the Pawtucket Heart Health Program Writing Group. The Pawtucket Heart Health Program: community changes in cardiovascular risk factors and projected disease risk. *Am J Pub Health* 1995;85:777–85

45. Salonen JT, Puska P, Mustaniemi H. Change in morbidity and mortality during comprehensive community program to control cardiovascular diseases during 1972–7 in North Karelia. *Br Med J* 1979;2:1178–83

46. Salonen JT, Puska P, Kotte TE, Tuomilheto J. Changes in smoking, serum cholesterol and blood pressure levels during a community-based cardiovascular disease prevention program: The North Karelia Project. *Am J Epidemiol* 1981;114:81–94

47. Tuomilehto J, Geboers J, Salonen JT, *et al.* Decline in cardiovascular mortality in North Karelia and other parts of Finland. *Br Med J* 1986;293:1068–71

48. Sacco RL, Wolf PA, Gorelick PB. Risk factors and their management for stroke prevention: outlook for 1999 and beyond. *Neurology* 1999;53(Suppl 4):S15–S24

49. Meyers L, Coughlin SS, Webber LS, *et al.* Prediction of adult cardiovascular multifactorial risk status from childhood risk factor levels. The Bogalusa Heart Study. *Am J Epidemiol* 1995;142:918–24

50. Twisk JWR, Kemper HCG, van Mechelen KW, Post GB. Tracking of risk factors for coronary heart disease over a 14-year period: A comparison between lifestyle and biologic risk factors with data from the Amsterdam Growth and Health Study. *Am J Epidemiol* 1997;145:888–98

51. Lewis CE, Smith DE, Wallace DD, *et al.* Seven-year trends in body weight and associations with lifestyle and behavioral characteristics in black and white young adults: the CARDIA Study. *Am J Pub Health* 1997;87:635–42

52. Tate RB, Manifreda J, Krahn AD, Cuddy TE. Tracking of blood pressure over a 40-year period in the University of Manitoba follow-up study, 1948–1988. *Am J Epidemiol* 1995;142:946–54

53. Hornberger J. A cost-benefit analysis of a cardiovascular disease prevention trial, using folate supplementation as an example. *Am J Pub Health* 1998;88:61–7

54. Reed DW, Foley DJ, White LR, *et al.* Predictors of healthy aging in men with high life expectancies. *Am J Pub Health* 1998;88:1463–8

55. Gorelick PB. Can we save the brain from the ravages of midlife cardiovascular risk factors? *Neurology* 1999;52:1114–15

Chapter 11

Stroke prevention in managed care: a five-dimensional health improvement model™

Meredith L. Tipton, PhD, MPH, and Michael Fleming, MA, MS

INTRODUCTION

Over the past decade, the managed care industry has been able to take credit for significant improvements in the rates of preventive health screenings, chronic disease management, improved clinical outcomes and more knowledgeable health care consumers. A variety of external forces and industry approaches including purchasers, National Committee for Quality Assurance (NCQA), and Health Employers' Data and Information Set® (HEDIS®), have contributed to this success. As a result of these external quality measures, health plans are required to improve members' health care when compared against a variety of standardized national HEDIS® measures, including the following that are specifically related to the prevention of stroke: beta blocker tracking following an acute myocardial infarction, cholesterol management following an acute cardiovascular event, comprehensive diabetes care, advising smokers to quit and controlling high blood pressure.

This Five-Dimensional Health Improvement Model™ was developed to secure improved health outcomes derived from public health practice that rely heavily upon population-based strategies as well as utilization of identified and effective interventions. Accomplishments from the managed care industry clearly contribute to stroke prevention at both the primary and secondary prevention levels. A health plan committed to improving the health of its membership would identify opportunities through epidemiological and demographic analysis of the membership and by comparing their results against state and national statistics. Disease categories are then ranked in a manner that reflects the burden of illness from the member's perspective. The most prevalent conditions are ranked by age and sex, and tracked utilizing the classic public health surveillance tool: disease registries. Interventions are based on the Five-Dimensional Health Improvement Model™ designed to cover the entire spectrum of illness in the affected populations, from conditions like hypertension amenable to primary prevention, to illness in the mild stage and severe illness within each disease category. Interventions designed with the overall objective of improving the health of

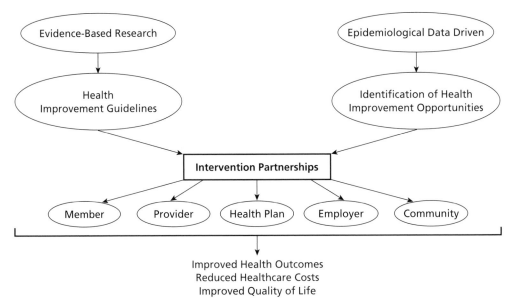

Figure 1 Five-Dimensional Health Improvement Model™

members and improving poor health outcomes call for an integrated and systematic approach for which the Five-Dimensional Health Improvement Model™ is an example. The process from identification of illness to earlier timely intervention to improve outcomes is depicted in Figure 1.

KEY SUCCESS FACTORS

Evidence-based, data driven initiatives

Nationally directed, multi-disciplinary health improvement guidelines are developed and serve as the basis of the Five-Dimensional Health Improvement Model's™ intervention strategies. Guidelines are developed to facilitate review by designated health plan quality committees that include practitioners from the health plan's health care delivery network. As new scientific evidence becomes available, quality committees evaluate the evidence against the health plan's current health improvement guidelines, assess its relevance to the target population, and make recommendations for changes

as appropriate. The guidelines also serve as the basis for all of the health plan's clinical activities including utilization management, member education, covered benefits among others delineated in the health plan's quality operating policies and procedures.

Population health principles

Health improvement initiatives utilize the framework of the Five-Dimensional Health Improvement Model™ to build upon a population-based approach to health care that involves a shift from disease-based, individual event-driven health care to a model that considers both the biological and non-biological (behavioral, socioeconomic, environmental) determinants that influence health status. Specific interventions based upon the epidemiology of the targeted population are used to effect changes in the health–illness spectrum. Population-based health improvement relies heavily on public health surveillance tools and epidemiological analysis to determine and manage the disease burden, predictors and prevalence, as well as measures of the success of interventions. Incorporated into the Five-Dimensional Health Improvement Model™ is a triage system that determines levels of intervention ranging from educational mailings for the entire affected population to case management for the more severely ill. All interventions are based on the scientific evidence supporting health improvement guidelines for primary and secondary prevention of stroke.

Multi-disciplinary

Health improvement opportunities are identified by multi-disciplinary teams that include representatives from each Five-Dimensional Health Improvement Model™.

Integration into the health care system

Workgroups, with representation from five key areas of the health plan, discuss operational changes resulting from initiatives based on the model. The guidelines significantly shape and drive the design of strategies that target specific illnesses. An example is the modification of the smoking cessation initiative that applied the recommendation from the *1996 AHCPR Smoking Cessation Guidelines*.

The Five-Dimensional Health Improvement Model™ of health care

The five dimensions of the model are:

(1) The patient; the single most important individual who influences health status is the patient who is motivated to improve his/her own state of health.

(2) The health care provider; physicians provide the medical expertise that influences individuals to change behavior in a way that is likely to improve health.

(3) The employer; because employees spend the majority of their waking hours at a worksite, employers have an opportunity to educate and influence healthy behavior in their workers.

(4) The community/environment; cultural influences affect community norms, and environmental policies that impact health status are encouraged.

(5) The health plan; the managed care organization is responsible for integrating interventions that improve the health status of individuals and populations.

Intervention options for primary and secondary stroke prevention

Within the context of the Five-Dimensional Health Improvement Model™, it is important to consider which population-based interventions are likely to be most effective in the prevention of primary and secondary stroke. There are many options for multiple stakeholder dimensions. The interventions have been categorized from the viewpoint of the health plan, which has responsibility for the health of the defined population but which does not itself provide direct health care services. Interventions are grouped according to which stakeholder group the lead agency works through to achieve the desired effects on patient care and outcomes.

Patient interventions

Patient interventions are those that the health plan can initiate by direct interaction with patient members of the target population. Such interventions can occur through mailings, telephone contacts, or various forms of electronic communication. The leading types of patient interventions include reminders, systematic personal outreach, health education materials like newsletters, and patient self-management tools. Patient reminders have generally been shown to be effective interventions. In particular, review articles have found that such reminders can be used successfully to improve rates of mammography and immunization[1,2]. Tailored letters and telephone reminders appear to be the most effective interventions[3]. However, reminders may not be an efficient use of resources for patients who have a history of consistent compliance or, conversely, a history of no compliance[4,5].

Another patient intervention is systematic personal outreach. The characteristic of this category of intervention is that trained staff educate and remind patients regarding care needs, usually through multiple personal contacts[6,7], home visits[8], and contacts at locations within the community[9]. In the managed care context systematic personal outreach has often been combined with other interventions (such as electronic monitoring and various types of health education materials) to produce wrap-around programs termed 'disease management'. Commercial vendors of such programs have reported dramatic improvements in outcomes and reductions in health-related costs[10]. The success of such programs has lead Rudd[11] to state that 'The emergence of rule-based … mediated interventions may add clinical reinforcement for improved adherence and better clinical outcomes…'. Health education materials and newsletters are among the most commonly used patient interventions. Health education materials designed for persons of low literacy (for example, special attention to written content[2], or through the use of audio-visual material[12]) are thought to have the broadest impact on patient knowledge and behavior change. Design of materials tailored to a patient's stage of change increases effectiveness[13].

Patient self-management tools are interventions that are designed to assist individuals in their own care. These tools include, but are not limited to, tracking logs (e.g. for weight loss), checklists and monitoring devices (e.g. home blood pressure cuffs), reminder calendars and compliance-enhancing medication organizers. A systematic review of studies concerning adherence to antihypertensive medication has found that electronic vial caps, calendar packaging and medication-tracking cards can have significant positive effects[14]. With more sophisticated tools, their effectiveness can be enhanced through patient education. For example, a program based on structured treatment, patient teaching and in-home self-monitoring was found to improve the quality of anticoagulation control[15].

Provider interventions

Provider interventions can be enhanced by working with physicians and health care facilities. The purpose of these interventions is to alter the behavior of providers so as to encourage practices that follow evidence-based health improvement guidelines. From the point of view of the health plan, working through providers adds the crucial element of face-to-face clinical encounters with individuals who need health services. Marlies *et al.* have categorized provider interventions into information transfer, social influence, data feedback, reminders, organizational interventions and regulatory interventions[16]. Feedback from patients to providers is also important. Information transfer covers all types of educational materials for individuals as well as groups (e.g. Continuing Medical Education). Simply distributing educational materials to providers appears not to be effective in changing patterns of practice[17–19]. Similarly, didactic group education, when tested, seems to lack effectiveness[20]. However, health educational materials, are used as part of a systematic, multifaceted approach to the education of providers[18], and can contribute to measurable improvements in health[20].

Interventions that involve learning through social influence include visits to a provider's office by trained personnel, small group meetings, activities designed to implement improved quality of care and the use of opinion leaders. Office visit training has been shown to influence practice in a number of studies[17]. The promotion of small group discussions, as part of practice improvement initiatives that address quality of care is also successful even though actual activities differ greatly from site to site[18]. The effectiveness of using opinion leaders to influence provider behavior also varies, but can have a significant impact[21]. Feedback, as a learning technique, informs providers of their performance after care has been delivered. It is important that feedback be acknowledged as valid and reliable by the providers themselves. It should be perceived as non-threatening and specific to individual practice rather than the aggregate of practices, and provided in a format that is easy to interpret[22]. Effective feedback interventions have been studied in a range of different practice environments[16]. In addition to interventions designed to improve care by professionals, feedback at the individual facility level, in particular by Medicare peer review organizations, has been shown to be effective[23].

Reminders alert providers to conduct targeted actions prior to the time those actions are expected to occur. Such reminders can be as sophisticated as a computerized decision support system or as simple as a well-designed paper form in a medical chart. Where reminders have been employed and their effects studied, they have been shown to improve practice performance[16].

Organizational interventions are those that are designed to change the organization of services, its processes, structure and/or content. These interventions often involve the day-to-day workflow and relationships among health care workers. Simple organizational interventions, for example, changing just one or two elements of practice, sometimes produces significant improvements in selected measures of care[16]. A number of studies describe instances where different categories of provider interventions have been combined effectively[16–26].

Employer interventions

Employers often have incentives to undertake health improvement intervention because it reduces health care costs, increases productivity and enhances employee morale. A health plan can influence employers to participate by communicating information concerning prospective health interventions and their potential benefits. It can provide training in healthy behavior and it can add incentives for employee participation.

Although enlisting employers to undertake health improvement interventions can raise concerns about employer/employee confidentiality, there are important advantages in this approach because employers have multiple communication channels to employees. Some are passive in that they simply provide resources to employees to promote their own health, for example fitness centers and health information resource centers. Others consist of environmental improvements at the worksite, such as reducing or eliminating smoking in the cafeteria. Interventions that have been shown to be effective are those that engage employees directly, through health education classes[25], or targeted support with groups or employees[26]. Systematic assistance in compliance with adherence to antihypertensive medication produces significant positive results[14]. Screening and referral programs and provision of on-site treatment such as immunization are also effective[28–30].

Potential incentives available to employers to promote participation in health improvement interventions include financial awards, insurance discounts, and flexible benefit credits. Some employers have structured financial disincentives for non-participants. Although offering employees reductions in insurance premiums can increase participation in programs and reduce risk factors[31], some employers consider disincentives to be nonproductive or counterproductive.

Community interventions

Community interventions are those in which the health plan works with community-based health agencies to implement health improvement agendas. Common goals and identified resources are pooled to achieve health improvement. Because many health plans do not directly provide health services, partnerships with community agencies offer opportunities to provide services to targeted groups of employees. In addition, community health agencies can provide community-wide health education activities. They can mount media campaigns and form advocacy groups to implement health policies, new regulations and laws, thereby enhancing their own health plan members' chances of acquiring better health care[32]. Community-wide health education efforts can also improve general awareness, knowledge and health behaviors in the general public as well as in the members of the health plan. These interventions have demonstrated their effectiveness in changing the community culture and environment, thereby complementing interventions targeted to specific groups of concern to the health plan. Intensive community health education efforts over a long period of time can reduce cardiovascular risks[33], and decrease smoking rates which increases health[34–35]. Health-related laws and regulations are another way in which environmental changes can improve health behaviors. Examples are the seat belt laws reducing mortality from motor vehicle accidents and reduction in smoking rates by increasing cigarette taxes.

Plan interventions

The health plans, through their management of health benefits and reimbursement and their access to relevant databases, allow the design and implementation of effective interventions but there must be an explicit commitment to improving the health of the plan's members. The plan can provide educational classes or pay for certain pharmaceuticals, make health professionals available who can provide specialized care, or it can provide higher levels of reimbursement for specific services. The health plan can discuss benefits and reimbursement with employees and help market benefits in the standard benefit schedule and/or add supplemental benefit riders. Health plans typically have access to a wide range of health-related data, for example information on the utilization of health care and pharmaceutical services, demographic characteristics based on the enrollment information, provider data that describes the utilization of professional services and facilities and employer data identifying organizations that help finance patient health insurance.

CONCLUSIONS

Health plans have a significant capacity to implement interventions that will improve the health of their members. Patients, providers, employers and community agencies all have relationships with health plans that further the mutual goal of improving health. The Five-Dimensional Health Improvement Model™ has been developed using the systems theory, medical research and insights from social and behavioral science. Health plans have applied this model to secure significant improvements in health outcomes that can be related to the primary and secondary prevention of stroke in targeted populations.

References

1. Wagner TH. The effectiveness of mailed reminders on mammography screening: a meta-analysis. *Am J Prev Med* 1998;14:64–70

2. Szilagy PG, Bordley C, Vann JC, *et al*. Effect of patient/recall interventions on immunization rates: a review. *J Am Med Assoc* 2000;284:1820–7

3. Lipkins IM, Rimer BK, Halabi S, *et al*. Can tailored interventions increase mammography use among HMO women? *Am J Prev Med* 2000;18:1–10

4. Clayton AE, McNutt L-A, Homestead HL, *et al*. Public health in managed care: a randomized controlled trial of the effectiveness of postcard reminders. *Am J Publ Health* 1999;89:1235–7

5. Costanze ME, Stoddard AM, Luckman R, *et al*. Promoting mammography: result of a randomized trial of tele-counseling and a medical practice intervention. *Am J Prev Med* 2000;19:39–46

6. DeBusk, Miller NH, Superko HR, *et al*. A case management system for coronary risk factor modification after acute myocardial infarction. *Ann Int Med* 1994;120:721–9

7. Lang M, Ed. Process improvement: built an effective patient education program. *Cardiovasc Dis Manage* 1998;4:7–9

8. Levine DM, Green LW, Deeds SG, *et al*. Health education for hypertensive patients. *J Am Med Assoc* 1979;241:170–3

9. Krieger J, Collier C, Long L, *et al*. *Improving Hypertension Control: A Patient Care Coordination Approach*. State Hypertension Intervention Project: The Seattle-King County Dept. of Public Health, WA, USA, in collaboration with the Center for Multicultural Health, Country Doctor/Carolyn Downs Community Clinics, Medalia Health Care, Group Health Cooperative and Pacific Medical Center. Primary funding NHLBI. Undated slide presentation.

10. PR Newswire via News Edge Corporation. *United Health Care Launches First Nationwide Cardiovascular Risk Reduction Program to Fight Heart Disease*. Sept 30, 1998. First! e-mail current intelligence service, INDIVIDUAL, Inc.

11. Rudd, P. Compliance with hypertensive therapy: raising the bar of expectations. *Am J Mgd Care* 1998;4:957–66

12. Man-Sun-Hing M, Laupacis A, O'Connor AM, *et al*. A patient decision aid regarding antithrombotic therapy for stroke prevention in atrial fibrillation: A randomized control trial. *J Am Med Assoc* 1999;292:737–43

13. Proschaska JO, DiClemente CC, Velicer WF, *et al*. Standardized, individual, interactive, and personalized self-help programs for smoking cessation. *Health Psychol* 1993;12:399–405

14. Morrison A, Wertheimer A, Berger M. Interventions to improve antihypertensive drug adherence: a quantitative review of trials. *Formulary* 2000;35:234–49

15. Sawicki PT, Working Group for the Study of Patient Self Management of Oral Anticoagulation. A structured teaching and self-management program for patients receiving oral anticoagulation: a randomized controlled trial. *J Am Med Assoc* 1999;28:145–50

16. Marlies EJL, Hulscher L, Wensing M, *et al*. Interventions to improve delivery of preventive services in primary care. *Am J Pub Health* 1999;89:737–46

17. Epps RP, Manley MW, Husten CG, *et al*. Transfer of preventive health program to physicians' practices through medical organizations. *Am J Prev Med* 1999;14:25–30

18. Well KB, Sherbourne C, Schoenbaum M, *et al*. Impact of disseminating quality improvement programs for depression in managed primary care: a randomized control trial. *J Am Med Assoc* 2000;283:212–20

19. Leviton LC, Goldenberg RL, Baker CS, *et al*. Methods to encourage the use of antenatal corticosteriod therapy for fetal maturation: a randomized controlled trial. *J Am Med Assoc* 1999;281:46–52

20. Davis D, O'Brien MA, Freemantle N, *et al*. Impact of formal continuing medical education: do conferences, workshops, rounds, and other traditional continuing education activities change physician behaviors or health care outcomes? *J Am Med Assoc* 1999;282:867–74

21. Heming JM. The role of clinical practice guidelines in disease management. *Am J Managed Care* 1998;4:1715–21

22. Sennet C. Implementing the new HEDIS hyperetension performance measure. *Managed Care* 2000;9:1–17

23. Marciniak TA, Ellerbeck EF, Radford MJ, *et al.* Improving the quality of care for Medicare patients with acute myocardial infarction results from the Cooperative Cardiovascular Project. *J Am Med Assoc* 1998;279:1351–7

24. Dickey LI, Gemson DH, Carney P, *et al.* Office systems interventions supporting primary care-based health behavior change counseling. *Am J Prev Med* 1999;17:299–308

25. Shi L. A cost-benefit analysis of a California county's back injury prevention program. *Public Health Reports* 1993;108:204–11

26. Burton WN, Connerty CM. Evaluation of a worksite-based patient education intervention targeted at employees with diabetes mellitus. *J Occupat Environ Med* 1996;4:702–6

27. Hartnett T, ed. Employers, health plans, docs join fight against HBP. *Healthcare Demand Dis Management* 1999;5:17–22

28. Nichol KL, Lind A, Margolis K, *et al.* The effectiveness of vaccination against influenza in healthy working adults. *New Engl J Med* 1995;333:889–93

29. Dille JH. A worksite influenza immunization program. *Am Assoc Occ Health Nurs* 1999:47:301–9

30. Bridges CB, Thompson WW, Meltzer MI, *et al.* Effectiveness and cost-benefit of influenza vaccination of healthy working adults: a randomized controlled study. *J Am Med Assoc* 2000;284:1655–62

31. Stein AD, Shakour SK, Zuidema RA. Financial incentives, participation in employer-sponsored health promotion, and changes in employees health and productivity: Healthplus Health Quotient program. *J Occupat Environ Med* 2000;42:1148–55

32. Krieger J, Collier C, Song L, *et al.* Linking community-based blood pressure measurement to clinical care: a randomized controlled trial of outreach and tracking by community health workers. *Am J Publ Health* 1999;89:856–61

33. Farquar JW, Fortmann SP, Flora JA, *et al.* Effects of community wide education cardiovascular risk factors: The Stanford Five-City Project. *J Am Med Assoc* 1990;264:359–65

34. Fitchberg CM, Glantz SA. Association of the California Tobacco Control Program with declines in cigarette consumption and mortality from heart disease. *New Engl J Med* 2000;343:1772–7

35. Pierce JPO, Gilpin EA, Emery SL, *et al.* Has the California tobacco control program reduced smoking? *J Am Med Assoc* 1998;280:893–9

Chapter 12

National, state and local opportunities for stroke prevention

Darwin R. Labarthe, MD, MPH, PhD, and Miriam M. Fay, MPH

THE PUBLIC HEALTH PERSPECTIVE

Because the purpose of this chapter is to address opportunities for stroke prevention at the national, state and local levels, a public health perspective will be taken. Illustrative examples will be drawn from the United States alone, although the importance of global efforts is also recognized.

What does the public health perspective mean? It refers primarily to the activities of official health agencies, whose three core functions, as articulated in the 1988 report from the Institute of Medicine, *The Future of Public Health*, are assessment, policy development and assurance[1]. Fulfillment of these core functions is expected to promote and protect the health of communities and populations through (1) collection, analysis and reporting of health-related data, (2) formulation and implementation of programs and policies designed on the basis of these data to protect and improve health, and (3) monitoring of activities and outcomes to verify, in turn, that these policies and programs are implemented with the intended effects.

The implications of these public health functions for stroke prevention, both in principle and in practice, are the central topic of this chapter. While societal responsibility for these functions resides formally in the official health agencies at national, state and local levels, there is much opportunity for contributions to these functions to be made by voluntary health organizations and others. Thus, examples from both official and voluntary health agencies and organizations will illustrate the range of current public health activities in stroke prevention. Also, prospects for future public health efforts will be considered.

GOALS AND OBJECTIVES

In the United States, current national public health goals and objectives for stroke prevention are presented in *Healthy People 2010*, Chapter 12: Heart Disease and Stroke[2]. The overall health goals to be achieved by 2010 are (1) to increase quality and years of healthy life, and (2) to eliminate health disparities that occur by gender, race or ethnicity, education or income, disability, residence (urban, suburban or rural), or sexual orientation. Stroke is an important contributor to the reduced life expectancy among blacks relative to that of whites in the United States, and death rates from stroke are substantially higher for blacks than are those reported for other racial or ethnic groups[3,4]. Thus, stroke prevention is directly relevant to each of these overall health goals for the nation.

Chapter 12 of *Healthy People 2010* presents four additional goals, each of which applies to both heart disease and stroke: prevention of risk factors, detection and treatment of risk factors, early identification and treatment of heart attacks and strokes and prevention of recurrent cardiovascular events. The chapter also includes 16 specific objectives, each potentially measurable through nationally collected data, of which two relate directly to stroke. The first of these two objectives is to reduce deaths from stroke (section 12.7). The target is 48 deaths per 100 000 population, a 20% improvement over the 60 deaths from stroke per 100 000 population recorded in 1998 (preliminary data, age-adjusted to the year 2000 standard population; source, National Vital Statistics System (NVSS), Centers for Disease Control and Prevention (CDC), National Center for Health Statistics (NCHS)). The second objective is to increase the proportion of adults who are aware of the early warning symptoms and signs of a stroke (section 12.8; developmental; potential data source, National Health Interview Survey (NHIS), CDC, NCHS)[2]. Numerous additional objectives are presented through which to reduce the national burden of coronary heart disease, congestive heart failure, high blood pressure and other risk factors for heart disease and stroke. To the extent that these national goals and objectives shape the priorities of national, state and local health agencies and organizations concerned with stroke prevention, they suggest something of the profile of activities one would expect to identify in reviewing current practices.

PRINCIPLES

Still broader principles applicable to stroke prevention suggest the potential for additional relevant public health activities in this area. It is useful to consider first the progressive development of stroke and other cardiovascular diseases (CVD), because this process itself suggests multiple potential points of intervention. The deepest roots of epidemic cardiovascular diseases are found in unfavorable social and environmental conditions. These conditions are unfavorable insofar as they foster adverse behavioral patterns, such as dietary imbalance, physical inactivity and widespread use of commercial tobacco products. Largely through the resulting major established risk factors such as high blood pressure, dyslipidemia and smoking, the progression of cardiovascular disease (CVD) continues through preclinical or subclinical phases to the appearance of the first clinical event, such as an acute stroke. This first clinical event may or may not have a rapid fatal outcome. Survival from the first event is commonly associated with significant disability and a greatly increased risk of a recurrent event. Late death – not necessarily in terms of life expectancy, but in relation to the long progression of underlying disease – is often due to one or another form of cardiovascular disease more or less directly related to the prior stroke.

The corresponding opportunities for cardiovascular health (CVH) promotion and CVD prevention are directly related to the foregoing progression. Policy and environmental change, at its most fundamental level of application, bears on social and environmental factors that support favorable conditions or fostering changes in unfavorable ones. (This approach may also apply in later phases of disease, as in settings for patient care, through policy changes affecting utilization of care, implementation of treatment guidelines, and in other ways.) Behavior change, similarly, supports patterns of behavior favorable to health or seeks to improve adverse ones. Risk factor detection and control, mainstays of CVD prevention in recent decades, are intended to reduce or eliminate the increased risk of stroke and other CVD through identification and treatment of affected individuals. Emergency care and acute case management apply once the first event has occurred, unless death comes too soon for any intervention. Rehabilitation and long-term care for survivors of the first event and end-of-life care for those with progressive disability and death from CVD complete the array of phases of intervention.

In principle, therefore, there are multiple opportunities for stroke prevention, and connections with the *Healthy People 2010* goals and objectives can readily be seen. Goal 1 in Chapter 12, to prevent risk factors, can be approached by promoting cardiovascular health – that is, by policy and environmental change and behavior change at the population level; goal 2, detection and treatment of risk factors, by risk factor detection and control; goal 3, early identification and treatment of heart attacks and strokes, by emergency care and acute case management; and goal 4, prevention of recurrent cardiovascular events, though long-term care and rehabilitation.

Given this comprehensive array of opportunities for stroke prevention that exist, in principle, examples of current practice at the national, state, and local levels can be considered.

PRACTICE

National level

In an important sense, all health – like all politics – is local, in that the health of any population reflects the health of its individual members. Correspondingly, activities at the national (or state) level are ultimately effective in promoting health and preventing disease only insofar as the possibility of good health is advanced for individuals. At the same time national agencies and organizations, official and voluntary, can have considerable influence over local determinants of health.

Leaders in stroke prevention at the national level include the National Center for Chronic Disease Prevention and Health Promotion (NCCDPHP) of the Centers for Disease Control and Prevention (CDC); the National Institute of Neurological Disorders and Stroke (NINDS), of the National Institutes of Health; the American Stroke Association (ASA), a Division of the American Heart Association (AHA); the National Stroke Association (NSA). Formal strategic partnerships, such as the *Healthy People 2010* Strategic Partnership, the Brain Attack Coalition (BAC) and others, that include these and other national organizations. No exhaustive inventory of these activities in stroke prevention exists. Compilation even within particular programs is made difficult by the very wide array of opportunities for prevention that might be pursued. Even though every program that focuses on high blood pressure, for example – whether on its prevention or its detection and treatment, and whether in primary or secondary prevention – contributes potentially to stroke prevention, many such programs are not explicitly identified in this way. Thus, current activity in stroke prevention can best be illustrated, then, by selected examples that should not necessarily be taken as representing the entire field.

One of the largest targeted federal programs in stroke prevention in the USA is the Cardiovascular Health State Program, conducted under the aegis of the Cardiovascular Health Branch, Division of Adult and Community Health (NCCDPHP). Initiated in fiscal year (FY) 1998, this program addresses the *Healthy People 2010* focus area of heart disease and stroke, reviewed above. It now supports 28 states with limited funding to develop core capacities (the 'Core Capacity Program' states) or to implement prevention programs (the 'Comprehensive Program' states). The federal role in this instance is to define eligibility requirements for the states that may apply, specify the program requirements, conduct peer review of proposals, and provide technical assistance, training and collaboration to the participating states.

Through this program, the Core Program states are directed to pursue the following activities: (1) develop and co-ordinate partnerships, (2) develop scientific capacity to define the cardiovascular disease problem, (3) develop an inventory of policy and environmental strategies, (4) develop or update a state plan, (5) provide training and technical assistance, (6) develop population-based strategies, and (7) develop culturally-competent strategies for priority populations.

The Comprehensive Program states are directed, in addition, to (1) implement population-based intervention strategies consistent with the state plan, (2) implement strategies addressing priority populations, (3) specify and evaluate intervention components, (4) implement professional education activities, and (5) monitor secondary prevention strategies. The states determine how to carry out the interventions with considerable flexibility and creativity. Still this is a national program, one that includes extensive communication among participating states.

Another targeted stroke program of the Cardiovascular Health Branch is the Paul Coverdell National Acute Stroke Registry. This is a newly established effort, in the name of the US senator from Georgia who suffered a fatal stroke in the year 2000, to develop and evaluate prototypes for registry of acute stroke cases. The ultimate objective is to establish a national registry to track and improve the delivery of care to patients with acute stroke. The study is being conducted in four sites and will be evaluated by a separate collaborating organization. It is hoped that this program will be a stimulus for still broader stroke prevention activities in all states.

The mission of NINDS is to reduce the burden of neurological disease, principally through conducting and supporting research. In keeping with this mission, one of the agency's nine overall goals is to 'enhance our program in clinical research and epidemiology to develop more effective therapies and prevention strategies'[5]. Perhaps the most important interface of NINDS with the practice of stroke prevention lies in its strategic initiatives to reduce health disparities in the burden of stroke and to promote early stroke treatment[6]. These initiatives are clearly concordant with the *Healthy People 2010* goals as indicated above. Other federal programs supporting public health efforts in stroke prevention operate primarily at the state and local level and are described below.

CDC and NINDS interact closely with national partners in stroke prevention, principally the ASA and the NSA, both voluntary associations. The ASA 'exists to reduce disability and death from stroke through research, education, fund raising and advocacy'[7]. One example of the many programs of the ASA is Operation Stroke, 'a community-based program to raise awareness of the stroke warning signs and the critical need to react quickly and get immediate emergency treatment'[7]. Scheduled to be active in 125 cities by 2003, the program is operated by coalitions of health care professionals and civic leaders. Extensive public and professional education activities are also undertaken by the ASA to address primary prevention, acute case management and secondary prevention of stroke.

The mission of the NSA is 'to reduce the incidence and impact of stroke'[8]. Programs in prevention, acute treatment and rehabilitation/recovery are offered and indicate a wide range of intervention activity. The NSA has announced the National Public Health Stroke Prevention Initiative, seeking to achieve the following goals: to develop a national public health program plan for the primary prevention of stroke; to implement the plan in each state and territory; and to develop specific reporting mechanisms for stroke[9]. The NSA has also established the Stroke Center Network, to foster implementation of the concept of acute stroke treatment centers to improve the acute care of stroke patients[10].

The CDC, through its Healthy People 2010 Strategic Partnership, is party to a memorandum of understanding with the AHA/ASA, the Center for Medicare & Medicaid Services (CMS), NHLBI, NINDS, and the Office of Disease Prevention and Health Promotion (ODPHP) of the Department of Health and Human Services. The purpose of this partnership is 'to catalyze progress toward the goals and targets set forth in the *Healthy People 2010* heart disease and stroke focus area'[11]. The partnership meets quarterly, with interim work carried out by three teams, of which two are charged to address the four prevention goals and one is responsible for overall co-ordination. The partnership seeks to accomplish these goals through six kinds of activities:

(1) population- and community-based health education and health promotion activities;

(2) co-ordination of a public awareness campaign and media activities, including signs and symptoms of heart attack and stroke, leading health indicators that address the reduction and elimination of risk factors and the promotion of healthy behaviors to reduce CVD and stroke;

(3) activities to effect environmental and policy and system changes;

(4) joint efforts to promote professional education and training, including joint presentations, co-hosting of national conferences, dissemination of best practices and joint efforts to provide consultation on cardiovascular issues for conferences and workshops;

(5) facilitation of relationship development, support, data collection, and resource sharing; and

(6) sharing among organizations of scientific and information resources[11].

The NSA is similarly engaged with the CDC in a partnership to achieve the *Healthy People 2010* goals, with two important additional areas of activity: collaboration on national and state public health stroke activities, including those related to addressing gender, geographic, and racial/ethnic disparities, and collaboration on developing a national public health stroke prevention plan[12].

Another example of collaboration among agencies and organizations at the national level is the BAC, a group representing multiple disciplines involved especially in the care of acute stroke patients. Members include the American Academy of Neurology, American Association of Neurological Surgeons, American Association of Neuroscience Nurses, American College of Emergency Physicians, American Society of Neurology, ASA, CDC, NINDS, NSA, and the Stroke Belt Consortium[13]. One product of this partnership is the development of recommendations for the establishment of primary stroke centers, to improve the medical care of patients with stroke[14]. This is the same program being fostered by the NSA that was mentioned earlier in this section.

State level

State-level activities, like national ones, have their ultimate impact locally. But this impact is achieved through the adoption of policies and implementation of programs at the state level. Both multi-state and single-state stroke prevention activities will illustrate this point.

Regional organizations

Two regional, multi-state collaborations illustrate the potential for sharing of expertise and resources in stroke prevention at the state level. One is the Stroke Belt Consortium (SBC), formed in 1994, encompassing the eight states in the Southeastern US with the highest stroke incidence and mortality[15]. The objectives of the SBC are to improve public and professional education about stroke, to promote improvements in stroke prevention, diagnosis and treatment, to provide pilot grants, and to support its member groups. Within the SBC states (Alabama, Arkansas, Georgia, Louisiana, Mississippi, North Carolina, South Carolina and Tennessee), three states with the highest stroke mortality are considered to be the 'stroke buckle' – Georgia, North Carolina and South Carolina. These three states have formed the Tri-state Stroke Network, under whose auspices the Tri-state Stroke Summit was convened in September, 1999. The document emerging from this conference is a valuable resource for information on state and local stroke prevention activities in this region[16].

Single-state Organizations

The Cardiovascular Health State Program of the CDC, described above, at present comprises 28 states, of which 22 have core capacity programs and 6 have comprehensive programs. Their activities represent a wide range of state and local efforts to plan and implement stroke prevention programs. Numerous additional state-level programs supported by the CDC address high blood pressure, nutrition and physical activity, smoking and other areas that contribute to stroke prevention. One other state-level program administered by the CDC, the Preventive Health and Health Services Block Grant, deserves special emphasis, as it reaches all states and gives wide discre-tion as to the program emphasis adopted by each one.

Preventive Health and Health Services Block Grant

The Preventive Health and Health Services (PHHS) Block Grant is an annual grant awarded to all states and territories by Congress. Each grantee identifies the health status objectives (HSOs) they will address with their funds; the HSOs correspond to *Healthy People 2000* objectives[17]. Additionally, the states outline a description of their health problems as identified by the HSOs and propose a budget for each HSO. The states outline their health status outcome objectives, risk reduction objectives and annual objectives and activities in their application for funds. At the end of each fiscal year, the states submit an annual report derived from the HSOs submitted in the prior fiscal year application. Each HSO includes a section for progress on activities. These data sources are very likely to underestimate the amount of stroke-related activities being conducted at the state level through the block grant.

The HSOs that most directly relate to CVD and stroke are 15.1 – reduce coronary heart disease deaths – and 15.2 – reduce stroke deaths. In fiscal year (FY) 2000, 29 states and territories addressed HSO 15.1 and three addressed HSO 15.2. Eight additional states and territories addressed both HSOs. Of these, a total of 28 states and territories mentioned in their FY 2000 annual report that they are addressing stroke. Many of the states conducted blood pressure screening, while others built capacity and formed key partnerships with groups such as the state stroke associations. While it is not possible to determine the specific amount of block grant funds dedicated to stroke-related activities, the amount these 28 states and territories were awarded to address HSOs 15.1 and 15.2 for FY 2000 was $19 011 803. There are very likely to be additional states that are addressing stroke with their block grant – some may be addressing stroke that did not say so in their progress report, and others may be addressing it indirectly through other HSOs. Two examples of the types of programs that addressed stroke in FY 2000 include Puerto Rico's hypertension program and Georgia's stroke and heart attack prevention program.

Puerto Rico, like many other states and territories, has prepared and displayed announcements and educational materials on hypertension, nutrition and early warning signs of heart attack and stroke in the offices of many primary care providers. General education programs about CVD and stroke are offered at shopping centers, churches, schools and other public and private agencies. Puerto Rico is also hoping to affect existing policies regarding patient evaluation in at least three important ways. First, those involved with the hypertension program are working to require that mandatory blood pressure readings be included in the norms and procedures for general patient evaluation. Second, advocates for policy change are working with primary health care providers to ask all patients over age 40 about their family history of hypertension. Third, the hypertension program is working with an organization called Health Companies under Health Reform to urge screening of all adults aged 40–60 for hypertension.

Georgia's stroke and heart attack prevention program (SHAPP) undertook efforts to identify the appropriate populations for programmatic intervention and to incorporate program evaluation into service delivery to measure the effectiveness of its activities. As a result, the Community Cardiovascular Council in the city of Savannah developed an outreach initiative through local fire departments, barbershops and hair salons to address the needs of people with hypertension. In addition, SHAPP formed partnerships with the Georgia chapter of the ASA and with Operation Stroke in Atlanta. SHAPP staff conducted clinic quality assessment activities in all health districts, during which clinicians were observed and medical records reviewed to determine adherence to protocols. Education and training in major CVD and stroke topics were provided to all SHAPP staff; training was also

conducted for nurses who were members of the nurses' guilds in 32 African-American churches. These nurses assisted blood pressure monitoring and medication assessment. SHAPP programs provided case management services and the promotion of risk reduction through lifestyle changes to 15 041 diagnosed hypertensives. For those unable to afford medicines and compliance with drug regimens, SHAPP ensured access to blood pressure-reducing drugs purchased with state funds. The SHAPP program in Georgia, then, addressed stroke in a number of ways – through community involvement, through the formation of key partnerships and through the education of healthcare professionals and the general community.

Local level

The plethora of local activities in stroke prevention, many of which are conducted under the national and state programs discussed above, can be illustrated by only a few examples. Several such projects are related to the REACH 2010 demonstration program or to the Prevention Research Centers Program.

REACH 2010 demonstration program

Racial and Ethnic Approaches to Community Health (REACH 2010) is a demonstration project aimed at eliminating disparities in health status experienced by ethnic minority populations. This initiative – which began in 1999 – addresses racial and ethnic disparities by developing culturally appropriate, community-based programs that focus on six priority health areas: CVD, immunizations, breast and cervical cancer screening and management, diabetes, HIV infections/AIDS, and infant mortality. The racial and ethnic groups targeted by REACH 2010 are African-Americans, Alaska natives, American Indians, Asian-Americans, Hispanic Americans, and Pacific islanders.

REACH 2010 is a two-phase, five-year project that supports community coalitions in designing, implementing and evaluating community-driven strategies to eliminate health disparities. Each coalition comprises a community-based organization and three other organizations, of which at least one is either a local or state health department or a university or research organization. During a 12-month planning phase, REACH 2010 grantees use local data to develop a community action plan that addresses one or more of the six priority areas and targets one or more of the racial and ethnic minority groups. During the four-year implementation phase, community coalitions carry out activities outlined in their community action plans and evaluate program activities.

In FY 2000, Congress appropriated $30 million to support REACH 2010. With this funding, CDC supported 14 new planning-phase projects and 24 projects in the implementation and evaluation phase. In FY 2001, Congress appropriated $35 million to continue REACH 2010 projects and to add a new emphasis on projects in American Indian and Alaska native communities. There are 39 projects to be supported during FY 2002. Of these, five address the American Indian and Alaska native communities in a core capacity building program. Two of these projects address CVD – the Chugachmiut of southeast Alaska and the Choctaw Nation of Oklahoma. The remaining 34 projects are all in the implementation and evaluation phase. Five of these programs address CVD as the only health priority area; another three projects address CVD as the primary priority area, with diabetes as the secondary focus.

Of the ten programs that have identified CVD as a health priority area, at least eight are also addressing stroke. The projects are accomplishing this in several ways. Several programs are designed to educate the community about CVD and stroke risk factors. The Chugachmiut will develop a state-wide registry of heart disease

and stroke among Alaska natives. Three programs will address stroke by providing screening for hypertension. Other programs are intended to improve access by their target population to clinical preventive services. One program is addressing stroke through a policy intervention designed to advocate improved quality and availability of healthy food in local restaurants, markets and schools.

The African-American Health Coalition, based in Portland, Oregon, will begin the implementation and evaluation phase of their project in FY 2002. Having addressed the greater rates of CVD and stroke among the African-American population, they propose to provide health education, strengthen social support networks and advocacy skills to combat racism, and to support changes to create a healthy environment. Their plan also aims to build capacity by training local community health workers to sustain improved health behavior. Of the five interventions the coalition has proposed, two appear to address stroke: 'steps to soulful living', which will promote increased access to clinical preventive services, including screenings, and 'reach community education', which is designed to provide information about CVD risk factors and health screenings available to African-Americans in the Portland metropolitan area.

Another example of how REACH 2010 projects are addressing stroke is represented by the Community Health Councils of Los Angeles. The focus of this project is to address the behavioral and systemic factors that contribute to the disparities in cardiovascular health. The primary risk factors addressed by the councils community action plan are physical inactivity and poor nutrition. The strategy they use to address the risk factors is a combination of community education, empowerment and economic development. Several interventions among African-Americans aged 21–65 living in south central Los Angeles, North Long Beach and Inglewood are potentially addressing stroke. The councils conducting information sessions regarding CVD, sponsor wellness/healthy living workshops to discuss prevention, treatment and disease management, and are advocating improved quality and availability of healthy food in local restaurants, markets and schools.

Health Promotion Disease Prevention Research Centers Program

The Health Promotion Disease Prevention Research Centers Program has been administered by the CDC since 1984. There are twenty-six prevention research centers (PRCs) that work with communities to reduce priority health risks and to promote healthy behavior. The centers are concerned with improving the quality of life of special populations, including persons who are elderly or under-served, and curbing the illness and premature death that drive the nation's health care costs. The funding for FY 2001 was approximately $23 million.

Of the 69 projects that identified CVD as a keyword, three could be readily identified as addressing stroke from brief descriptions of the projects' focus and aims. This is not to say that these are the only programs addressing CVD or stroke. For example, additional (but not readily identifiable) stroke prevention projects may address physical activity, nutrition, diabetes and smoking.

The theme of the PRC at the University of Alabama at Birmingham is 'Bridging the gap between public health science and practice in risk reduction across the lifespan among African-Americans and other underserved communities'. The primary focus is not on any particular disease but, rather, on risk reduction. The specific risk factors they address are tobacco use, dietary intake and physical activity. The primary objective is to develop methods to promote community capacity to adopt and sustain broad, multiple-component risk reduction programs and to evaluate the long-term benefit of these programs in terms of community capacity-building, risk factor changes, disease outcome changes and changes in quality of life indices. Support and Training for African-American Women in Networking and Disease Prevention (STAND) addresses CVD and cancer risk factors. In addition to forming key partnerships, this project aims to build a longitudinal database to examine long-term changes in county-wide risk factors, disease outcomes and quality of life. Rather than implementing and evaluating this project throughout the state, STAND is implemented only in Wilcox County, Alabama. In this way, the nature and extent of the behavior changes that are realized may be evaluated more fully and over a more extended period than with other designs.

In Atlanta, Georgia, the project 'Impact of race-related stress and coping on CVD', at Morehouse School of Medicine, was designed to better understand the role of life constraints and potential mediation efforts in the prevention and control of essential hypertension among adult African-Americans. The investigators hope to address whether the disparity of hypertension and CVD among African-American men and women when compared with their white counterparts may be due to consequential interaction of effects between life-constraining psychosocial stressors and adverse coping behaviors.

PROSPECTS

National, state and local opportunities for stroke prevention are widespread and can potentially have favorable impacts on stroke incidence and mortality as well as on a broader range of cardiovascular disease outcomes. Taken together, the activities at all three levels that are identifiable with stroke prevention appear to address the full range of opportunities and illustrate approaches to the three core functions of public health. Yet investment in these programs remains far below that required to realize their full potential.

The national and regional partnerships organized in support of the *Healthy People 2010* goals for heart disease and stroke, or for stroke prevention more specifically, may have a growing impact. The efforts of the NSA and CDC to develop long-range public health strategic plans for stroke prevention, with the mutual aim of reaching every state and territory of the US, provide an impetus for expanded public health intervention to prevent stroke. Increased investment in support and evaluation of programs currently planned or in progress, and in research to continue advancing policy and program development, would be expected to multiply the opportunities further.

References

1. Committee for the study of the future of public health, division of health care services, Institute of Medicine. *The Future of Public Health.* Washington, DC: National Academy Press, 1988
2. U.S. Department of Health and Human Services. *Healthy People 2010* (Conference edition, in two volumes). Washington, DC, January 2000
3. Influence of homicide on racial disparity in life expectancy – United States, 1998. *Morbid Mortal Weekly Rep* 2001;36:780–3
4. American Heart Association. *2001 Heart and Stroke Statistical Update.* Dallas: American Heart Association, 2000
5. National Institute of Neurological Disorders and Stroke. *Neuroscience at the New Millennium.* Bethesda: National Institute of Neurological Disorders and Stroke, National Institutes of Health, NIH Publication No. 99-4566, August 1999
6. National Institute of Neurological Disorders and Stroke. *Neuroscience at the New Millennium.* Implementation Update May 2000. (unpublished document)
7. American Stroke Association webpage. http:/www.StrokeAssociation.org
8. National Stroke Association webpage. http:/www.stroke.org
9. National Stroke Association. The national public health stroke prevention initiative of the National Stroke Association (unpublished document)
10. National Stroke Association. The stroke center network (unpublished document)
11. *Healthy People 2010* strategic partnership. Memorandum of understanding (unpublished document)
12. Stroke prevention partnership. Memorandum of understanding (unpublished document)
13. The brain attack coalition website. http://www. stroke-site.org
14. Alberts MJ, Hademenos G, Latchaw RE, *et al.* Recommendations for the establishment of primary stroke centers. *J Am Med Assoc* 2000; 283:3102–9
15. The stroke belt consortium webpage. http:// www.neurology.mc.duke.edu/mainsbc.html
16. Huston SL, Lengerich EJ, Pratap S, Puckett E, eds. *Unexplained Stroke Disparity: Report and Recommendations from Three Southeastern States.* Full report, division of public health, North Carolina department of health and human services. For The North Carolina heart disease and stroke prevention task force and the state health officers of Georgia, North Carolina, and South Carolina. Raleigh, North Carolina, 2000
17. US Dept of Health and Human Services. *Healthy People 2000*: national health promotion and disease prevention objectives: full report with commentary. Washington, DC: Public Health Service, US Dept of Health and Human Services, 1991. DHHS publication (PHS) 91-50212

Chapter 13

Quality improvement in stroke prevention

Robert G. Holloway, MD, MPH, and Steven R. Rush, MA

INTRODUCTION

The evidence base for stroke prevention is clear, unambiguous and large. Pharmacological, behavioral and surgical interventions are available that can substantially reduce one's risk of future stroke. Despite these clear indications of best practices, many of which have been codified into guidelines, they are often not being implemented[1].

UNDERUSE, OVERUSE AND MISUSE OF STROKE PREVENTION SERVICES

Reasons for not achieving optimal quality stroke prevention care include underuse, overuse, or misuse of interventions or services (Table 1)[2]. Underuse is the failure to provide a stroke-prevention service when it would have produced a favorable health outcome. Overuse

Table 1 Potential quality of care problems in treating patients at risk for stroke

Service Area	Underuse	Overuse	Misuse
Outpatient	Hypertension management Lipid management Tobacco product management Screen and manage atrial fibrillation Screen and manage diabetes Antithrombotic management Screen for carotid stenosis Diet and exercise recommendations Adequate physician-to-physician communication	Carotid Doppler studies (?) Imaging studies (head, neck, cardiac) (?)	Anticoagulation management
Inpatient	Screen for carotid stenosis Measurement of lipids Screen for diabetes Diet and exercise recommendations Screen and manage ischemic heart disease Adequate physician-to-physician communication	Carotid Doppler studies (?) Imaging studies (head, neck, cardiac) (?) Carotid endarterectomy	Anticoagulation management Inadequate technical skills in performing carotid endarterectomy

occurs when a service is provided in which the potential harm exceeds the benefits. Misuse occurs when an appropriate service has been selected but a preventable complication occurs and the patient does not receive the full benefit of the therapy.

The most common cause for stroke-prevention practices often falling short of the ideal is underuse[3]. There are many reasons for the underuse of stroke prevention services. Patients may lack knowledge regarding stroke risk factors or may not be compliant with care. Physicians also may lack up-to-date knowledge, or they may not consider prevention services part of their responsibility. Lack of training in performance improvement methods and increasing demands on provider time without adequate reimbursement also contribute.

Overuse and misuse of services can also occur. An overuse problem would occur if, for example the risk of angiography and carotid endarterectomy exceeded the benefits to be gained[4]. A misuse problem would occur if warfarin was properly selected for an individual, but improper dosing and follow-up management resulted in an anticoagulation-related hemorrhage[5]. Misuse problems stem mainly from medical error and unsafe practice conditions. Overuse of stroke prevention services, and overuse of medical technologies in general, often occur in situations where uncertainty exists regarding the proper role of the service coupled with an incentive to perform the service (e.g., financial gain, fear of litigation, high patient demand).

Past improvement efforts

Performance improvement in stroke care is an evolving science and has received increasing attention in the literature[6]. Previous terms used to describe quality improvement activities, most adopted from non-health care sectors, include continuous quality improvement (CQI), total quality management (TQM), Six Sigma methods, and the Plan-Do-Study-Act (PDSA) cycle of improvement[7]. A central theme throughout all of these initiatives is to improve performance by implementing changes and measuring outcomes, either processes or outcomes of care. An increasing number of quality improvement projects in stroke-prevention care have been published. These projects have focused on risk factor identification and management, either in the hospital or outpatient setting, or on improving the appropriateness of carotid endarterectomy[8–13]. No clear consensus has emerged as to the ideal strategies or methods that optimize the quality of stroke-prevention care.

CHALLENGES IN QUALITY IMPROVEMENT

There are many challenges to improving the quality of stroke-prevention care, some of which are outlined below.

Quality measurement

Measuring the quality of medical care is difficult. Administrative data often lack the clinical detail required for planning improvements. The hospital or office medical record, although more detailed, still often lacks details of services rendered. Patient satisfaction data, although important, do not always permit a judgment on the adequacy of services. Adding to the challenge are the additional time and effort required to perform the measurement and then acting upon it, if necessary. Stroke-specific quality measures are being developed[14] and measurement systems, as found within Health Plan Employer Data and Information Set (HEDIS) and Joint Commission on Accreditation of Healthcare Organizations (JCAHO) core measures, have or will have direct relevance for improving stroke prevention[15,16].

Lack of knowledge about current practice patterns

Given the paucity and insensitivity of current quality measures, it is not surprising that information regarding current practice patterns for stroke-prevention care are insufficient. Although 'needs assessments' do occur prior to continuing medical education (CME) activities, such assessments are based on self-reported areas of need, rather than on identified suboptimal delivery of care.

From passive dissemination to active implementation

Passive dissemination of information, as in published guidelines or traditional CME, have no or minimal impact on changing provider practices. To be effective, evidence needs to be actively channeled using multiple strategies such as the use of local opinion leaders, one-on-one educational sessions, computerized reminders, mass media campaigns and performance feedback using audits or physician knowledge assessments[17,18]. Specific methods to actively disseminate and implement strategies to ensure the uptake of evidence-based stroke-prevention practices should be based on behavior change theories (e.g., social influence, adult learning, diffusion of information and social marketing) and will depend on the characteristics of the message, recognition of barriers to change and the readiness to change of the targeted providers.

Debate over risk adjustment

There has been debate over the proper role and use of risk adjustment for performance improvement initiatives. Adjusting for differences in the case mix of patients is important when publicly comparing patient outcomes across providers[19]. Risk adjustment is not necessary, however, for local or regional improvement purposes to compare one's performance over time. The lack of a valid risk-adjusted method should never preclude performance of improvement activities.

Many solutions beyond immediate control of providers

Many solutions to improving the quality of stroke-prevention services are beyond the immediate control of providers. One example would be the health policy initiatives needed to align the financial incentives of payers and providers to reduce services that are overused and to increase services that are underused in ways that achieve a lower stroke risk in populations of patients[20]. Another example would be the lack of knowledge and experience in medical error and patient safety research. New research teams are being formed that include educational psychologists, industrial engineers and safety experts from other industries, to understand and prevent medical errors and the misuse of medical and surgical therapies[21].

A dearth of quality improvement champions

There is a dearth of individuals who can serve as stroke quality improvement champions, 'beating the drum' constantly for performance excellence. Performance improvement projects should be an integral part of all service programs that care for patients at risk for stroke.

STRATEGIES TO IMPROVE STROKE-PREVENTION CARE

Despite the challenges, there are strategies that can readily be applied to improve the quality of stroke-prevention services[1].

Provider strategies

Providers need to promote a culture of continuous improvement, provide a supporting environment and identify stroke risk factors in all patients, regardless of the complaint. Written office policies should detail the importance of screening for risk factors and the procedures for their management. Simple office tools such as preventive care chart reminders, computerized reminders, in-office visual prompts and patient-mediated material can improve the delivery of stroke-prevention practices. Tracking forms and computerized reminder systems for follow-up can assist in tracking progress over time. Providers also need to develop effective communication strategies with other providers, and effective advice and counseling strategies that will improve patient compliance.

Hospital strategies

Hospitals should admit patients to dedicated stroke units, given the evidence that such units improve patient outcomes and lower costs, and a structured quality improvement program should be a component of all multidisciplinary stroke teams. Efficient risk-factor assessment should be routine on all patients who are admitted. These assessments should be incorporated into hospital-based critical care pathways. Standard order sheets could also facilitate the ordering of routine laboratory studies such as a lipid profile within the first 24 hours of presentation. Providers and the stroke team need to ensure effective communication and co-ordination of care as the patient progresses from the inpatient setting to rehabilitation, and into the outpatient setting.

Educator strategies

Educators have a unique opportunity to provide an upstream solution to improving the quality of stroke-prevention care. This opportunity occurs in the context of the Accreditation Council for Graduate Medical Education (ACGME) Outcome Project[22]. The ACGME Outcome Project is an initiative to emphasize educational outcomes in accrediting residency education programs. One of the six core competencies requiring implementation and evaluation is 'practice-based learning and improvement', in which residents will be expected to investigate and evaluate their patient care practices, appraise and assimilate scientific evidence, and improve their patient care practices over time. These parallel practice and educational agendas will provide increasing opportunities to give physicians early exposure to performance improvement projects early in their training.

STROKE IMPROVEMENT CASE EXAMPLE

'Dr Prevent' is a faculty member in a university department of neurology. He is also on the staff of the 750-bed university hospital. Each year, approximately 250 ischemic strokes and 50 transient ischemic attacks (TIAs) are admitted to his hospital. Of the total number of strokes and TIAs admitted, the neurology faculty cares for about 60%. The remaining patients with stroke are cared for by other physician groups, mostly internists and family practitioners. Dr Prevent read with interest the article that ranked states by the quality of care given to Medicare beneficiaries[23]. He noted that the state where he practices had one of the lowest adherence rates of any state for prescribing an antithrombotic agent at hospital discharge for patients with a TIA or stroke. Therefore, he undertook a focused 'mini-study' to see how his hospital ranked over the past year. He spoke with the manager of the medical record department. Together, they identified all medical records of patients discharged with a TIA or stroke over the past year with the following International Classification of Disease, version 9 (ICD-9) diagnoses: 435 (TIA), 434 and 436 (stroke). He asked the medical records manager to provide the number of

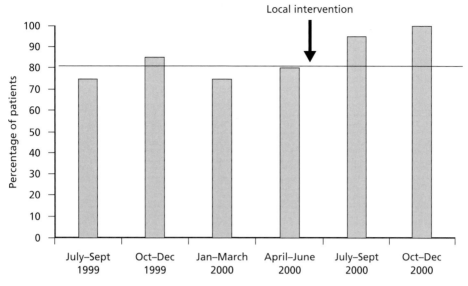

Figure 1 Percentage of ischemic stroke and TIA patients discharged on an antiplatelet agent

total discharges with the above diagnoses for the past four quarters and found the following numbers: July–September 1999, 74; October–December 1999, 83; January–March 2000, 74; April–June 2000, 78. Dr Prevent decided to review a sample of 20 records per quarter. With his nurse practitioner, he developed a one-page chart abstraction form to evaluate how many of the TIA/stroke patients were taking an antithrombotic agent when discharged. He and his nurse reviewed five charts together to make sure that their understanding of appropriate indications for an antiplatelet agent after TIA/stroke was identical. They also clarified their interpretation of the abstraction form. The nurse practitioner then abstracted the remaining 75 charts, each chart taking approximately 3–5 minutes. The task was accomplished in three one-and-a-half-hour sessions over a two-week period.

Dr Prevent's colleagues thought that he needed institutional review board (IRB) approval for the project, so he called the IRB project specialist, who informed him that his project did not need such approval because its goal was quality improvement. He proceeded to analyze his data. Although he had not received prior formal training in statistics, he found a trend graph of the percentage of TIA/stroke patients who appropriately were prescribed antiplatelet agents at discharge very helpful in displaying his data (Figure 1). This graph showed that only 75–85% of all patients who should have received an antiplatelet agent at discharge were so treated. Dr Prevent met with the Chief Quality Officer of the hospital, as well as the Chair of the Department of Medicine. They decided to present the results of this study at grand rounds in both the Departments of Neurology and Medicine. Dr Prevent also informally discussed the importance of antiplatelet agents with his peers. This information was shared with the nursing staff, as well as with the neurology and medicine residents. Finally, he posted his graph in locations where stroke care was delivered.

Six months after his grand rounds presentation, Dr Prevent abstracted another similar sample of charts for the two successive quarters and was delighted to see that the percentage of patients that had received an antiplatelet agent had increased to 95% and 100%, respectively. He again shared the results with the medical and nursing staff. Subsequently, every six months he undertook a focused 'ministudy' on a sample of stroke and TIA patients admitted to the hospital targeting different areas of care – e.g. smoking cessation counseling and lipid management – and this too was successful.

CONCLUSION

Quality stroke care means more than narrowing the evidence–practice gap. Quality stroke care is care that is safe, effective, patient-centered, timely, efficient, and equitable[24]. Well-intentioned, dedicated and highly motivated individuals can make a difference, as illustrated by the above example, and can go a long way towards achieving performance excellence in stroke-prevention care.

References

1. Holloway RG, Benesch C, Rush SR. Stroke prevention: narrowing the evidence-practice gap. *Neurology* 2000;54:1899–906
2. Schuster MA, McGlynn EA, Brook RH. How good is the quality of health care in the United States? *Milbank Q* 1998;76:517–63
3. Morgenstern LB, Steffen-Batey L, Smith MA, *et al.* Barriers to acute stroke therapy and stroke prevention in Mexican Americans. *Stroke* 2001; 321:360–4
4. Winslow CM, Solomon DH, Chassin MR, *et al.* The appropriateness of carotid endarterectomy. *N Engl J Med* 1988;318:721–7
5. Hamby L, Weeks WB, Malikowski C. Complications of warfarin therapy: causes, costs, and the role of the anticoagulation clinic. *Eff Clin Pract* 2000;3:179–84
6. Quality of Care and Outcomes Research in CVD and Stroke Working Groups. Measuring and improving quality of care: a report from the American Heart Association/American College of Cardiology first scientific forum on assessment of healthcare quality in cardiovascular disease and stroke. *Stroke* 2000;31:1002–12
7. Langley GJ, Nolan KM, Nolan TW, *et al. The Improvement Guide. A Practical Approach to Enhancing Organizational Performance.* San Francisco: Jossey-Bass Publishers, 1996
8. Joseph LN, Babikian VL, Allen NC, Winter MR. Risk factor modification in stroke prevention: the experience of a stroke clinic. *Stroke* 1999; 30:16–20
9. Kalra L, Perez I, Melbourn A. Stroke risk management: changes in mainstream practice. *Stroke* 1998;29:53–7
10. Gordon DL, Cobb AB, McIlwain JS, *et al.* Cooperative stroke management project by a peer-review organization. *J Stroke Cerebrovasc Dis* 1996;6:45–53
11. Weir N, Dennis MS. Towards a national system for monitoring the quality of hospital-based stroke services. *Stroke* 2001;32:1415–21
12. Asch SM, Sloss EM, Hogan C, *et al.* Measuring underuse of necessary care among elderly Medicare beneficiaries using inpatient and outpatient claims. *J Am Med Assoc* 2000;284: 2325–33
13. Wong JH, Lubkey TB, Suarez-Almazor ME, *et al.* Improving the appropriateness of carotid endarterectomy: results of a prospective city-wide study. *Stroke* 1999;30:12–15
14. Holloway RG, Vickrey BG, Benesch CG, *et al.* Development of performance measures for acute ischemic stroke. *Stroke* 2001;32: 2058–74
15. http://www.ncqa.org/Programs/HEDIS/index. htm
16. http://www.jcaho.org
17. Haines A, Donald A. *Getting Research Findings into Practice.* London: BMJ Publishing Group, 1998
18. Cohen SJ, Halvorson HW, Gosselink CA. Changing physician behavior to improve disease prevention. *Prev Med* 1994;23:284–91

19. Iezzoni LI, Shwartz M, Ash AS, *et al.* Using severity-adjusted stroke mortality rates to judge hospitals. *Int J Qual Health Care* 1995;7:81–4

20. Committee on Quality of Health Care in America. Aligning payment policies with quality improvement. In *Crossing the Quality Chasm. A New Health System for the 21st Century.* Washington: National Academy Press, 2001: 193–219

21. Committee on Quality of Health Care in America. Errors in health care. A leading cause of death and injury. In *To Err is Human. Building a Safer Health System.* Washington: National Academy Press, 2000:26–48

22. http://www.acgme.org/Outcome/

23. Jencks SF, Cuerdon T, Burwen DR, *et al.* Quality of medical care delivered to medicare beneficiaries: a profile at state and national levels. *J Am Med Assoc* 2000;284:1670–6

24. Committee on Quality of Health Care in America. Formulating new rules to redesign and improve care. In *Crossing the Quality Chasm. A New Health System for the 21st Century.* Washington: National Academy Press, 2001:65–94

Gaps in professional and community knowledge about stroke prevention and treatment

Larry B. Goldstein, MD

A variety of strategies can be employed to improve the care of stroke patients and to reduce the incidence of stroke and ameliorate its consequences. For example, new risk factors can be identified and novel methods of risk reduction and treatment can be developed. However, a large body of evidence exists to guide current clinical stroke prevention and treatment practices. Optimizing the utilization of these existing, proven modes of prevention and therapy offers an important opportunity for reducing the societal and individual impact of stroke.

Both clinical trials and epidemiological studies provide unambiguous evidence supporting the efficacy of a series of diverse primary and secondary stroke preventive therapies[1–3]. Despite this evidence, it is apparent that these approaches are under-utilized. For example, of eligible patients in the US without a prior history of stroke or transient ischemic attack (TIA), only 24–64% of hypertensives and 25–64% of those with hyperlipidemia are appropriately treated[4]. Less than half of those with atrial fibrillation who are candidates for anticoagulant therapy receive warfarin[5–7] and only 40% of patients with atrial fibrillation who are anticoagulated have international normalized ratios (INRs)

in the recommended therapeutic range[5]. Antithrombotic therapy is under-utilized in patients discharged from a hospital following a TIA or stroke[4]. Nearly one-third of patients presenting to a primary care physician's office with a first-ever TIA or minor stroke have no diagnostic studies over the ensuing month[8], the period of highest risk[9]. In addition, only small proportions of ischemic stroke patients receive intravenous thrombolytic therapy under clinical guidelines, as approved by the US Food and Drug Administration[10].

The potential reasons for these discrepancies between evidence and observed practice are probably varied. Physicians may not be sufficiently motivated to change their practices as new study results become available. There may be both recognized and unrecognized external barriers to providing services. Patient-related factors, time pressures, reimbursement issues and administrative obstacles can also influence the provision of preventive care, acute treatments and rehabilitative services. However, several lines of evidence suggest that gaps in professional and public stroke-related knowledge exist that contribute to this problem.

A US national survey of physician practices carried out long after the results of several randomized trials demonstrating the benefit of carotid endarterectomy for symptomatic high-grade carotid artery stenosis had been published[11-13] found that only about half of non-internist primary care physicians and internists would always or often use carotid endarterectomy for such patients[14]. Almost 25% of non-internist primary care physicians and approximately 20% of internists responded that they would seldom or never use carotid endarterectomy in this setting. In addition, 39% of the non-internist primary care physicians and 22% of internists who responded that they would seldom or never use carotid endarterectomy also reported that they always or often use anticoagulants for these patients[15]. Further, 80–90% of these physicians also reported that they were comfortable with their current practices and were not anticipating change[16]. These findings illustrate a potential problem with the effective dissemination of information. Some physicians continued to use an unproven therapy (anticoagulation) in place of a therapy of proven value (endarterectomy) and were comfortable with that approach, suggesting that they were relatively unaware of the results of relevant clinical trials. Another possible example of a professional knowledge gap comes from a practice audit that found primary care physicians frequently did not evaluate patients with new onset TIA urgently[4]. Although the reasons are uncertain, lack of knowledge of the significance of TIA may also be contributing to this discrepancy between optimal and observed practices.

In contrast to these knowledge gaps, more than 99% of surveyed physicians reported that they use platelet antiaggregants for secondary and tertiary stroke prevention[17]. Yet only 50–80% of patients discharged from a hospital after TIA or stroke receive antithrombotic therapy[4]. Similarly, only 10% of physicians indicate that they seldom or never use anticoagulants for eligible patients with non-valvular atrial fibrillation[16]. However, several studies demonstrate that this therapy is underused[5-7]. Thus, in these examples, the gap is between knowledge and practice rather than a lack of knowledge of the efficacy of specific treatment approaches. This knowledge–practice gap can be due to a number of potential factors as suggested above, including factors related to the patients themselves.

Patient-related factors, including gaps in knowledge, represent another important barrier to effective stroke prevention and treatment. For example, a national survey identified patients at risk for stroke because they had a TIA (15%), a non-disabling stroke (33%), or specific stroke risk factors (cervical bruit, carotid artery stenosis, atrial fibrillation, etc., 52%)[18]. Only 41% of patients were aware of their increased risk of stroke, and only 27% recalled being informed of that risk by a physician. Importantly, 26% of those who recalled being informed of their increased stroke risk continued to indicate that they did not feel that they were at elevated risk. These individuals, although educated to the extent that they knew their increased stroke risk, were not effectively educated (i.e., they did not accept that risk).

A lack of stroke-related knowledge may also affect how patients and families respond to stroke symptoms. Several studies have now demonstrated a general lack of public knowledge regarding stroke, its risk factors, symptoms and potential treatment modalities[19-22]. This is true even among high-risk patients (the elderly and African-Americans) residing in high-risk regions of the country[19,21]. In one study, only approximately one-quarter of patients presenting to the hospital with acute stroke correctly interpreted their symptoms[20]. With time-sensitive treatments such as the use of thrombolysis, delay in seeking appropriate medical attention represents one factor contributing to its lack of utilization.

Addressing these gaps in both professional and public stroke-related knowledge is not

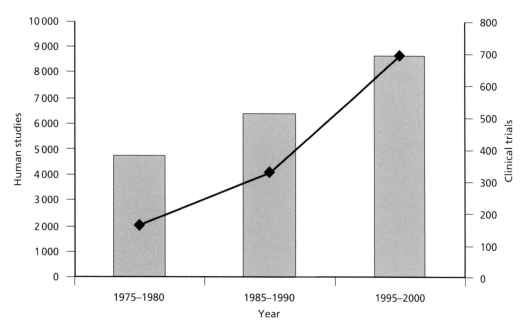

Figure 1 The numbers of stroke-related publications involving humans (bars) and stroke-related clinical trials (♦) listed in *Index Medicus* in three five-year periods

trivial. As shown in Figure 1, there were 4739 cerebrovascular disease-related clinical reports listed in *Index Medicus* during the five-year period from 1975 to 1980. This number nearly doubled to 8646 during the period from 1995 to 2000. The number of stroke-related clinical trial reports also increased dramatically over this period. There were 161 clinical trial reports published between 1975 and 1980, with 695 between 1995 and 2000. As has been pointed out previously[23], it is nearly impossible for generalist physicians to read and interpret this complex and growing literature. Clinical practice guidelines are designed to summarize available evidence in a format intended to facilitate its incorporation into clinical practice. However, even the number of stroke-related clinical practice guidelines listed in *Index Medicus* has mushroomed from four between 1975 and 1980 to 17 between 1995 and 2000. As stroke affects only a small proportion of patients in a typical generalist physician's practice, even keeping apprised of the

evolving relevant clinical guidelines is a daunting task. In addition, evidence that clinical practice guidelines have a significant impact on physician performance or patient outcomes are lacking[24,25]. Traditional continuing medical education courses tend to be ineffective[26] and outreach visits, chart audits, automated reminders, and patient-mediated programs have variable impacts on physician practices[26]. So-called 'academic detailing', in which educational programs are tailored to individual physicians or practices[27], and delivered by recognized opinion leaders is one of the most effective single strategies[26,28,29]. However, the use of multimodal educational strategies appears superior to any single method[26].

Different types of strategies will be required to address the stroke-related knowledge gap of the general public. Knowledge among stroke patients and their caregivers can be improved with targeted educational programs[30]; community-based surveys conducted before and after a public stroke education campaign demonstrated a significant improvement in public knowledge of stroke warning signs in at least some patient subgroups[31]. Another study found that knowledge significantly improved when measured immediately after a slide/audio community education program, but it is unknown how long the information was retained[32]. It is of concern that other studies have found that patient knowledge of stroke symptoms is not necessarily associated with early presentation to an emergency department (i.e. an uncoupling of knowledge and action)[20,33]. This discrepancy between knowledge and action was also demonstrated in an analysis carried out as part of the Asymptomatic Carotid Atherosclerosis Study (ACAS)[34]. Patients enrolled in this randomized trial of endarterectomy received formal education regarding stroke warning signs, and were repeatedly instructed to report any symptoms immediately. Despite this intensive education in a group of highly motivated patients, fewer than 40% of events were reported within three days, with less than 25% reported within 24 hours.

Notwithstanding these challenges to effective professional and public stroke-related educational programs, encouraging data are emerging. At least two studies suggest that multifaceted public/professional educational campaigns can increase the proportion of patients presenting to hospitals soon after the onset of symptoms[35,36]. The first study was carried out prior to the advent of thrombolytic therapy and measured the number of patients coming to the hospital within 24 hours of the onset of symptoms. The second study divided five East Texas counties into comparison and intervention communities. Intervention consisted of the dissemination of informational brochures and posters in addition to radio and television public service announcements and targeted seminars aimed at the public, with continuing medical education courses, newsletters and care protocols designed to improve professional awareness and knowledge. There was a significant increase in the proportion of eligible candidates treated with intravenous tissue plasminogen activator (t-PA) in the intervention community (14% at baseline vs. 52% after the intervention) whereas there was no change in the comparison community (7% vs. 6% over the same time period).

Identifying and understanding gaps in physician and public stroke-related knowledge considered in the context of the social milieu and healthcare system can lead to the development of effective educational strategies (i.e. educational strategies that lead to improved health outcomes). The available data suggest that these approaches will need to be both multifaceted and sustained. Interventional programs such as the American Heart Association's Operation Stroke as well as proposed legislative initiatives (e.g. the Stroke Ongoing Treatment and Prevention Act) are in part based on these data and will, it is hoped, result in a reduction in the burden of stroke.

References

1. Goldstein LB, Adams R, Becker K, *et al.* Primary prevention of ischemic stroke. *Circulation* 2000; 103:163–82
2. Gorelick PB, Sacco RL, Smith DB, *et al.* Prevention of a first stroke: a review of guidelines and a multidisciplinary consensus statement from the National Stroke Association. *J Am Med Assoc* 1999;281:1112–20
3. Wolf PA, Clagett PA, Easton JD, *et al.* Preventing ischemic stroke in patients with prior stroke and transient ischemic attack. *Stroke* 1999;30:1991–4
4. Holloway RG, Benesch C, Rush SR. Stroke prevention. Narrowing the evidence–practice gap. *Neurology* 2000;54:1899–906
5. Samsa GP, Matchar DB, Goldstein LB, *et al.* Quality of anticoagulation management among patients with atrial fibrillation: results from a review of medical records from two communities. *Arch Intern Med* 2000;160:967–73

6. Cohen N, Almoznino-Sarafian D, Alon I, *et al.* Warfarin for stroke prevention still underused in atrial fibrillation. Patterns of omission. *Stroke* 2000;31:1217–22

7. Gage BF, Boechler G, Flaker G, *et al.* Utilization of antithrombotic therapy in Medicare beneficiaries with nonvalvular atrial fibrillation: an opportunity lost. *J Gen Intern Med* 1997;12(Suppl 1):71

8. Goldstein LB, Bian J, Samsa GP, *et al.* New TIA and stroke: outpatient management by primary care physicians. *Arch Intern Med* 2000; 160:2941–6

9. Johnston SC, Gress DR, Browner WS, Sidney S. Short-term prognosis after emergency department diagnosis of TIA. *J Am Med Assoc* 2000;284:2901–6

10. Katzan IL, Furlan AJ, Lloyd LE, *et al.* Use of tissue-type plasminogen activator for acute ischemic stroke: the Cleveland area experience. *J Am Med Assoc* 2000;283:1151–8

11. European Carotid Surgery Trialists' Collaborative Group. MRC European carotid surgery trial: interim results for symptomatic patients with severe (70–99%) or with mild (0–29%) carotid stenosis. *Lancet* 1991;337:1235–43

12. Mayberg MR, Wilson E, Yatsu F, *et al.* Carotid endarterectomy and prevention of cerebral ischemia in symptomatic carotid stenosis. *J Am Med Assoc* 1991;266:3289–94

13. North American Symptomatic Carotid Endarterectomy Trial Collaborators. Beneficial effect of carotid endarterectomy in symptomatic patients with high-grade carotid stenosis. *N Engl J Med* 1991;325:445–53

14. Goldstein LB, Bonito AJ, Matchar DB, *et al.* U.S. National survey of physician practices for the secondary and tertiary prevention of ischemic stroke: carotid endarterectomy. *Stroke* 1996;27:801–6

15. Goldstein LB, Bonito AJ, Matchar DB, *et al.* U.S. National survey of physician practices for the secondary and tertiary prevention of stroke: medical therapy in patients with carotid artery stenosis. *Stroke* 1996;27:1473–8

16. Goldstein LB, Cohen SJ, Matchar DB, *et al.* Physician-reported readiness to change stroke prevention practices. *J Stroke Cerebrovasc Dis* 1998;8:358–63

17. Goldstein LB, Bonito AJ, Matchar DB, *et al.* U.S. National survey of physician practices for the secondary and tertiary prevention of stroke: design, service availability, and common practices. *Stroke* 1995;26:1607–15

18. Samsa GP, Cohen SJ, Goldstein LB, *et al.* Knowledge of risk among patients at increased risk for stroke. *Stroke* 1997;28:916–21

19. Pancioli AM, Broderick J, Kothari R, *et al.* Public perception of stroke warning signs and knowledge of potential risk factors. *J Am Med Assoc* 1998;279:1288–92

20. Williams LS, Bruno A, Rouch D, Marriott DJ. Stroke patients' knowledge of stroke. Influence on time to presentation. *Stroke* 1997;28:912–15

21. Goldstein LB, Gradison M. Stroke-related knowledge among patients with access to medical care in the Stroke Belt. *J Stroke Cerebrovasc Dis* 1999;8:349–52

22. Smith MA, Doliszny KM, Shahar E, *et al.* Delayed hospital arrival for acute stroke: The Minnesota Stroke Survey. *Ann Intern Med* 1998;129:190–6

23. Goldstein LB. Evidence-based medicine and stroke. *Neuroepidemiology* 1999;18:120–4

24. Lomas J. Words without action? The production, dissemination, and impact of consensus recommendations. *Annu Rev Pub Health* 1991; 12:41–65

25. Worrall G, Chaulk P, Freake D. The effects of clinical practice guidelines on patient outcomes in primary care: a systematic review. *Can Med Assoc J* 1997;156:1705–12

26. Davis DA, Thomson MA, Oxman AD, Haynes RB. Changing physician performance. A systematic review of the effect of continuing medical education strategies. *J Am Med Assoc* 1995;274:700–5

27. Soumerai SB, Avorn J. Principles of educational outreach ('academic detailing') to improve clinical decision making. *J Am Med Assoc* 1990;263:549–56

28. Lomas J, Enkin M, Anderson GM, *et al.* Opinion leaders vs. audit and feedback to implement practice guidelines. Delivery after previous cesarean section. *J Am Med Assoc* 1991;265:2202–7

29. Soumerai SB, McLaughlin TJ, Gurwitz JH, *et al.* Effect of local medical opinion leaders on quality of care for acute myocardial infarction: a randomized controlled trial. *J Am Med Assoc* 1998;279:1358–63

30. Rodgers H, Atkinson C, Bond S, *et al.* Randomized controlled trial of a comprehensive stroke education program for patients and caregivers. Stroke 1999;30:2585–91

31. Dornan WA, Stroink AR, Pegg EE, *et al.* Community stroke awareness program increases public knowledge of stroke. *Stroke* 1998;29:288

32. Stern EB, Berman M, Thomas JJ, Klassen AC. Community education for stroke awareness: an efficacy study. *Stroke* 1999;30:720–3

33. Cheung RTF. Patients' knowledge of stroke does not influence time to hospital presentation. *Stroke* 2001;32:365

34. Castaldo JE, Nelson JJ, Reed JFI, *et al*. The delay in reporting symptoms of carotid artery stenosis in an at-risk population. *Arch Neurol* 1997;54:1267–71

35. Alberts MJ, Perry A, Dawson DV, Bertels C. Effects of public and professional education on reducing the delay in presentation and referral of stroke patients. *Stroke* 1992;23:352–6

36. Morgenstern LB, King M, Staub L, *et al*. Community and professional intervention to increase FDA-approved acute stroke therapy: final main results of the TLL Temple Foundation Stroke Project. *Neurology* 2001; 56(Suppl 3):A77

Chapter 15

Stroke and public policy: the role of stroke advocacy groups

Patti Shwayder, MPA

THE CHALLENGE OF STROKE PREVENTION AND ADVOCACY

Stroke is the third leading cause of death in America and the leading cause of adult disability; it kills twice as many women each year as breast cancer[1]. We know that many strokes are preventable, yet the need for more education and better intervention remains critically high. A recent nationwide poll revealed that public awareness of the warning signs of stroke is alarmingly poor – 40% of adults do not know that stroke occurs in the brain and only 20% know that stroke can be prevented[2]. The public has an extremely limited view of what can be done to prevent stroke. Although high blood pressure is a leading risk factor for stroke, only 17% of people polled knew that lowering their blood pressure would reduce their risk of stroke. Furthermore, 70% of the public are not getting a clear stroke prevention message from their health care provider[2].

There is consensus in the medical community that stroke is one of the most preventable of all life-threatening health problems. Treatment of certain medical conditions and modification of high-risk lifestyle factors have

been shown to reduce the risk of stroke. In 1999, the National Stroke Association published an article in the *Journal of the American Medical Association* outlining guidelines for the prevention of a first stroke that included treatment of both medical and lifestyle factors[3].

Despite the fact that many strokes are preventable and that new therapies are being developed for acute treatment of stroke, 750 000 Americans will experience a stroke each year and two-thirds of them will survive, many with disability. In addition to the often-devastating personal toll that strokes take on survivors, families and caregivers, stroke costs the nation at least $43 billion annually[4]. A few states and communities in the USA have developed and implemented stroke awareness programs and comprehensive stroke care systems, but no uniform standard for stroke screening exists. Moreover, there is little information about the nationwide effects of stroke or the availability of acute care for stroke.

The public is not demanding the level of research that will reduce stroke frequency and improve care; they require more education to make an impact on this often-debilitating disease. The systems and infrastructure for management and prevention of stroke that have been instrumental in reducing other diseases are developing but still can be improved.

Stroke advocacy in the United States lags behind that of other chronic and infectious diseases and government programs for stroke prevention, research and rehabilitation are underfunded, given the magnitude of the problem. Development of comprehensive strategies to reduce stroke are needed.

PUBLIC HEALTH EXPENDITURE FOR STROKE

Every year chronic diseases such as stroke, heart disease, diabetes and cancer claim the lives of more than 1.7 million Americans, and account for seven of every ten deaths in the United States, according to the Centers for Disease Control and Prevention (CDC)[5]. Chronic disease is broadly defined as illnesses that are prolonged, do not resolve spontaneously and are rarely cured completely. The medical care costs for people with chronic diseases total more than $400 billion annually, or more than 60% of all medical expenditure[5]. However, in 1994, the public health expenditure targeting chronic diseases was only $1.21 per person[5]. The CDC's entire federal appropriation for chronic disease prevention programs was $749.7 million in 2001, with only $35 million (< 5%) dedicated to heart disease and stroke programs[6]. Until 1998, no federal funding had been given to states to target cardiovascular disease. Furthermore, less than 5% of state health department budgets have historically been directed at preventing and controlling chronic diseases[6]. Compounding the problem of poor funding is the fact that the few cardiovascular programs that have been implemented do not adequately address cerebrovascular prevention strategies

specific to stroke, but rather are related to cardiovascular prevention strategies.

Many chronic diseases are an extension of lifestyle choices and offer opportunities to reduce risk factors by changing these choices. Three risk factors in particular, tobacco use, inadequate physical activity and poor nutrition are major contributing factors to cardiovascular disease, cancer and stroke[6]. Promoting healthier behavior through public education and community programs is essential to reducing the burden of chronic disease in the United States and reducing the escalation of health care costs. For example, each $1 spent on diabetes outpatient education saves $2–3 in hospitalization costs, according to the CDC. And cervical cancer screening among low-income elderly women is estimated to save 3.7 years of life and nearly $6000 for every 100 Pap tests performed[6]. Presumably, similar savings could be achieved by investing in stroke prevention education.

Many health organizations, such as the CDC and the World Health Organization, combine stroke with heart disease under the category of 'cardiovascular disease'. This fosters the belief that stroke is a heart condition rather than a brain condition and subordinates stroke to heart disease. This is confusing to the public, to policy makers and even to some health professionals. It has also limited the action that must be directed to reduce the specific burden of stroke.

In addition to underfunding at the federal level, many states have not developed detailed strategic plans or prevention and health promotion programs to reduce stroke. A recent survey by the National Stroke Association indicated that only one state has a comprehensive strategic plan for stroke[7], though several states are beginning to address stroke by expanding nascent cardiovascular programs. Other states use programs aimed at reducing risk factors for a multitude of diseases and promoting primary prevention strategies in general, believing that in this way stroke too can be reduced. Yet, there are special high risk factors for stroke, most notably atrial fibrillation, personal or family history of a stroke or transient ischemic attack (TIA) and carotid stenosis, that are not as effectively addressed by using only generic cardiovascular health promotion programs to reduce stroke. Both primary and secondary prevention programs geared specifically to stroke risk factors are more cost-efficient and effective in reducing stroke morbidity and mortality.

FOCUSED ADVOCACY IS IMPERATIVE

Better organization of those interested in reducing stroke would help to focus more attention at all levels of government on this health problem. The 'community' of interest is broad and comprises professionals, patients, families, caregivers and non-profit-making organizations. Uniting the efforts of this broad community would offer excellent opportunities to advance public policy to undertake the effort necessary to prevent stroke. An advocate is one who supports or defends a cause, or who pleads a cause on behalf of another. Patient advocacy organizations have had an important impact on health care policy in the United States in the past few decades. By raising their voices with a common message and giving a human face to a disease, advocacy groups have raised awareness among the general public and policymakers about stroke and what can be done to reduce its frequency and improve its outcomes.

Advocacy groups advance their cause on many fronts. They promote compelling, memorable public information campaigns to educate people about the disease and encourage individuals not only to take care of their health, but also to get involved with the cause – by volunteering time, donating money and writing letters to Congress, as well as using other techniques to attract attention. They

may lobby elected officials on health care policy, coordinate professional development programs, work with business partners to champion the cause, and provide funding for medical research, to cite but a few of the activities used. Until recently, activities that drove change in public policies were all but absent in stroke. Concerted efforts by the professional stroke community, working side by side with patient and family advocates, will ultimately improve stroke care and reduce the burden of stroke[8].

Until the year 2000, when the National Stroke Association (NSA) assumed a leadership role for stroke advocacy, there was not a single group devoted solely to advocating for stroke on behalf of stroke professionals, patients and their families. The NSA is a leading independent, national non-profit organization dedicated solely to reducing the incidence and impact of stroke. One-hundred percent of its resources and efforts are devoted to stroke. The NSA develops and implements innovative approaches and programs to advance stroke prevention, treatment and recovery. In addition to educating the public and professionals, the NSA works to improve the quality of stroke care through public policy and advocacy efforts. Public policy on stroke has shifted toward increasing education, funding and support of programs for reducing the burden of stroke.

STROKE PUBLIC POLICY CHOICES

There are many public policy issues that must be researched carefully and a multitude of public policy choices that can be made concerning stroke. For example, a variety of public health screening programs exist for cancer, heart disease, HIV/AIDs and other chronic and infectious diseases. These programs are paid for by federal funds and private insurers and have been implemented in order to curb disease and reduce the debilitating costs of illness. Yet, there is no risk factor assessment and screening program for stroke, despite its being, as already mentioned, the third leading cause of death and the leading cause of disability. Promotion of early detection of risk factors for stroke may enhance early intervention, and thereby reduce the risk of stroke. Furthermore, there is a need for better education for health care professionals who treat stroke. Increasingly, strokes are treated by neurologists, internists and family physicians assisted by emergency medical personnel, nurses and other allied professionals[8]. Emergency medical technicians are a critical link in improving stroke outcomes. All of these health professionals need specific training in stroke-risk reduction and effective treatment. In fact, a recent national survey indicated that less than one-third of physicians discuss what a stroke is, options for stroke-risk reduction and individual stroke risk with their patients[2]. In contrast, the same survey indicates that 55% of physicians discuss the risk of breast or prostate cancer with patients[8].

Physicians are not optimally equipped to prevent stroke nor has the United States developed the health care infrastructure to effectively treat stroke. Efforts to improve this situation are reflected by the guidelines for stroke centers published by the NSA in 1997[9]. The Brain Attack Coalition refined these recommendations in 2000 and published a consensus statement in the *Journal of the American Medical Association*[10]. These guidelines could be the basis for future efforts to identify or designate stroke centers that are best equipped to give optimal patient care.

A recent survey of neurologists, neurosurgeons, emergency medicine physicians and hospitals who are members of the NSA's stroke center network indicates that, while 80% agree on the need for stroke centers and the same proportion would like to become a primary stroke center, only 7% of hospitals would meet all the criteria for such a designation[11]. Even more troubling is the fact that 76% of hospital physicians surveyed believed that they already have the systems and protocols in place to qualify as a stroke center[11]. A national blue ribbon task force has been set up to determine how best to implement these guidelines. While the public strongly supports designation of stroke centers[2], this effort has been inhibited by disagreements among Brain Attack Coalition members.

There is no reimbursement for stroke prevention and screening efforts and there is only low reimbursement for acute care and rehabilitation for stroke. Current reimbursement levels for acute stroke care are inadequate and act as a disincentive for effective treatment. Medicare, which covers the age group that constitutes 75% of stroke patients, reimburses hospitals at a rate of $5429 per patient, far short of the actual cost of care[12]. Medicare payments to physicians for treatment of stroke are about $100 per patient[13]. Additional research on the costs and benefits of treatment are needed but it is clear that stroke care is undervalued in the health care marketplace. Reimbursement for post-stroke rehabilitation is also underfunded. The Balanced Budget Act of 1997 placed a $1500 cap on rehabilitation therapy services for stroke patients delivered in nursing homes and other settings. Yet, the average cost per patient for the first 90 days post stroke is $15 000, and in 10% of cases costs exceed $35 000[14]. A moratorium on raising this cap has been extended several times. A national effort is needed to increase reimbursement at all stages of stroke prevention, acute treatment and rehabilitation services. Inadequate reimbursement provides disincentives for health professionals and hospitals to place a high priority on effective stroke care.

MODELS OF EFFECTIVE ADVOCACY

There are several models of advocacy that have been quite successful in raising the profile of a particular disease and have stimulated increased action by health care professionals and the public. For example, polio vaccine grew out of research funded primarily by the 'March of Dimes'. In the early 1980s, little federal money was spent on AIDS research. By the early 1990s, after a massive grassroots lobbying effort by activists, 10% of the National Institutes of Health's (NIH) $8.9 billion budget was spent on AIDS research[15]. That funding has grown to $2.2 billion today[16].

Lobbying efforts by women's health groups resulted in the creation of the NIH's Office of Research on Women's Health. In 1992, breast-cancer activists sent more than 600 000 letters to Congress demanding more research into the disease. Funding for breast cancer research increased from $60.9 million to $132.7 in five years[15] and totals $553 million today[17]. Similarly, local chapters for multiple sclerosis and breast cancer have raised millions of dollars in walks, races and events that focus attention on survivors and their families. Through doing so, the added media attention has increased public awareness and stimulated a resolve to fight these diseases.

Another successful strategy for raising awareness of a disease involves enlisting the help of high-profile celebrities. For example, Christopher Reeve is an effective supporter of research in spinal-cord injury, Michael J. Fox is an eloquent advocate for Parkinson's disease and Mary Tyler Moore campaigns timelessly for diabetes education. Della Reese, Robert Guillaume and recently Kirk Douglas have begun to increase the focus of the public on stroke.

Diabetes advocates have been very effective in working with federal agencies to implement programs to reduce that disease. The CDC has taken a national leadership role in reducing the impact of diabetes by sponsoring several coordinated public service education campaigns, supporting scientific studies into the disease and investigating best practices for care, and provides $58.3 million in funding to states and territories for diabetes control programs. Many states have effectively used the money to prevent and treat diabetes. In New York state provider and community-focused interventions over the past two years have reduced diabetes hospitalization rates by 35% and decreased lower-extremity amputation rates in diabetics by 39%[18]. The success of coordinated advocacy and investments in federal and state programs could be replicated to produce real gains in reducing stroke.

Compelling, personal stories and commitment by dedicated volunteers is another strength of lay organizations. Groups such as the American Cancer Society and the Alzheimer's Association have worked effectively with the media to bring these diseases down to a personal level of attention, often highlighting individual patients and survivors. The Race for the Cure for breast cancer grew from one woman's desire to honor her affected sister. That effort grew into one of the nation's most well known fundraising activities. As advocacy groups have shown, there is power in numbers. Building coalitions is an effective tool in advancing an issue. An organization like the National Stroke Association has chapters in many communities across the country, and is in contact with numerous stroke survivor support groups. In partnerships with other public health organizations, other neurological associations, medical professionals, pharmaceutical companies and other concerned groups, public awareness can be raised to elevate stroke to a higher level on the public health agenda.

Coordination of the multitude of professional disciplines that treat stroke patients – including neurologists, family practice physicians, obstetricians and gynecologists, physical therapists, emergency medical technicians, occupational therapists and nurses – is needed for them to participate in stroke advocacy. Successful models of advocacy indicate that people – those directly affected – tug at the heart and purse strings of Congress. It is the stroke survivors, coupled with expert professionals and strategic non-profit-making organizations that have the best chance of capturing the media and public attention needed to effect change. Spouses, family members, loved ones, caregivers and friends also make compelling spokespeople and can help change the awareness of stroke from a perception of passivity to one of action in their offices, their neighborhoods, their states and ultimately the country at large.

Public health policy regarding stroke has gained momentum recently with legislative attention in Congress and the formation of the Paul Coverdell National Acute Stroke Registry to track the delivery of stroke care[19]. In 2001, the first comprehensive stroke legislation was introduced and would set up systems of stroke care and implement an extensive public information campaign across the USA[20]. These efforts, in combination with sustained public education and intense research initiatives, will save lives and reduce disability from stroke.

There is much to do to reduce stroke worldwide. Focused efforts in prevention, public education, emergency response, designating stroke centers and educating stroke teams will make a difference for stroke patients and ultimately for stroke survivors. Effective policies aimed at adequate reimbursement for stroke prevention and care must be implemented. A grass roots advocacy effort built by those most affected by stroke – patients, families, caregivers and compassionate professionals – can have a favorable impact. It is time for stroke to take its rightful place as a public health issue worthy of discussion and action. It is time for the nation to build the infrastructure to ensure that stroke is effectively prevented, treated and survived by the hundreds of thousands who suffer a brain attack each year.

ACKNOWLEDGEMENT

Special thanks go to Jennifer McCarty, Manager of Communications, National Stroke Association, for her important work on this chapter.

References

1. Hoyert DL, Kochanek KD, Murphy SL. Deaths: Final Data for 1997. *National Vital Statistics Reports*, Vol. 47 no. 19. Hyattsville, Maryland: National Center for Health Statistics, 1999
2. Awareness of Stroke Symptoms, Treatment and Support Organizations, National Stroke Association, Sell Communications, 2001
3. Gorelick PB, Sacco RL, Smith DB, *et al.* Prevention of a first stroke: a review of guidelines and a multidisciplinary consensus from the national stroke association. *J Am Med Assoc* 1999; 281(12):1112
4. Taylor TN, Davis PH, Torner JC, *et al.* Lifetime cost of stroke in the United States, *Stroke* 1996; 27:1459–66
5. Centers for Disease Control and Prevention. *Chronic Diseases and Their Risk Factors: The Nation's Leading Causes of Death.* December 1999
6. Chronic Disease Directors. *General Chronic Fact Sheet.* www.chronicdiseases.org; June 2001
7. National Stroke Association. *Survey of Public Health Officials.* NSA, 2000
8. AstraZeneca Stroke Specialists Advisory Board. *Report of the AstraZeneca Stroke Specialists Advisory Board.* July 21–23, 2000
9. Furlan A, Murdock M, Spilker J, *et al.* NSA stroke center network stroke center recommendations. *J Stroke Cerebrovascular Dis* 1997;6: 299–302

10. Alberts, MJ, Hademos G, Latchaw RE, *et al. J Am Med Assoc* 2001;283(23):3102

11. Kidwell C. *Recommendations for the Establishment of Primary Stroke Centers: US Survey of Physician Attitudes and Hospital Resources.* UCLA Stroke Center, Presentation to Brain Attack Coalition, August 1, 2000, Washington, DC

12. Strauss MJ. *Presentation to AstraZeneca Stroke Specialists Advisory Meeting.* November 12–14, 1999

13. Scott PA. *Presentation to AstraZeneca Stroke Specialists Advisory Board Meeting.* November 12–14, 1999

14. Natchar DB, Duncan PW. Cost of stroke. National Stroke Association. *Stroke Clinical Updates* 1994;5:9–12

15. Washington DT. Your money or their lives: patient advocates learning from AIDS advocates how to work the system. *Time Magazine,* October 12, 1992

16. *Budget Justification 2001.* Office of AIDS Research, National Institutes of Health, US House of Representatives Appropriations Committee Report (106–645) and FY2001 Conference Appropriations Committee Report (106–1033)

17. *Shaping the Future of Breast Cancer Awareness, Research, Diagnosis and Treatment.* FY 2001 Budget Information, US Department of Health and Human Services fact sheet, October 2000

18. Centers for Disease Control and Prevention. *Diabetes: A Serious Public Health Problem at a Glance.* Bethesda, MD: CDC, National Center for Chronic Disease Prevention and Health Promotion, 2001

19. US Federal Legislation, H.R. 4577, Labor-Health and Human Services, Education Appropriations, 106th Congress, 2nd Session

20. US Federal Legislation, Senate Bill 1274, 107th Congress, 1st Session

Chapter 16

I. Hypertension treatment

William J. Elliott, MD, PhD, Jay Garg, MD, and
Munavvar Izhar, MD

OVERVIEW

Blood pressure lowering has been recognized, even in the popular press, as a very important and effective strategy for both primary and secondary prevention of stroke. According to the July 1999 *Consumer Reports*, 'Controlling hypertension is the single most important step most people can take to prevent stroke'. Data from many epidemiologic surveys and cohort studies (for example, The Framingham Heart Study) indicate that stroke is about 2–4 times more common among hypertensive than normotensive people; the higher the blood pressure, the greater the risk. Many randomized clinical trials have shown a substantial reduction in the risk of stroke when antihypertensive medications are provided. A 1990 meta- analysis of such studies estimated that stroke rates were reduced by $42 \pm 6\%$ (mean ± standard deviation) when active antihypertensive drugs were used, as compared to placebo. Although lifestyle modifications have a place in hypertension treatment, they are less effective than antihypertensive pills in both lowering blood pressure and preventing stroke. As a result, people at high risk for stroke and other cardiovascular disease should seldom be treated without pills for more than a year. Diuretics, beta-blockers, calcium antagonists and angiotensin-converting enzyme (ACE)-inhibitors have been used as initial antihypertensive drug therapy in clinical trials in

which stroke has been significantly reduced (compared to placebo). Which of these agents is the best initial antihypertensive drug is a controversy that may be resolved when Antihypertensive and Lipid Lowering Heart Attack Trial (ALLHAT) and other large clinical trials are completed. The role of angiotensin II receptor blockers as initial therapy is also being studied; they can be recommended when an angiotensin-converting enzyme ACE-inhibitor causes cough.

For many years neurologists had been reluctant to lower blood pressure after stroke, owing to a fear of increasing the ischemic penumbra. A large clinical trial has recently been reported in which 6105 patients with a stroke or transient ischemic attack in the preceding five years were randomized to an ACE-inhibitor (with or without a diuretic) or matching placebo(s). The mean blood pressure across groups over four years was lower in the group receiving active antihypertensive drugs by 9/4 mmHg (systolic/diastolic), and was accompanied by a 28% reduction in the risk of recurrent stroke. This benefit was seen across all levels of both systolic and diastolic blood pressures. Although the study design did not allow identification of any benefit of the drug regimen that was unrelated to blood pressure lowering, this study provides strong evidence in favor of reducing blood pressure to prevent a second stroke.

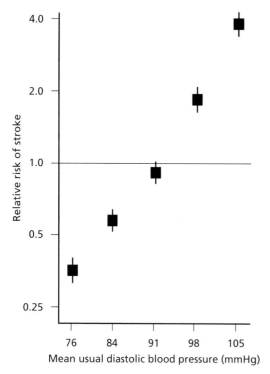

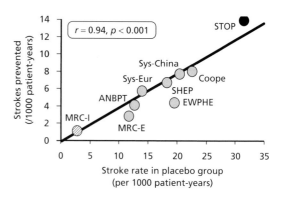

Figure 2 Plot of large primary prevention trials in hypertension showing a significant relationship between baseline risk of stroke (x-axis) vs. absolute benefit of treatment (strokes avoided per 1000 patient-years). MRC-I, Medical Research Council Trial # 1; MRC-E, Medical Research Council Trial in Elderly; ANBPT, Australian National Blood Pressure Trial; Sys-Eur, Systolic Hypertension in Europe Trial; Sys-China, Systolic Hypertension in China Trial; SHEP, Systolic Hypertension in the Elderly Program; Coope, Coope & Warrender Trial; STOP, Swedish Trial in Older Patients

Figure 1 The relative risk of stroke, estimated from the combined results of several prospective observational studies including 843 strokes in over 420 000 people, for each of five categories of diastolic blood pressure (DBP). Estimates of the usual DBP in each baseline DBP category are taken from mean DBP values obtained 4 years after the baseline examination in the Framingham Heart Study. The 95% confidence intervals for the estimates of relative risk are denoted by vertical lines. (Redrawn from Mac Mahon et al.[1])

EVIDENCE

Elevated blood pressure has been recognized as an important risk factor for stroke for nearly 100 years. Large epidemiological and cohort studies have consistently shown a strong graded increase in the risk of stroke as blood pressure increases (Figure 1)[1]. More important than the epidemiological evidence supporting hypertension as a risk factor for stroke is clinical trial evidence proving that antihypertensive treatment is effective in preventing stroke. In

an overview of 14 randomized clinical trials in which more than 37 000 hypertensive people were given either placebo or antihypertensive drug therapy, active treatment reduced the risk of a first stroke by 42 ± 6%[2]. This conclusion has been confirmed and extended by more recent meta-analyses that include several clinical trials that used newer drugs[3]. Significant reductions in stroke have been seen in: hypertensive patients older than 60 years (36 ± 7% reduction in fatal and non-fatal stroke; 39 ± 11% reduction in fatal stroke[4]); hypertensive patients 80 years and older (34% reduction[5]); and patients with 'isolated systolic hypertension' (30% reduction[6]). Recent analyses of data from the Systolic Hypertension in the Elderly Program (SHEP) have shown a beneficial effect of antihypertensive therapy on essentially all subtypes of stroke[7]. A major public health implication of these clinical trials is that, although the usual relative reduction in

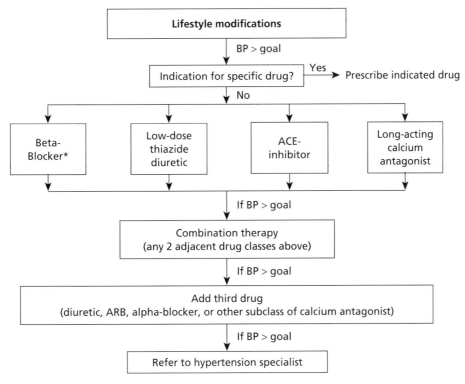

Figure 3 A simple algorithm for choosing antihypertensive drug therapy to prevent a first stroke. *An initial beta-blocker is not recommended for hypertensive patients over age 60. The combination of a diuretic and a calcium antagonist may lower blood pressure, but has not yet been shown in clinical trials to reduce morbidity and mortality in hypertensives. One attractive feature is that, if an initial choice does not lower blood pressure to goal, an appropriate choice for the second-line agent is found adjacent to the initially-chosen drug. ARB, angiotensin II receptor blocker

stroke seen with antihypertensive drug therapy is about 35–40%, the number of strokes prevented depends on the absolute risk to the patient (Figure 2, updated from Lever and Ramsay[8]). Thus, the patients in the Swedish Trial in Older Patients (STOP)-Hypertension trial (average age 77 years; dark circle in Figure 2) had, at baseline, about 12 times the risk of stroke compared to the much younger patients (aged 35–64 years) in the first Medical Research Council trial (cross-hatched circle in Figure 2). These data support the recommendation of the Sixth Report of the Joint National Committee on Prevention, Detection, Evaluation, and Treatment of High Blood Pressure

(JNC VI[9]) to treat high-risk patients intensively, and to attempt to control blood pressure in people at lower risk with less expensive 'lifestyle modifications'.

The independent effect of lifestyle modifications in preventing stroke, if any, will probably never be demonstrated. Lifestyle modifications that can lower blood pressure include (in order of effectiveness): weight loss, sodium restriction, potassium supplementation, alcohol restriction, stress reduction, calcium and/or magnesium supplementation and fish oil consumption. All of these are difficult to maintain over the long term; they are, however, often recommended, as either definitive, adjunctive,

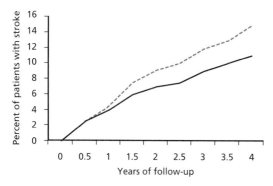

Figure 4 Primary results of the Perindopril Protection Against Recurrent Stroke Study (PROGRESS). Active treatment in this randomized clinical trial consisted of perindopril, with the optional addition of indapamide, based on investigator's preference at randomization. Over the 4 years of follow-up the 28% relative risk reduction in stroke was accompanied by a very significant 9/4 mmHg difference in blood pressure across the randomized groups. Relative risk reduction 28% (95% CI, 17–38%; $p < 0.001$). solid line, active treatment; dashed line, placebo

or alternative therapies to antihypertensive drugs. In the only trial (Treatment of Mild Hypertension Study[10]) that compared lifestyle modifications with and without antihypertensive drug therapy, there was a significantly greater risk of all major events (including stroke) among those randomized to lifestyle modifications alone. Even in the 'mildest' of cases (e.g. average BP 142/91 mmHg), therefore, it may be wise to supplement lifestyle modifications with drug treatment, especially if the target blood pressure is difficult to maintain.

The issue of which antihypertensive drug is most effective in preventing stroke is controversial. Many head-to-head studies of different classes of drugs have been organized; some of the larger ones will soon be reported. In recent meta-analyses, there is a trend toward better stroke prevention with a calcium antagonist than with a diuretic, beta-blocker, or ACE-inhibitor[3], but this benefit may be outweighed by opposite effects on myocardial infarction and heart failure[11]. Since diuretics, calcium

antagonists, and ACE-inhibitors have all been used as initial therapy in successful clinical trials to prevent stroke, any of these may be chosen. The role of beta-blockers and angiotensin II receptor blockers as initial therapy is less clear, as fewer studies have reported prevention of stroke with these drugs as initial therapy. A simple algorithm for choosing antihypertensive drug therapy to prevent a first stroke is shown in Figure 3.

A more important issue than the initial choice of antihypertensive agent is achieving the appropriate blood pressure target. For most hypertensives, a blood pressure goal of less than 140/90 mmHg is recommended, but infrequently achieved. Among Americans aged 18–74, only 27.4% of the hypertensives had a blood pressure lower than 140/90 mmHg in 1988–91[12]. In JNC VI, for the first time, a lower goal blood pressure was recommended for diabetics and patients with renal impairment. The United Kingdom Prospective Diabetes Study #38 supported this recommendation, and showed a significant, 44% lower, stroke rate among the diabetics randomized to the lower goal blood pressure[13]. In the Hypertension Optimal Treatment (HOT) study, the lowest stroke rate was seen in the group randomized to a diastolic blood pressure goal of less than 80 mmHg, but this did not achieve statistical significance[14]. One possible reason that the SHEP trial[7] did not show a significant reduction in stroke among those achieving a systolic blood pressure less than 140 mmHg was that only 1356 of the 4736 patients in the study reached this now-recommended blood pressure level.

Blood pressure lowering during an acute stroke is generally not recommended because of the risk of acutely increasing the ischemic penumbra, and extending the neurological defect[15]. The effects of lowering blood pressure in survivors of either a stroke or transient ischemic attack (TIA) up to five years after the initial neurological event were recently reported[16]. Over the four years of follow-up, active treatment with perindopril, an ACE-inhibitor (with or without indapamide, a diuretic) reduced blood pressure by 9/4 mmHg, stroke by 28% (Figure 4) and all cardiovascular events by 26% (compared to placebo). Similar, significant reductions in recurrent stroke were seen across all entry blood pressures, including in those participants not considered hypertensive at baseline (27% reduction in stroke, 95% CI: 8–42%, $p < 0.01$). These data indicate that, in survivors of acute neurological events, antihypertensive therapy is beneficial in preventing not only another stroke, but cardiovascular events as well.

CONCLUSION

These data from studies of both primary and secondary prevention of stroke using antihypertensive agents corroborate the important conclusion drawn by one of America's leading consumer magazines[17]: 'Controlling hypertension is the single most important step most people can take to prevent stroke'.

RECOMMENDATIONS FOR SPECIFIC LIFESTYLE AND PHARMACOLOGIC INTERVENTIONS

Authoritative recommendations for controlling elevated blood pressure have been disseminated recently by the National Stroke Association[18], the Stroke Council of the American Heart Association[19] and the Joint National Committee on Prevention, Evaluation, and Treatment of High Blood Pressure[9]. These and other policy-making bodies recommend controlling blood pressure to lower than 140/90 mmHg in everyone, lower than 130/80 mm Hg in diabetics and renally-impaired people, and lower than 125/75 mmHg in people with more than a gram of proteinuria per day. Lifestyle modifications are an important adjunctive (and occasionally definitive) treatment, but intensive drug therapy is recommended early during the treatment of high-risk patients. A diuretic, ACE-inhibitor, and perhaps a calcium antagonist can be recommended for primary prevention of stroke, although the latter's effects on heart disease may make it a less desirable option. An ACE-inhibitor can be recommended (especially with a diuretic) for secondary prevention of stroke, based on the Perindopril Protection Against Recurrent Stroke Study (PROGRESS) trial data.

ACKNOWLEDGEMENT

Dedicated to the memory of Vincent DeQuattro, MD, friend, colleague, and world-renowned hypertension expert, who was originally invited to write this chapter.

References

1. MacMahon S, Peto R, Cutler J, *et al*. Blood pressure, stroke, and coronary heart disease. Part 1. Prolonged differences in blood pressure: prospective observational studies corrected for the regression dilution bias. *Lancet* 1990;335: 765–74

2. Collins R, Peto R, MacMahon S, *et al*. Blood pressure, stroke, and coronary heart disease. Part 2. Short-term reductions in blood pressure: overview of randomised drug trials in their epidemiological context. *Lancet* 1990;335: 827–38

3. Blood Pressure Lowering Treatment Trialists' Collaborative. Effects of ACE-inhibitors, calcium antagonists, and other blood-pressure-lowering drugs: results of prospectively designed overviews of randomised trials. *Lancet* 2000;356: 1955–64

4. Elliott WJ. Treatment of hypertension in the elderly: an updated meta-analysis (abstract). *Am J Hypertens* 2001;14:145A

5. Gueyffier F, Bulpitt C, Boissel JP, *et al.* Antihypertensive drugs in very old people: a subgroup meta-analysis of randomised clinical trials. INDANA Group. *Lancet* 1999;353: 793–6

6. Staessen JA, Gasowski J, Wang JG, *et al.* Risks of untreated and treated isolated systolic hypertension in the elderly: meta-analysis of outcome trials. *Lancet* 2000;355:865–72

7. Perry HM Jr, Davis BR, Price TR, *et al.* Effect of treating isolated systolic hypertension on the risk of developing various types and subtypes of stroke. The Systolic Hypertension in the Elderly Program (SHEP). *J Am Med Assoc,* 2000; 284:465–71

8. Lever AF, Ramsay LE. Treatment of hypertension in the elderly. *J Hypertens* 1995;13: 571–9

9. The Sixth Report of the Joint National Committee on Prevention, Detection, Evaluation, and Treatment of High Blood Pressure (JNC VI). *Arch Intern Med* 1997;157: 2414–46

10. Neaton JD, Grimm RH Jr, Prineas RJ, *et al.* Treatment of Mild Hypertension Study: final results. *J Am Med Assoc* 1993;270:713–24

11. Pahor M, Psaty BM, Alderman MH, *et al.* Blood-pressure lowering treatment [letter]. *Lancet* 2001;358:152–3

12. Burt VL, Cutler JA, Higgins M, *et al.* Trends in the prevalence, awareness, treatment, and control of hypertension in the adult US population. Data from the health examination surveys, 1960 to 1991. *Hypertension* 1995;26:60–9

13. Turner R, Holman R, Stratton I, *et al.* for the United Kingdom Prospective Diabetes Study Group. Tight blood pressure control and risk of macrovascular and microvascular complications in type 2 diabetes: UKPDS 38. *Br Med J* 1998;317:707–13

14. Hansson L, Zanchetti A, Julius S, *et al.,* on behalf of the HOT Study Group. Effects of intensive blood pressure lowering and low-dose aspirin in patients with hypertension: principal results of the Hypertension Optimal Treatment (HOT) randomised trial. *Lancet* 1998;351: 1755–62

15. Hankey GJ, Warlow CP. Treatment and secondary prevention of stroke: evidence, costs, and effects on individuals and populations. *Lancet* 1999;354:1457–63

16. Randomised trial of a perindopril-based blood-pressure-lowering regimen among 6105 individuals with previous stroke or transient ischaemic attack. PROGRESS Collaborative Group. *Lancet* 2001;358:1033–41

17. 'Brain attack' breakthrough: Doctors can stop a stroke—if you get help fast. *Consumer Reports*, July 1999:62–3

18. Gorelick PB, Sacco RL, Smith DB, *et al.* Prevention of a first stroke: a review of guidelines and a multidisciplinary consensus statement from the National Stroke Association. *J Am Med Assoc* 1999;281:1112–20

19. Goldstein LB, Adams R, Becker K, *et al.* Primary prevention of ischemic stroke: a statement for healthcare professionals from the Stroke Council of the American Heart Association. *Circulation* 2001;103:163–82

II. Smoking cessation

Philip B. Gorelick, MD, MPH, FACP

SMOKING CESSATION

Background information

Cigarette smoking and other forms of tobacco use remain a major public health problem. Cigarette smoking has been cited as the leading preventable cause of mortality in the United States and is a substantial contributor to the economic costs related to cardiovascular and pulmonary diseases[1]. It is estimated that, in the United States, tobacco use will claim the lives of 430 000 direct users and up to 67 000 individuals who are exposed to tobacco smoke in the environment each year[2]. Worldwide, up to 4 million persons may die of tobacco-related illness annually, and this figure may increase to 10 million persons within the next several decades[3]. The majority of these deaths will occur in developing countries. China, the largest tobacco-producing country in the world, has over 300 million smokers, the largest of any country in the world[4,5]. It is estimated that at least 500 000 persons die from smoking in China annually.

Although it is estimated that the prevalence of smoking among adults in the United States will decline from its current level of 25% to 15–16% by the second quarter of this century[6], the prevalence of smoking remains high among 18–24-year-olds (28.7%) and 25–44 year olds (28.6%)[7]. Furthermore, the percentage of cigarette smokers among high school students in the United States increased from 12.7% in 1991 to 16.8% in 1999[8]. The Surgeon General reports that the highest prevalence of tobacco use for adults in the United States occurs among American Indians and Alaska natives, with the next highest groups being African-Americans and South-east Asian men. Asian American and Hispanic women have the lowest prevalence of tobacco use[9].

The FDA tobacco rule makes it a federal violation to sell cigarettes or chewing tobacco to anyone younger than 18 years of age (FDA Medical Bulletin, Summer 1998). Even though it is illegal, young persons continue to be exposed to a barrage of cigarette advertising[10]. The negative effects of such advertising campaigns may be especially detrimental to Blacks or other groups who have higher cotinine blood levels. Cotinine is an indicator of higher nicotine intake or differential pharmacokinetics, and may serve as a marker of difficulties in quitting smoking as well as higher rates of smoking-related diseases such as lung cancer[11]. To help combat this and other adverse effects of smoking, substantial and sustained government-supported public health efforts are needed to offset the forces of the tobacco marketing lobby.

Epidemiology

The epidemiology of smoking is discussed in more detail in Chapter 3. Overall, there is about a 1.5–2.0-fold greater relative risk of stroke among smokers[12,13]. The population attributable risk from smoking is estimated to be 12–18%[13]. Environmental tobacco smoke may be associated with a relative risk of stroke as high as 1.82[14]. After cessation of smoking, the risk of stroke may return to that of the non-smoking individual within 2–5 years. Mechanisms by which smoking may lead to stroke and other cardiovascular diseases include enhancement of the atherosclerotic process, increases in coagulability, blood viscosity, and fibrinogen levels, increased platelet aggregation, elevation of blood pressure, increase in hematocrit and decrease of high-density lipoprotein cholesterol[12,13].

Smoking cessation strategies

The main strategies to affect cigarette smoking cessation include counseling, nicotine replacement therapy and bupropion hydrochloride[12,13,15]. Hard-core smokers (i.e. heavy smokers with a history of unsuccessful quitting) remain a substantial challenge to smoking cessation programs, as they may underestimate the consequences of cigarette exposure, are unaffected by public health messages that stress the benefit of stopping tobacco use, do not choose to quit or are discouraged by past failures[16]. For those smokers who are interested in giving up smoking, counseling by physicians and nurses and behavioral interventions (individual counseling or group therapy) may be effective. According to the Cochrane Tobacco Addiction Review Group[15], even simple advice given by physicians increases quit rates by a weighted odds ratio of 1.7. Similarly, counseling given by nurses enhances stopping rates. In the same Cochrane review, individual counseling or group therapy was also deemed effective. Physician and nurse counseling was more effective than brief advice, usual care, or distribution of self-help materials. Although physician-delivered interventions are effective[17,18], physicians often do not engage their smoking patients in discussions about smoking and, generally, are not trained in medical school to treat nicotine dependence[19,20]. Information is available online at *www.surgeongeneral.gov/tobacco*[21] regarding effective strategies to identify smoking status, to provide 'stop-smoking' advice and to assess the smoker's readiness to take the appropriate action, as well as recommendations for brief counseling and follow-up.

According to the Cochrane Tobacco Addiction Review Group[15], nicotine replacement treatment, in all forms, is effective for smoking cessation by a weighted odds ratio of 1.7. In the year 2000, a systematic review of evidence by the United States Public Health Service (USPHS) identified four nicotine replacement products as being effective: gum, patch, inhaler, and nasal spray[22]. Bupropion, an antidepressant, was also found to be effective by this group. According to the Cochrane Group[15], the antidepressants bupropion and nortriptyline increased smoking cessation rates. Although clonidine showed effectiveness, its use was limited by the side-effect profile, whereas acupuncture, hypnotherapy and exercise showed limited effectiveness. Furthermore, treatment of nicotine dependence is cost-effective[12,23].

Recommendations for smoking cessation

Overall, both the Cochrane Group and the USPHS reports conclude that all forms of nicotine replacement therapy are about equally effective; sustained-release bupropion[24] is also efficacious; all forms of counseling are effective; self-help materials are of limited usefulness; and anxiolytic agents are not effective[25]. The United States Public Health Service report favored combination nicotine replacement therapy, and aversive therapy, whereas the Cochrane Group report did not favor these modalities. Therefore, administration of the mainstays for smoking cessation – counseling, nicotine replacement therapy and bupropion – should be individualized for each patient guided by the patient's past experience, preference for therapy, and the adverse event profile of the pharmacologic agents that are being considered for use[26]. New strategies are needed as the abstinence rate after 12 months with combination therapy (e.g. counseling, nicotine-patch and bupropion) may be only 22.5% (*vs.* placebo, 5.6%; nicotine-patch, 9.8%; and bupropion, 18.4%)[24]. Public health policy initiatives are another important way to discourage smoking among youths and young adults, and to provide education about the dangers of smoking to all tobacco users.

References

1. Kannel WB. Curbing the tobacco menace (editional). *Circulation* 1997;96:1070
2. Houston T, Kaufman NJ. Tobacco control in the 21st century. Searching for answers in a sea of change (editorial). *J Am Med Assoc* 2000;284:752–3
3. Brundtland GH. Achieving worldwide tobacco control (editorial). *J Am Med Assoc* 2000;284:750–1
4. Lam TH, He Y, Li LS, *et al.* Mortality attributable to cigarette smoking in China. *J Am Med Assoc* 1997;278:1505–8
5. Yang G, Fan L, Tan J, *et al.* Smoking in China. Findings of the 1996 National Prevalence Survey. *J Am Med Assoc* 1999;282:1247–53
6. Mendez D, Warner KE, Courant PN. Has smoking cessation ceased? Expected trends in the prevalence of smoking in the United States. *Am J Epidemiol* 1998;148:249–58
7. Cigarette smoking among adults – United States, 1997. Reprinted in *J Am Med Assoc* 1999;282:2115–16 from *MMWR* 1999;48:993–6
8. Trends in cigarette smoking among high school students – United States, 1991–1999. Reprinted in *J Am Med Assoc* 2000;284:1507–8 from *MMWR* 2000;49:755–8
9. Publication of Surgeon Generals's Report on Smoking and Health. Reprinted from *J Am Med Assoc* 1998;279:1776 from *MMWR* 1998;47:335–6
10. King C III, Siegel M. The master settlement agreement with the tobacco industry and cigarette advertising in magazines. *N Engl J Med* 2001;345:504–11
11. Caraballo RS, Giovino GA, Pechacek TF, *et al.* Racial and ethnic differences in serum cotinine levels of cigarette smokers. Third National Health and Nutrition Examination Survey, 1988–1991. *J Am Med Assoc* 1998;280:135–9
12. Gorelick PB, Sacco RL, Smith DB, *et al.* Prevention of a first stroke. A review and a multidisciplinary consensus statement from the National Stroke Association. *J Am Med Assoc* 1999;281:1112–20
13. Goldstein LB, Adams R, Becker K, *et al.* Primary prevention of ischemic stroke. A statement for healthcare professionals from the Stroke Council of the American Heart Association. *Stroke* 2001;32:280–99
14. Bonita R, Duncan J, Truelsen T, *et al.* Passive smoking as well as active smoking increases the risk of acute stroke. *Tob Control* 1999;8:156–60
15. Lancaster T, Stead L, Silagy C, Sowden A, for the Cochrane Tobacco Addiction Review Group. Effectiveness of interventions to help people stop smoking: findings from the Cochrane Library. *Br Med J* 2000;321:355–8
16. Emery S, Gilpin EA, Ake C, *et al.* Characterizing and identifying "hard-core" smokers: implications for further reducing smoking prevalence. *Am J Pub Health* 2000;90:387–94
17. Der DE, You Y-Q, Wolter TD, *et al.* A free smoking intervention clinic initiated by medical students. *Mayo Clin Proc* 2001;76:144–51
18. Ockene JK. Physician-delivered interventions for smoking cessation: strategies for increasing effectiveness. *Prev Med* 1987;16:723–37
19. Goldstein MG, Niaura R, Willey-Lessne C, *et al.* Physicians counseling smokers. A population-based survey of patients' perceptions of health care provider-delivered smoking cessation

interventions. *Arch Intern Med* 1997;157: 1313–19

20. Ferry LH, Grissino LM, Runfola PS. Tobacco dependence curricula in US undergraduate medical education. *J Am Med Assoc* 1999;282: 825–9

21. Rigotti NA, Thorndike AN. Reducing the health burden of tobacco use: what's the doctor's role? *Mayo Clin Proc* 2001;76:121–3

22. Tobacco Use and Dependence Clinical Practice Guideline Panel, Staff and Consortium Representatives. A clinical practice guideline for treating tobacco use and dependence: a US Public Health Service report. *J Am Med Assoc* 2000;283:3244–54

23. Croghan IT, Offord KP, Evans RW, *et al.* Cost-effectiveness of treating nicotine dependence: the Mayo Clinic experience. *Mayo Clin Proc* 1997;72:917–24

24. Jorenby DE, Leischow SJ, Nides MA, *et al.* A controlled trial of sustained-release bupropion, a nicotine patch, or both for smoking cessation. *N Engl J Med* 1999;340:685–91

25. Luckmann R. Commentary. *ACP Journal Club* 2001 March/April:60

26. Hughes JR, Goldstein MG, Hurt RD, Shiffman S. Recent advances in the pharmacotherapy of smoking. *J Am Med Assoc* 1999;281:72–6

Chapter 17

Hyperlipidemia and diabetes mellitus

Ambika Babu, MD, Chakravarthy Kannan, MD, and Theodore Mazzone, MD

INTRODUCTION

Stroke is a common cause of disability and death[1], but it can be prevented. The prevention advisory board of the National Stroke Association has recently identified a group of potent, yet modifiable, risk factors for stroke that include hyperlipidemia and diabetes mellitus[2]. In the past, considerable controversy existed regarding the relationship of hyperlipidemia to stroke. However, important recent data appear to confirm a relationship between the two. Middle-aged men from Finland who died of stroke had higher cholesterol levels when compared to subjects who were alive at the end of the study[3]. The Multiple Risk Factor Intervention Trial (MRFIT) study[4] and the Honolulu Heart Study[5] have clearly demonstrated that higher cholesterol levels are associated with an increase in stroke mortality. In the MRFIT study the adjusted relative risk for developing a non-hemorrhagic stroke was 1.8 when serum cholesterol levels were between 240 and 279 mg/dl and 2.6 for levels greater than 280 mg/dl compared to subjects with total cholesterol levels less than 160 mg/dl. In addition, an independent association between low-density liprotein cholesterol (LDL-C) and risk of dementia with stroke has been reported[6]. Recently a protective role of high-density lipoprotein cholesterol (HDL-C) in reduction of stroke risk, similar to that in coronary artery disease (CAD), has been found. HDL-C level was inversely associated with the risk for non-fatal stroke in both smokers and non-smokers, and was apparent more in lean men, in men with CAD and in patients with hypertension (HTN)[7]. In the Northern Manhattan Stroke (NOMAS) study, a similar finding of reduced risk for ischemic stroke was observed in elderly subjects of varying ethnic backgrounds with higher levels of HDL-C[8].

The incidence of stroke in diabetics is 2–3 times higher than in non-diabetics and stroke is a major macrovascular complication of diabetes. Stroke in diabetic patients is seen at a younger age, and is associated with a higher mortality and a slower recovery. In a prospective study of middle-aged subjects followed over a mean of 16.4 years, men who had diabetes at baseline had a sixfold increased risk of death from any cause compared to men who developed diabetes during follow-up. The relative risk in women who were diabetic at baseline, followed for a similar length of time, was 8.2 compared to women who developed diabetes later. When the specific cause of mortality was analyzed, 16% of stroke deaths in men and 33% in women were attributed to diabetes[3]. In the Honolulu Heart Study, asymptomatic subjects with high normal fasting glucose or impaired glucose tolerance showed an increased risk for thromboembolic stroke[5]. In another study from Finland, each increase in blood glucose level of 1 mmol/l increased the relative risk of fatal stroke by 1.13[9].

PATHOPHYSIOLOGICAL CONSIDERATIONS

Hyperlipidemia

Increased circulating levels of non-HDL cholesterol (i.e LDL and VLDL) have been postulated to lead to increased retention and modification (e.g. oxidation or aggregation) of cholesterol-containing particles in the vessel wall. Retention of these modified lipoproteins may underlie many of the features of atherosclerotic plaques. Modified LDL in the vessel wall is chemotactic for circulating leukocytes, helping to promote a local inflammatory reaction. The local production of cytokines, growth factors and proteases follows. The local accumulation of these factors produces growth of plaque lesions by stimulating cell growth, extracellular matrix production and a prothrombotic environment. These same factors produce endothelial cell dysfunction and reduced production of endothelial nitric oxide. An increased amount of cholesterol ester in vessel wall plaques is associated with an increased tendency to fissure and rupture with a resultant superimposed clot. HDL may oppose initiation and growth of the atherosclerotic plaque by mobilizing lipoprotein-derived cholesterol out of the vessel wall back to the liver for catabolism to bile acids.

Diabetes mellitus

The mechanism by which diabetes accelerates atherogenesis remains controversial. The lipoprotein abnormalities that accompany diabetes, specifically type 2 diabetes, certainly contribute (increased non-HDL cholesterol, low HDL cholesterol). Hypertension, another potent cardiovascular risk factor, is also common in type 2 diabetes patients. Insulin resistance, highly prevalent in patients with type 2 diabetes, produces a systemic procoagulant environment including increased platelet aggregation, increased fibrinogen and plasminogen activator inhibitor-1 (PAI-1) levels. Potential direct roles for hyperinsulinemia or hyperglycemia on atherogenesis are more controversial. Insulin stimulates the growth of arterial wall cells *in vitro*[10]. Hyperglycemia leads to the accumulation of glycosylated proteins in the vessel wall, and these glycosylated proteins are recognized by receptors on vessel wall cells leading to pro-inflammatory functions[11]. Coronary atherectomy specimens from diabetic patients when compared with those from non-diabetics show a larger total area occupied by lipid rich atheroma (7% *vs.* 2%) and by macrophages (22% *vs.* 12%), and an increased tendency for thrombus formation (62% *vs.* 40%)[12].

RISK REDUCTION

Hyperlipidemia

The effectiveness of lipid lowering therapy for the reduction of stroke risk can be evaluated from two perspectives – clinical event rate reduction or improvement in surrogate markers, specifically carotid intimal-medial thickness (IMT). A meta-analysis of 41 randomized controlled trials involving a total of 80 000 subjects followed for an average of four years showed a 16% reduction in the incidence of fatal and non-fatal strokes among patients treated with lipid lowering therapy compared to controls[13]. Other meta-analyses of statin-only trials showed an even greater reduction in risk that ranged from 23 to 30%[13–15]. These observations and data from animal experiments suggest that statins may reduce stroke by working directly at the vessel wall as well as by lowering cholesterol levels.

There have been a number of major secondary prevention trials in which stroke was a secondary end point. These include the Scandinavian Simvastatin Survival Study (4S), the Cholesterol and Recurrent Events (CARE) study, the Long-term Intervention with Pravastatin in Ischemic Disease (LIPID) study and the Veterans Administration – HDL Intervention Study (VA-HIT) trial. In the 4S trial[16] patients treated with simvastatin showed a statistically significant reduction of new or worsening carotid bruit along with a 28% reduction in the risk of fatal and non-fatal strokes. In the CARE study[17] a similar population of patients treated with pravastatin showed a 32% reduction in fatal and non-fatal strokes, and in the LIPID trial[18] treatment with pravastatin produced an 18% reduction in total cholesterol (TC), a 25% reduction in LDL-C, an 11% reduction in triglycerides (TG) and a 5% increase in HDL-C, associated with a 19% reduction in the incidence of stroke compared to the placebo group. The VA-HIT study[19] used fibrates to treat patients with a HDL-C less than 40 mg/dl and an LDL-C under 140 mg/dl. Treatment with gemfibrozil led to a 25% relative risk reduction for strokes, a 59% reduction for transient ischemic attack (TIA) and a 65% reduction in the frequency of carotid endarterectomy.

The clinical benefit of lipid lowering is also supported by observations that statins can reverse the progression of ultrasonographically assessed carotid IMT. This has been demonstrated in multiple major randomized controlled trials, including Monitored Atherosclerosis Regression Study (MARS), Cholesterone Lowering Atherosclerosis Study (CLAS), Pravastatin, Lipids and Atherosclerosis in the Carotid Arteries (PLAC-2), Asymptomatic Carotid Artery Progression Study (ACAPS), and LIPID trials. The MARS trial[20] used lovastatin

and diet, while colestipol–niacin was used in the CLAS study[21]. Both included only patients with early pre-intrusive atherosclerosis, a stage where atherosclerosis is limited to the arterial wall without significant intrusion into the arterial lumen. In the CLAS trial the rate of progression of carotid IMT in the treated group was –0.026 mm/yr compared to 0.018 mm/yr in the placebo group. The MARS trial reported similar results (–0.028 mm/yr and 0.015 mm/yr in treated versus untreated). At the end of four years a difference of 0.062 mm between patients treated with pravastatin and placebo was reported in the LIPID arteriosclerosis sub study[22]. The PLAC-2[23] and the ACAPS[24] trials included patients with ultrasonographically demonstrable carotid artery disease with lesions of at least 1.3 mm and 1.5 mm, respectively. PLAC-2 reported a significant 35% reduction in the progression of carotid IMT in the distal common carotid artery in the pravastatin-treated group with CAD over three years. In the ACAPS study, asymptomatic patients with modest hypercholesterolemia and increased carotid IMT were treated with lovastatin and warfarin. The progression rate was –0.009 mm/yr in the treated group versus 0.006 mm/yr in the placebo group. This was the first trial to demonstrate the benefit of lipid lowering therapy in asymptomatic subjects who had baseline LDL-C below recommended National Cholesterol Education Program (NCEP) treatment guidelines. A similar beneficial effect of lipid lowering on carotid atherosclerosis in asymptomatic subjects with moderate hypercholesterolemia was reported in the Carotid Atherosclerosis Italian Ultrasound (CAIUS) study[25].

Diabetes mellitus

Many aspects of the diabetic state may increase the risk for stroke, therefore reduction of the risk in these patients must utilize a multifactorial approach. This section will examine the role for glucose control, blood pressure control, lipid control and therapeutic lifestyle changes.

Glucose control

The Framingham[26] and other epidemiological studies show that diabetes increases the risk for stroke by approximately 2–3-fold, but very few studies have evaluated risk reduction by lowering blood glucose levels. Earlier prospective studies had implied that hyperglycemia predicts stroke events more strongly than it does CAD events[27]. The UK Prospective Diabetes Study (UKPDS) is one of the largest and longest studies on patients with type 2 diabetes[28]. Patients were assigned to either intensive glucose control or conventional control, with an 11% difference in HbA1c between the two groups over ten years. Even though there was a reduction in total diabetic complication endpoints in the intensively treated group, there was a non-significant change in stroke incidence, suggesting that intensive glycemic control does not reduce the risk of stroke. The results were similar in the Lehigh Valley study, which involved a large cohort of individuals with an initial stroke who were followed prospectively twice annually for stroke recurrence and monitored for diabetic control with HbA1c[29]. This is in accordance with another analysis of the UKPDS study that showed a lack of association between hyperglycemia and the risk of stroke[30].

However, an independent association between high glyco-hemoglobin levels and stroke is well documented[31]. In the Multicenter Isradipine Divretic Atherosclerosis Study (MIDAS) trial[32] the relative risk for major cardiovascular events including stroke was 2.8 for HbA1c of more than 6.7% compared to 1.1 when the HbA1c was less than 6.7%. The Helsinki Policemen Study[33] followed healthy middle-aged men over a period of 22 years. At 5, 10, 15 and 22 years follow-up there were 7, 21, 33 and 70 fatal and non-fatal strokes respectively. When compared to the reference group, men with strokes were older, had higher body mass index (BMI), and higher blood pressure and TG levels. Their fasting glucose, 2-hour post-load glucose and area under the curve insulin levels were higher compared to those of controls. The Epidemiology of Diabetes Interventions and Complications (EDIC) trial[34] represents a follow-up study of the Diabetes Control and Complications Study (DCCT) cohort, where carotid IMT was measured one and six years after the DCCT study ended. The common carotid IMT difference between year six and year one was 0.026 mm in the intensively-treated group and 0.040 mm in the conventionally-treated group, while the internal carotid IMT was 0.078 mm and 0.096 mm respectively. It was concluded that intensive glycemic treatment retarded carotid atherosclerosis in the DCCT cohort.

A significant proportion of patients with acute stroke are hyperglycemic. Of these, 20–30% have either previously unrecognized diabetes or impaired glucose tolerance[35]. There is considerable debate regarding the significance of hyperglycemia. It may represent an acute stress response to cerebral ischemia, and is often considered an independent predictor of poor outcome[36]. The Diabetes and Insulin-Glucose Infusion in Acute Myocardial Infarctions (DIGAMI) study[37] has clearly established hyperglycemia as a risk factor for poor outcome following MI, and further suggested that tight control of blood sugar in the peri-infarct period can improve outcomes. While there is evidence to suggest that hyperglycemia perpetuates the neurologic damage after an acute stroke, the benefits of lowering blood glucose levels during the acute phase of a stroke remain unknown.

The Glucose Insulin in Stroke Trial (GIST)[38], a randomized controlled trial, was designed to determine whether glucose/insulin-induced euglycemia in patients with acute stroke can improve the post-stroke outcome. The group titrated with insulin/glucose infusion had lower plasma glucose levels compared to the control group, and a four-week mortality of 28% compared to 32% in the control group.

Hypertension in diabetes

Hypertension (HTN) is common in patients with diabetes, with a prevalence of 40 to 60%[39]. The Systolic Hypertension in Europe (Syst-Eur) trial[40,41] and the Systolic Hypertension in the Elderly Program (SHEP)[42,43] showed a reduction in fatal and non-fatal strokes by 42% and 36%, respectively, with control of systolic HTN. When HTN coexists with diabetes the risk of stroke increases dramatically; about 75% of all diabetes related complications are attributed to HTN. This observation has led to recommendations for more aggressive lowering of blood pressure (BP) by the Joint National Committee on Prevention, Detection, Evaluation and Treatment of High Blood Pressure (JNC-6) to less than 130/85 mmHg[44].

The Syst-Eur trial included 492 diabetics and the SHEP trial included 583; these represented 10.5% and 12.3% of their study cohorts, respectively. Active treatment of HTN in the Syst-Eur trial was associated with a 73% decrease in fatal and non-fatal strokes in diabetic patients compared to a 38% decrease in the non-diabetic group. The SHEP trial reported a 50% absolute risk reduction in major cardiovascular events, including strokes, in diabetics compared to non-diabetics. The UKPDS observed that a decrease in systolic pressure by 10 mmHg was associated with a reduction in risk of 12% for any complication related to diabetes, 11% for MI and 13% for microvascular complications[45]. In 1148 patients with HTN in the UKPDS trial[39] who were randomly assigned to tight BP control (< 150/85 mmHg) *vs.* less tight control (< 180/105 mmHg) there was a 44% relative risk reduction for fatal and non-fatal strokes with tight blood pressure control.

The Hypertension Optimal Treatment (HOT) trial assessed whether tighter control of diastolic BP (< 80 mmHg) would benefit patients with diabetes[46]. The best results among 1501 diabetics were seen in those randomized to a diastolic BP goal of less than 80 mmHg. In this group the stroke reduction was 30% compared to the group with diastolic BP no greater than 90 mmHg. Recent evidence from the Heart Outcomes Prevention Evaluation (HOPE) trial has also conclusively demonstrated that diabetics benefit from BP reduction[47]. Diabetics on ramipril demonstrated a 33% reduction in stroke compared to diabetics in the placebo group.

Hyperlipidemia in diabetes

The most common pattern of dyslipidemia in type 2 diabetes is increased levels of TC, LDL-C and TG and low HDL-C. Even if the LDL-C level is normal there is a preponderance of small dense LDL-C which may have increased atherogenicity. New NCEP-3 guidelines have classified diabetes as a CAD equivalent and reco mended lowering LDL-C to less than 100 mg/dl in diabetic patients[48]. There have been no clinical trials prospectively designed to assess the effects of lipid lowering therapy exclusively in diabetics. Most major trials, however, have included patients with diabetes and retrospective subgroup analyses have shown that diabetic patients demonstrate reduced cardiovascular end-points with lipid lowering therapy. In a subgroup analysis of diabetics in the 4S study there was a reduction in the risk for major cerebrovascular events, although it was not statistically significant[49]. In the VA-HIT trial 627 of 2531 patients had diabetes[50]. This group benefited from therapy, with a 24% risk reduction for the expanded endpoint of fatal and non-fatal MI and definite strokes.

Lifestyle factors in diabetes

Lifestyle modification in diabetes has always been the first-line approach to metabolic control and risk factor reduction. Smoking is associated with accelerated carotid artery disease and an increased incidence of ischemic strokes. Arteriosclerosis obliterans in type 2 diabetics is associated with longer duration of diabetes, higher incidence of nicotine use, a higher prevalence of CAD and a higher incidence of insulin requirement and a more severe insulin resistance compared to diabetics without arteriosclerosis obliterans[51]. In white patients with cerebral ischemia smoking was independently associated with severe carotid disease in both the NOMAS and Berlin Cerebral Ischemia Databank (BCID) trials[52].

In patients with type 2 diabetes the insulin resistance syndrome is considered an important risk factor for diabetic complications. The beneficial effects of exercise and weight loss on metabolic control may relate to improvements in insulin sensitivity. In the Finnish diabetes prevention study group[53] patients with impaired glucose tolerance, when given counseling regarding diet and increased physical activity over 3.2 years, had a lower incidence of developing diabetes compared to the control group (11% *vs.* 23% respectively)[53]. Older, overweight African-American diabetic patients randomized to weight reduction and increased physical activity were twice as likely to have a 1% decrease in HbA1c compared to the control group[54]. The Aerobics Center Longitudinal Study (ACLS) study, a prospective observational trial, reported 180 deaths in 1263 men with type 2 diabetes over an average follow up of 11.7 years[55]. This study evaluated the relationship between physical fitness and mortality. Based on exercise testing, expressed as maximal metabolic units (MET), there was a 2.1-fold higher risk of death in unfit men compared to fit men at baseline. Each 1 MET increase in cardiorespiratory fitness was associated with a 25% lower risk for all-cause mortality. In another report 5125 female nurses with diabetes had a total of 98 strokes over a 14-year follow up. In this study the degree of physical activity was inversely related to the risk for ischemic strokes[56].

RECOMMENDATIONS

Based on the large body of evidence discussed above, recommendations for managing cardiovascular risk in hyperlipidemic and diabetic patients have been developed. In patients with hyperlipidemia, the current recommendations of the Adult Treatment Panel III define three categories of risk that modify LDL cholesterol goals[48]. For the highest risk patients (those with diabetes, evidence of vascular disease, or coronary heart disease risk equivalents) an LDL cholesterol goal of less than 100 mg/dl is recommended. For those patients at intermediate risk (those with multiple risk factors) an LDL cholesterol goal of less than 130 mg/dl is the target. For the treatment of elevated LDL cholesterol the statins are now the most widely used drugs. In addition to lowering LDL cholesterol level, these drugs can also lower triglyceride levels in most patients, and can modestly raise HDL cholesterol level. The American Diabetes Association produces recommendations for diabetics for modifying cardiovascular risk which are updated yearly[57]. The current recommendations call for the aggressive management of hypertension to a blood pressure goal of less than 130/80 mmHg. At the present time angiotensin converting enzyme inhibitors and angiotensin II receptor blockers are preferred for the treatment of hypertension in patients with diabetes. The treatment of diabetic dyslipidemia should have an LDL cholesterol target level of less than 100 mg/dl as (noted above). In addition, the current recommendations call for an HDL cholesterol level higher than 45 mg/dl (higher than 55 mg/dl in women) and a triglyceride level of less than 200 mg/dl. For the treatment of diabetic dyslipidemia, the statin class of drugs is, again, the most frequently utilized. With respect to glucose control, the current guidelines recommend a HbA1c level of less than 7%, given that the normal range is less than 6%. In patients with type 2 diabetes, insulin, oral hypoglycemics, or a combination of agents may be used to obtain this goal.

CONCLUSIONS

There is now strong evidence from clinical trials that treatment of hyperlipidemia and aggressive risk factor modification for diabetic patients (including aggressive treatment of hypertension and hyperlipidemia) can significantly reduce the risk of stroke. The role of glucose control for stroke prevention in diabetic patients remains less clear. In hyperlipidemic and diabetic patients, the highly favorable benefit/risk and benefit/cost ratios for therapeutic lifestyle modification (including avoidance of smoking and obesity, and increasing physical activity) are worth emphasizing. With appropriate diligence and compliance the information and therapeutic tools now available will allow clinicians to significantly and favorably affect the risk for stroke in patients with hyperlipidemia or diabetes.

References

1. American Heart Association. *1998 Heart and Stroke Statistical Update*. American Heart Association, 1997
2. Gorelick PB, Sacco RL, Smith DB, *et al*. Prevention of a first stroke: a review of guidelines and a multidisciplinary consensus statement from the National Stroke Association. *J Am Med Assoc* 1999;281:1112–20
3. Tuomilehto J, Rastenyte D, Jousilahti P, *et al*. Diabetes mellitus as a risk factor for death from stroke: prospective study of the middle aged Finnish population. *Stroke* 1996;27:210–15
4. Iso H, Jacobs DR, Wentworth D, *et al*. Serum cholesterol levels and six-year mortality from stroke in 350,977 men screened for the multiple risk factor intervention trial. *N Engl J Med* 1989;320:904–10
5. Burchfiel CM, Curb JD, Rodriguez BL, *et al*. Glucose intolerance and 22-year stroke incidence: the Honolulu Heart Program. *Stroke* 1994;25:951–7
6. Moroney JT, Tang MX, Berglund L, *et al*. Low-density lipoprotein cholesterol and the risk of dementia with stroke. *J Am Med Assoc* 1999; 282:254–60
7. Wannamethee SG, Shaper AG, Ebrahim S. HDL-cholesterol, total cholesterol, and the risk of stroke in middle-aged British men. *Stroke* 2000;31:1882–8
8. Sacco RL, Benson RT, Kargman DE, *et al*. High-density lipoprotein cholesterol and ischemic stroke in the elderly. The Northern Manhattan Stroke Study. *J Am Med Assoc* 2001;285: 2729–35

9. Hahein LL, Holme I, Hjermann I, *et al*. Non fasting serum glucose and the risk of fatal stroke in diabetic and nondiabetic subjects. 18-year follow-up of the Oslo study. *Stroke* 1995;26:774–7
10. Stout RW. Insulin and atheroma – 20-year perspective. *Diabetes Care* 1990;13:631–54
11. Vlassara H. Recent progress in advanced glycation end products and diabetic complications. *Diabetes* 1997;46(S1):19–25
12. Moreno PR, Murcia AM, Palacios IF, *et al*. Coronary composition and macrophage infiltration in atherectomy specimens from patients with diabetes mellitus. *Circulation* 2000;102: 2180–4
13. Di Mascio R, Marchioli R, Tognoni G. Cholesterol reduction and stroke occurrence: an overview of randomized clinical trials. *Cerebrovasc Dis* 2000;10:85–92
14. Blauw GJ, Lagaay AM, Smelt AH, *et al*. Stroke, statins, and cholesterol: a meta-analysis of randomized, placebo controlled, double-blind trials with HMG-CoA reductase inhibitors. *Stroke* 1997;28:946–50
15. Crouse JR, Byington RP, Hoen HM, *et al*. Reductase inhibitor monotherapy and stroke prevention. *Arch Intern Med* 1997;157:1305–10
16. Pedersen TR, Kjekshus J, Pyorala K, *et al*. Effect of simvastatin on ischemic signs and symptoms in the Scandinavian Simvastatin Survival Study (4S). *Am J Cardiol* 1998;81:333–5
17. Plehn JF, Davis BR, Sacks FM, *et al*. Reduction of stroke incidence after myocardial infarction

with pravastatin: The Cholesterol and Recurrent Events (CARE) Study. *Circulation* 1999;99: 216–23

18. The Long-term Intervention with Pravastatin in Ischemic Disease (LIPID) Study Group. Prevention of cardiovascular events and death with pravastatin in patients with coronary heart disease and a broad range of initial cholesterol levels. *N Engl J Med* 1998;339: 1349–57

19. Rubins HB, Robins SJ, Collins D, *et al.* Gemfibrozil for the secondary prevention of coronary heart disease in men with low levels of high-density lipoprotein cholesterol. *N Engl J Med* 1999;341:410–18

20. Hodis HN, Mack WJ, LaBree L, *et al.* Reduction in carotid wall thickness using lovastatin and dietary therapy. A randomized, controlled clinical trial. *Ann Intern Med* 1996;124: 548–56

21. Mack WJ, Selzer RH, Hodis HN, *et al.* One year reduction and longitudinal analysis of carotid intima-media thickness associated with colestipol/niacin therapy. *Stroke* 1993;24: 1779–83

22. MacMahon S, Sharpe N, Gamble G, *et al.* Effects of lowering average or below-average cholesterol levels on the progression of carotid atherosclerosis: results of the LIPID Atherosclerosis Substudy. *Circulation* 1998;97: 1784–90

23. Crouse JR, Byington RP, Bond MG, *et al.* Pravastatin, Lipids and Atherosclerosis in the Carotid arteries (PLAC-2). *Am J Cardiol* 1995; 75:455–9

24. Furberg CD, Adams HP, Applegate WB, *et al.* Coronary heart disease/myocardial infarction: effect of lovastatin on early carotid atherosclerosis and cardiovascular events. *Circulation* 1994;90:1679–87

25. Mercuri M, Bond MG, Sirtori CR, *et al.* Pravastatin reduces carotid intima-media thickness progression in an asymptomatic hypercholesterolemic Mediterranean population: The carotid atherosclerosis Italian ultrasound study. *Am J Med* 1996;101:627–34

26. Kannel WB, McGee DL. Diabetes and cardiovascular disease: The Framingham Study. *J Am Med Assoc* 1979;241:2035–8

27. Moss SE, Klein R, Klein B, *et al.* The association of glycemia and cause-specific mortality in a diabetic population. *Arch Intern Med* 1994; 154:2473–9

28. UKPDS Group. Intensive glucose control with sulfonylureas on insulin compared with conventional treatment and role of complications in patients with type 2 diabetes (UKPDS 33). *Lancet* 1998;352:837–53

29. Alter M, Lai S-M, Friday G, Sobel E. Stroke recurrence in diabetics: does control of blood glucose reduce risk? *Stroke* 1997;28:1153–7

30. Adler AI, Neil HA, Manley SE, *et al.* Hyperglycemia and hyperinsulinemia at diagnosis of diabetes and their association with subsequent cardiovascular disease in the United Kingdom Prospective Diabetes Study (UKPDS 47). *Am Heart J* 1999;138:353–9

31. Lehto S, Ronnemaa T, Pyorala K, *et al.* Predictors of stroke in middle-aged patients with non-insulin-dependent diabetes. *Stroke* 1996;27:63–8

32. Byington RP, Craven TE, Furberg CD, *et al.* Isradipine, lowered glycosylated haemoglobin and risk of cardiovascular events. *Lancet* 1997;650:1075–6

33. Pyorala M, Miettinen H, Halonen P, *et al.* Insulin resistance syndrome predicts the risk of coronary heart disease and stroke in healthy middle-aged men: The 22-year follow-up results of the Helsinki Policemen Study. *Arterioscler Thromb Vasc Biol* 2000;20:538–50

34. Molitch ME, Cleary PA, Orchard TJ, *et al.* Changes in carotid artery wall thickness in the DCCT/EDIC cohort. Abstract 650-P. American Diabetes Association: Philadelphia, 2001

35. Gray CS, Taylor R, French JM, *et al.* The prognostic value of stress hyperglycemia and previously unrecognized diabetes mellitus in acute stroke. *Diabetic Med* 1987;4:237–40

36. Weir CJ, Murray GD, Dyker AG, *et al.* Is hyperglycemia an independent predictor of poor outcome after acute stroke? Results of a long term follow up study. *Br Med J* 1997;314: 1303–6

37. Malmberg K, for the DIGAMI Study Group. Prospective randomized trial of intensive insulin treatment on long-term survival after acute myocardial infarction in patients with diabetes mellitus. *Br Med J* 1997;314:1512–15

38. Scott JF, Robinson GM, French JM, *et al.* Glucose potassium insulin infusion in the treatment of acute stroke patients with mild to moderate hyperglycemia: the Glucose Insulin in Stroke Trial (GIST). *Stroke* 1999;30:793–9

39. UK Prospective Diabetes Study Group. Tight blood pressure control and risk of macrovascular

and microvascular complications in type 2 diabetes. *Br Med J* 1998;317:703–12

40. Staessen JA, Fagard R, Thijs L, *et al.* Randomised double-blind comparison of placebo and active treatment for older patients with isolated systolic hypertension: for the Systolic Hypertension in Europe (Syst-Eur) Trial Investigators. *Lancet* 1997;350:757–64

41. Staessen JA, Thijs L, Gasowski J, *et al.* Treatment of isolated systolic hypertension in the elderly: further evidence from the Syst-Eur trial. *Am J Cardiol* 1998;82:20R–22R

42. SHEP Cooperative Research Group. Prevention of stroke by antihypertensive drug treatment in older persons with isolated systolic hypertension: final results of the Systolic Hypertension in the Elderly Program (SHEP). *J Am Med Assoc* 1991;265:3255–64

43. Curb JD, Pressel SL, Cutler JA, *et al.* Effect of diuretic based anti HTN treatment on cardiovascular disease risk in older diabetic patients with isolated systolic HTN. *J Am Med Assoc* 1996;276:1886–92

44. The Sixth Report of the Joint National Committee on Prevention, Detection, Evaluation and Treatment of High Blood Pressure. *Arch Intern Med* 1997;157:2413–46

45. Adler A, Stratton IM, Neil HA, *et al.* Association of systolic blood pressure with macrovascular and microvascular complications of type 2 diabetes. (UKPDS36): prospective observational study. *Br Med J* 2000;321:412–19

46. Hansson L, Zanchetti A, Carruthers SG, *et al.* Effects of intensive blood-pressure lowering and low-dose aspirin in patients with hypertension: principal results of the Hypertension Optimal Treatment (HOT) randomised trial. *Lancet* 1998;315:1755–62

47. Heart Outcomes Prevention Evaluation (HOPE) Study Investigators. Effects of ramipril on cardiovascular and microvascular outcomes in people with diabetes mellitus: results of the HOPE study and MICRO-HOPE substudy. *Lancet* 2000;355:253–9

48. Executive Summary of the Third Report of the National Cholesterol Education Program (NCEP) Expert Panel on Detection, Evaluation, and Treatment of High Blood Cholesterol in Adults (Adult Treatment Panel III). *J Am Med Assoc* 2001;285:2486–97

49. Pyorala K, Pedersen TR, Kjekshus J, *et al.* Cholesterol lowering with simvastatin improves prognosis of diabetic patients with coronary heart disease: A subgroup analysis of the Scandinavian Simvastatin Survival Study (4S). *Diabetes Care* 1997;20:614–20

50. Rubins HB, Robins S. Conclusions from the VA-HIT Study. *Am J Cardiol* 2000;86:543–4

51. Matsumoto K, Miyake S, Yano M, *et al.* Insulin resistance and arteriosclerosis obliterans in patients with NIDDM. *Diabetes Care* 1997;20:1738–43

52. Mast H, Thompson JL, Lin IF, *et al.* Cigarette smoking as a determinant of high-grade carotid artery stenosis in Hispanic, Black, and White patients with stroke or transient ischemic attack. *Stroke* 1998;29:908–12

53. Tuomilehto J, Lindstrom J, Eriksson JG, *et al.* Prevention of type 2 diabetes mellitus by changes in lifestyle among subjects with impaired glucose tolerance. *N Engl J Med* 2001;344:1343–50

54. Agurs-Collins TD, Kumanyika SK, Ten Have TR, *et al.* A randomized controlled trial of weight reduction and exercise for diabetes management in older African-American subjects. *Diabetes Care* 1997;20:1503–11

55. Wei M, Gibbons LW, Kampert JB, *et al.* Low cardiorespiratory fitness and physical inactivity as predictors of mortality in men with type 2 diabetes. *Ann Intern Med* 2000;132:605–11

56. Hu FB, Stampfer MJ, Solomon C, *et al.* Physical activity and risk for cardiovascular events in diabetic women. *Ann Intern Med* 2001;134:96–105

57. American Diabetes Association. Standards of medical care for patients with diabetes mellitus. *Diabetes Care* 2001;24(Suppl):S33–S43

Chapter 18

Ethanol consumption and physical inactivity

William J. Elliott, MD, PhD

OVERVIEW

The effects (if any) of ethanol intake or physical inactivity on stroke are controversial. In most studies excessive alcohol intake increased stroke risk. This is presumably mediated, in part, by the acute rise in blood pressure associated with alcohol intake, and/or ethanol-induced cardiac dysrhythmias. Some studies have linked stroke with a recent excessive ingestion of alcohol; this is particularly common in hemorrhagic stroke, Asian populations, and locales where binge drinking is common. The issue of whether 'moderate' or 'light drinking' (≤ 90 or < 30 oz of ethanol/week, respectively) reduces stroke risk is more contentious. This has been observed in many case–control and cohort studies, as well as in the Physicians' Health Study. There is always the question of whether this level of consumption is highly associated with other advantageous health habits that independently reduce the risk of stroke and cardiovascular events. The finding that even one alcoholic drink a week significantly reduced the risk of stroke may be as close to a *reductio ad absurdum* as can be found in epidemiology. The only study so far done about increasing alcohol consumption from none to 'light drinking' suggests a benefit. Whether this can be accomplished in the general population is open to question.

The effect of physical activity on stroke is less well-studied. Such an effect was seen in many racial/ethnic groups, and across many ages in the North Manhattan Stroke Study. In several prospective cohort studies, a protective effect of chronic physical activity was seen on stroke, but this may again be confounded by many other characteristics of 'the healthy cohort'. Although it is unlikely that a randomized trial could be carried out to demonstrate the effects of either alcohol consumption or physical activity on stroke, current policy is consistent with the findings of many research studies. Alcohol consumption at a low level (< 2 drinks/day for men, half that for women), and routine physical activity are each likely to reduce the risk of stroke, as well as other cardiovascular events.

ETHANOL INTAKE

The answer to the question of whether the consumption of alcohol is related to stroke risk is complex, difficult and controversial[1,2]. The complexity arises partly because stroke is not a homogeneous disorder. Alcohol consumption appears to be directly correlated, in a graded fashion, with hemorrhagic stroke risk[3–6], but ischemic stroke is more complicated. When

Table 1   Recent or important case–control studies on ethanol intake and risk of stroke

Authors	Stroke cases, n	Control cases, n	ARR, 'moderate consumption'	ARR, 'heavy consumption'
Malarcher et al.[41]	224	392	0.57	Not given
Sacco et al.[34]	677	1139	0.51*	2.96*
Caicoya et al.[62]	467	477	0.58*	3.2*
Hillbom et al.[21]	212	274	NS	1.82* (recent)
You et al.[23]	201	201	Not given	15.3*
Beghi et al.[63]	200	372	2.2*	2.9*
Hillbom et al.[22]	75	133	Not studied	6.0–7.8* (just before stroke)

*, statistically significant compared with the non-drinking group, after adjustment for other covariables; ARR, adjusted relative risk; NS, not significant

analyses are done using ethanol intake as a dichotomous variable, there is typically no overall difference in stroke between those who drink and those who do not[7]. In more complex models that distinguish between different levels of alcohol intake, low levels appear to protect from stroke, but this effect disappears, and the risk of stroke becomes significantly greater (compared to not drinking), as more alcohol is consumed[8,9]. In addition to this dose-dependent complexity, current research study design and analyses are suboptimal to prove an association, even at the lower levels of consumption. In the hierarchy of 'evidence-based medicine', case–control and cohort study designs are considered inferior to randomized clinical trials, because they are more prone to bias[10]. Essentially all of our information about the possible relationship between alcohol consumption and stroke is derived from either case–control or cohort studies (Tables 1, 2). For ethical and economic reasons it is unlikely that a randomized clinical trial will ever be done to investigate the effects of ethanol on health. As a result, controversy will continue about the quality of, and potential biases present in, research about the possible effects of alcohol on stroke.

Even if there were incontrovertible evidence for a protective effect of alcohol consumption on stroke, it would still be difficult to recommend it to the general population. High levels of alcohol consumption have major adverse health effects on many organ systems[11]. According to the National Center for Health Statistics, 19 086 (or about 0.8% of the total) deaths in 1999 in the USA were attributed directly to alcohol[12]. In 1995, alcohol abuse and alcoholism in the USA cost an estimated $166.5 billion, according to the National Institute on Drug Abuse[13].

The major problem with alcohol consumption is that some individuals are unlikely to adhere to a recommendation for only 'light' consumption. Instead, they may increase their consumption and end up abusing alcohol, thereby overwhelming any public health benefit of 'light consumption'. The 'slippery slope' argument against a public health recommendation in favor of alcohol consumption has been difficult to overcome[14–16].

Excessive use (or abuse) of ethanol

The increase in stroke risk with high levels of alcohol ingestion was first recognized in 1725[17], and has been seen more recently with chronic alcohol abuse[18,19], acute (binge) drinking[18,20,21], and even in young people with an otherwise low risk of stroke[22–24]. All

Table 2 Recent or important cohort studies on ethanol intake and risk of stroke

Authors	Subjects, n	Strokes with 0 units/wk, n (%)	Subjects 0 units/wk, n	Strokes, 1–7 units/wk, n (%)	Subjects, 1–7 units/wk, n	ARR, 1–7 units/wk	Strokes, ≥ 42 units/wk, n (%)	Subjects, ≥ 42 units/wk, n	ARR, ≥ 42 units/wk
Berger et al.[36]	22 071 men	206 (3.62)	5696	264 (2.46)	10 731	~0.8*	Not studied	Not studied	Not studied
Leppälä et al.[35]	26 556 men	121 (4.13)	2931	741 (4.56)	16 258	0.9	64 (5.12)	1251	1.52*
Romelsjo and Leifman[64]	49 618 men	Not given	Not given	Not given	Not given	1.59	Not given	Not given	2.3
Truelsen et al.[42]	13 329 men & women	212 (6.83)	3106	260 (5.30)	4905	0.85*	61 (9.34)	653	1.15
Wannamethee and Shaper[18]	7 735 men	20 (4.85)	412	61 (1.76)	3472	~0.62*	32 (4.05)	791	1.6*
Lee et al.[65]	2600 men & women	174 (5.71)	3046	Not given	Not given	NS	16 (11.51)	139	1.73
Iso et al.[66]	2890 men	29 (4.96)	585	14 (3.80)	368	0.8	45 (9.13)	493	1.9*
Kiyohara et al.[67]	1621 men & women	Not given	1063	Not given	373	NS	Not given	184	~2.1*
Stampfer et al.[4]	87 526 women	49 (0.17)	28 096	53 (0.15)	35 798	0.6*	Not given	Not given	Not given

*, statistically significant compared with the non-drinking group, after adjustment for other covariables; ARR, adjusted relative risk; NS, not significant; 1 unit = one standard alcoholic drink

authorities[25,26], including the National Institute on Drug Abuse, agree that excessive intake of alcohol increases the risk of both hemorrhagic and ischemic strokes. The physiological mechanisms for the effect are likely to include alcohol-related hypertension[2,18], dysrhythmias[27], coagulation factors[28], homocysteine[29], antioxidants[30], or changes in cerebral blood flow[31] or plasma lipid fractions[32].

Limited ethanol consumption

Because of the many cultural, societal, religious, ethnic and gender-based differences in alcohol consumption, a universally-accepted scheme for quantifying alcohol ingestion has not been defined. Furthermore, since this research is largely based on self-reported alcohol consumption, confounded by individuals' recall of their behavior, there is concern that people who consume alcohol generally underestimate their actual intake[33], thereby reducing the 'minimally effective dose', and biasing the presumed protective effect toward even smaller quantities of alcohol. Nonetheless, the existing literature about all-cause mortality, coronary heart disease, and stroke suggests that consistently, low levels of alcohol consumption may protect against these events. The evidence from both case–control and large prospective cohort studies is relatively in agreement (Tables 1, 2). Probably the most convincing case–control study was from Upper Manhattan, which compared 677 first ischemic strokes with 1139 age, gender and race-matched controls[34]. Their conclusion was that 'moderate' alcohol consumption (less than two drinks/day) reduced the risk of stroke by 49%; the effect was similar across all sociodemographic groups. Three large prospective cohort studies arrived at the same conclusions, although the size of the protective effect of alcohol was smaller (~20%)[4,35,36]. Data from the Physicians' Health Study are particularly intriguing (Figure 1). Extremely low levels of self-reported alcohol

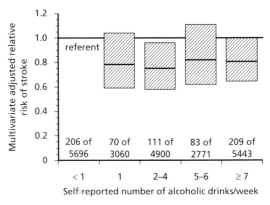

Figure 1 Multivariate adjusted risk of stroke, according to self-reported alcohol consumption (drinks/week) in the Physicians' Health Study (adapted from Berger *et al.*[36]). The dark line near the center of each cross-hatched box represents the point estimate, and the upper and lower bounds of the 95% confidence limits correspond to the top and bottom of each cross-hatched box. The number of Physicians' Health Study subjects with strokes and who reported alcohol intake at each level are given at the bottom of the figure. The '*P* value for trend' pertains to the comparison across all reported levels of alcohol intake and was 0.07. These data may be confounded by 'ascertainment bias' (e.g. under-reporting of actual alcohol consumption) that would lower the apparent minimal effective dose of alcohol. No data about the widely-recognized increase in stroke risk at higher levels of alcohol consumption are included

drinking (one drink each week) appear to have a beneficial effect on stroke, essentially equivalent to that seen with more typical 'light drinking' (defined as less than one alcoholic drink per day, on average)[36].

Change in alcohol consumption

One of the more powerful criteria of Sir Arthur Bradford Hill for establishing an association as causal is the 'experiment' in which individuals change their exposure to a putative risk factor, and observations are made as to whether the

Table 3   Recent or important case–control studies on exercise and risk of stroke

Authors	Strokes	Controls	ARR for physical activity	Dose-dependent?	Duration-dependent?
Sacco et al.[45]	369	678	0.37*	Strongly	Strongly
Shinton and Sagar[68]	125	198	0.33*	Somewhat	Across ages

risk of the outcome event changes thereafter. There are very few reports of a change in stroke risk after modification of alcohol intake. Some individuals with a recent stroke do not change their drinking, even if the drinking pattern was excessive prior to the stroke[37]. There is only one report regarding an increase in alcohol consumption from little or none to 'light or moderate'. Although stroke is not reported separately in this analysis, the 839 men in the Physicians' Health Study who reported increasing their consumption from less than one drink/week to 1–6 drinks/week over seven years had a 29% decrease (which is borderline significant) in all cardiovascular disease events, compared to the 46 413 who did not change their pattern of alcohol consumption[38].

Ethanol or other substances in wine?

Much public discussion has resulted from the 'French paradox' that suggests that consumption of wine may decrease the risk of cardiovascular disease, including stroke[39]. Wine contains many phenolic compounds and other antioxidants, in addition to ethanol, that are now beginning to be studied independently[40]. Some case–control studies[41] and one Danish cohort study[42] have found a better protective effect for wine consumption than for other forms of alcohol. Other investigators have attributed this effect to higher social status and better psychological functioning among Danish wine drinkers, compared to beer drinkers[43]. This Danish study points out an unrecognized confounder of previous analyses, and reinforces the limitations of conclusions drawn from case–control and cohort studies.

PHYSICAL INACTIVITY

Regular exercise protects against death and heart attack, but the relationship of exercise to stroke is less well-proven[44]. The larger of the two recent case–control studies found a significant 63% reduction in adjusted relative risk for stroke for leisure-time physical activity, as well as a significant dose–response relationship, for both intensity of exercise and duration (in hours/week)[45]. Many earlier and smaller case–control studies showed lower (and often non-significant) effects.

The complexity of the situation is perhaps better understood by closer examination of recent cohort studies (Tables 3, 4). In the Physicians' Health Study there was a very significant trend across intensity of exercise to protect against stroke, which was significantly better for even a single period of exercise per week. After full adjustment for all baseline differences, however, both the 'P value for trend' across the various intensities of exercise, and the individual comparisons against 'no exercise' became non-significant[46]. A more complex analysis of the Harvard Alumni Health Study showed a significant protective effect of mild to moderate exercise (especially walking), that became non-significant as the intensity of exercise increased[47]. Several earlier cohort studies also showed a protective effect of reported low levels of physical activity on stroke, both in men[48–51] and women[52]. Increased intensity of exercise, and the age at which exercise begins, may not play an important role in stroke prevention, although the prevalence of regular physical exercise among older people is low.

Table 4 Recent or important cohort studies on exercise and risk of stroke

Authors	Subjects, n	Strokes with no exercise, n (%)	Subjects with no exercise, n	Strokes, mild exercise, n (%)	Subjects, mild exercise, n	ARR, mild exercise	Strokes, heavy exercise, n (%)	Subjects, heavy exercise, n	ARR, heavy exercise
Lee et al.[46]	21 823 men	189 (3.12)	6055	172 (2.10)	8193	0.74*	85 (2.39)	3557	0.74*
Lee and Paffenbarger[47]	11 130 men	Not given	3450	Not given	2026	0.54*	Not given	1324	0.82
Gillum et al.[69]	1285 young white men	Not given	Not given	Not given	Not given	0.80	Not given	Not given	0.85
	1083 older white men	Not given	Not given	Not given	Not given	0.78	Not given	Not given	1.16
	1473 young white women	Not given	Not given	Not given	Not given	0.32	Not given	Not given	0.56
	1240 older white women	Not given	Not given	Not given	Not given	0.79	Not given	Not given	0.65
Abbott et al.[50]	8006 men	235 (9.29)	2529	209 (8.41)	2484	~0.90†	177 (7.03)	2519	~0.75*†
Kiely et al.[51]	1791 younger men	Not given	597	Not given	597	0.9	Not given	597	0.84
	1228 older men	Not given	409	Not given	409	0.41*	Not given	409	0.53*
	2099 younger women	Not given	700	Not given	699	1.21	Not given	700	0.89
	1676 older women	Not given	559	Not given	558	0.97	Not given	559	1.21
Haheim et al.[48]	14 403 men	25	Not given	47	Not given	0.64 (0.70* by Cox method)	9	Not given	0.36*
Lindenstrom et al.[52]	7060 women	227 (4.08)	5570	38 (2.55)	1490	0.69*	Not examined	Not examined	Not examined
Wannamethee and Shaper[49]	7735 men	21 (3.06)	686	15 (1.24)	1205	0.50*	2 (0.39)	513	0.30*

*, statistically significant compared to No Exercise group; †, Unadjusted (calculated *de novo* from data in paper); ARR, adjusted relative risk

A more difficult question is whether leisure-time physical activity has any 'return on investment'. Aside from the general good feelings associated with acute exercise-induced endorphin release, several mortality studies have suggested that the increase in life expectancy among those who exercise nearly exactly equals the time spent performing the exercise[53]. Because of 'discounting', some suggest that younger people are wasting their time exercising, because they recoup only this amount of time (and no more!) when they are older, presumably less healthy, and less able to enjoy their longer life. This argument may be less convincing if one considers the substantive reductions in quality of life after major cardiovascular events (especially stroke, heart attack and heart failure) that can be prevented with regular exercise[54].

The largely beneficial effect of exercise on reduction of stroke (and other cardiovascular events) may be confounded by, and even perhaps mediated by, its effects on other intermediate conditions. Exercise usually improves hypertension[55], diabetes[56], obesity[57], clotting factors[58], platelet dysfunction[59], and/or dyslipidemia[60], all of which are likely to reduce stroke risk. Whether physical activity is independent of these parameters is difficult to ascertain, but may not be important for recommending physical activity to the general population[61].

SPECIFIC LIFESTYLE AND PHARMACOLOGIC INTERVENTIONS

Authoritative recommendations for alcohol consumption and leisure time physical activity have been disseminated recently by the National Stroke Association[25], and the Stroke Council of the American Heart Association[26]. These and other policy-making bodies recommend limiting ethanol consumption to no more than 2 alcoholic drinks (or 2 oz of absolute ethanol) per day for men, and half that for non-pregnant women. Excessive and 'binge' drinking are particularly discouraged, as each has been linked to a substantially higher risk of all stroke subtypes, especially hemorrhagic stroke. Leisure time physical activity should consist of at least 30 minutes of moderate-intensity activity (e.g. brisk walking) on most, and preferably all, days of the week, or another equal-intensity exercise program designed by one's personal physician.

CONCLUSIONS

Although controversy about the relative importance of alcohol consumption and physical activity on the prevention of stroke may exist, many case–control and prospective cohort studies suggest that each can be beneficial. The preponderance of the evidence includes several of Sir Arthur Bradford Hill's classical criteria for causation. In most studies, the association is strong: the adjusted relative risk reduction is in the 20–70% range. Prospective and case–control studies show a temporal sequence of lower alcohol consumption before stroke and the effect is consistent across many studies (Tables 1–4). Because there is a persistence of a significant effect after statistical adjustment for potential confounders, the finding is not dependent on these other factors. Pathophysiological mechanisms have been proposed for the effect, lending biological plausibility. And, because the effect is seen across several types of alcohol-containing beverages, and several types of exercise, the effect may be specific. These data by no means prove that low-levels of alcohol consumption or physical activity help to prevent stroke, but recommendations to the general population in favor of each can be (and have been[25,26]) made, based on their proven beneficial effects on total cardiovascular events, quite apart from their putative beneficial effects on risk of stroke.

References

1. Hommel M, Jaillard A. Alcohol for stroke prevention? [Editorial]. *N Engl J Med* 1999; 341:1605–6
2. Hillbom M, Juvela S, Numminen H. Alcohol intake and the risk of stroke. *J Cardiovasc Risk* 1999;6:223–8
3. Donahue RP, Abbott RD, Reed DM, *et al.* Alcohol and hemorrhagic stroke: The Honolulu Heart Program. *J Am Med Assoc* 1986;255:2311–14
4. Stampfer MJ, Colditz GA, Willett WC, *et al.* A prospective study of moderate alcohol consumption and the risk of coronary disease and stroke in women. *N Engl J Med* 1988; 319:267–73
5. Zodpey SP, Tiwari RR, Kulkarni HR. Risk factors for haemorrhagic stroke: A case-control study. *Pub Health* 2000;114:177–82
6. Sankai T, Iso H, Shimamoto T, *et al.* Prospective study on alcohol intake and risk of subarachnoid hemorrhage among Japanese men and women. *Alcoholism: Clin Exp Res* 2000;24:386–9
7. Corrao G, Bagnardi V, Zambon A, Arico S. Exploring the dose-response relationship between alcohol consumption and the risk of several alcohol-related conditions: A meta-analysis. *Addiction* 1999;94:1551–73
8. Camargo CA Jr. Moderate alcohol consumption and stroke: The epidemiologic evidence. *Stroke* 1989;1989:20
9. Camargo CA Jr. Case-control and cohort studies of moderate alcohol consumption and stroke. *Clin Chim Acta* 1996;246:107–19
10. Sackett DL, Rosenberg WMC, Muir Gray JA, *et al.* Evidence based medicine: What it is and what it isn't [Editorial]. *Br Med J* 1996;312: 71–2
11. Papadakis JA, Ganotakis ES, Mikhailidis DP. Beneficial effect of moderate alcohol consumption on vascular disease: Myth or reality? *J Royal Soc Health* 2000;120:11–15
12. Kochanek KD, Smith BL, Anderson RN. Deaths: Preliminary data for 1999. National Vital Statistics Reports, Vol. 49, No. 1. Hyattsville, MD: National Center for Health Statistics, 2001
13. *Economic Costs of Alcohol and Drug Abuse in the United States, 1992.* Bethesda, MD: National Institute on Drug Abuse, 1998:253
14. Wannamethee SG, Shaper AG. Alcohol, coronary heart disease, and stroke: An examination of the J-shaped curve. *Neuroepidemiology* 1998;17:288–95
15. Meister KA, Whelan EM, Kava R. The health effects of moderate alcohol intake in humans: An epidemiologic review. *Crit Rev Clin Lab Sci* 2000;37:261–96
16. Marmot MG. Alcohol and coronary heart disease. *Int J Epidemiol* 2001;30:724–9
17. Sedgwick J. *A new treatise on liquors wherein the use and abuse of wine, malt drinks, water, etc. are particularly considered in many diseases, institutions and ages with proper manner of using them hot or cold either as physick, diet or both.* London: Rivington, 1725
18. Wannamethee SG, Shaper AG. Patterns of alcohol intake and risk of stroke in middle-aged men. *Stroke* 1996;27:1033–9
19. Hart CL, Smith GD, Hole DJ, Hawthorne VM. Alcohol consumption and mortality from all causes, coronary heart disease, and stroke: Results from a prospective cohort study of Scottish men with 21 years of follow up. *Br Med J* 1999;318:1725–9
20. Hansagi H, Romelsjo A, de Verdier MG, *et al.* Alcohol consumption and stroke mortality: 20-year follow-up of 15 077 men and women. *Stroke* 1995;26:1768–73
21. Hillbom M, Numminen H, Juvela S. Recent heavy drinking of alcohol and embolic stroke. *Stroke* 1999;30:2307–12
22. Hillbom M, Haapaniemi H, Juvela S, *et al.* Recent alcohol consumption, cigarette smoking, and cerebral infarction in young adults. *Stroke* 1995;26:40–5
23. You R, McNeil JJ, O'Malley HM, *et al.* Risk factors for stroke due to cerebral infarction in young adults. *Stroke* 1997;28:1913–18
24. Kwon SU, Kim JS, Lee JH, Lee MC. Ischemic stroke in Korean young adults. *Acta Neurol Scand* 2000;101:19–24
25. Gorelick PB, Sacco RL, Smith DB, *et al.* Prevention of a first stroke: A review of guidelines and a multidisciplinary consensus statement from the National Stroke Association. *J Am Med Assoc* 1999;281:1112–20
26. Goldstein LB, Adams R, Becker K, *et al.* Primary prevention of ischemic stroke: A statement for healthcare professionals from the

Stroke Council of the American Heart Association. *Circulation* 2001;103:163–82

27. Shanmugan M, Regan TJ. Alcohol and cardiac arrhythmias. In Zahari S, Wassef M, eds. *Alcohol and the Cardiovascular System*. Washington, DC: National Institute on Alcohol Abuse and Alcoholism, 1996:159–72

28. Djousse L, Pankow JS, Arnett DK, *et al*. Alcohol consumption and plasminogen activator type 1: The National Heart, Lung, and Blood Institute Family Heart Study. *Am Heart J* 2000;139: 704–9

29. Bleich S, Degner D, Kropp S, *et al*. Red wine, spirits, beer, and serum homocysteine [letter]. *Lancet* 2000;356:512

30. Trevithick CC, Chartrand MM, Wahlman J, *et al*. Shaken, not stirred: Bioanalytical study of the antioxidant activities of martinis. *Br Med J* 1999;319:1600–2

31. Yang ZW, Wang J, Zheng T, *et al*. Ethanol-induced contractions in cerebral arteries: Role of tyrosine and mitogen-activated protein kinases. *Stroke* 2001;32:249–57

32. Langer RD, Criqui MH, Reed DM. Lipoproteins and blood pressure as biological pathways for effect of moderate alcohol consumption on coronary heart disease. *Circulation* 1992;85:910–15

33. Poikolainen K. Underestimation of recalled alcohol intake in relation to actual consumption. *Br J Add* 1985;80:215–16

34. Sacco RL, Elkind M, Boden-Albala B, *et al*. The protective effect of moderate alcohol consumption on ischemic stroke. *J Am Med Assoc* 1999; 281:53–60

35. Leppälä JM, Paunio M, Virtamo J, *et al*. Alcohol consumption and stroke incidence in male smokers. *Circulation* 1999;100:1209–14

36. Berger K, Ajani UA, Kase CS, *et al*. Light-to-moderate alcohol consumption and the risk of stroke among U.S. male physicians. *N Engl J Med* 1999;341:1557–64

37. Redfern J, McKevitt C, Dundas R, *et al*. Behavioral risk factor prevalence and lifestyle change after stroke: A prospective study. *Stroke* 2000;31:1877–81

38. Sesso HD, Stampfer MJ, Rosner B, *et al*. Seven-year changes in alcohol consumption and subsequent risk of cardiovascular disease in men. *Arch Intern Med* 2000;160:2605–12

39. Rimm EB, Klatsky A, Grobbee D, Stampfer MJ. Review of moderate alcohol consumption and reduced risk of coronary heart disease: Is the effect due to beer, wine, or spirits? *Br Med J* 1996;312:731–36

40. Puddey IB, Croft KD. Alcohol, stroke, and coronary heart disease. Are there anti-oxidants and pro-oxidants in alcoholic beverages that might influence the development of atherosclerotic cardiovascular disease? *Neuroepidemiology* 1999;18:292–302

41. Malarcher AM, Giles WH, Croft JB, *et al*. Alcohol intake, type of beverage, and the risk of cerebral infarction in young women. *Stroke* 2001;32:77–83

42. Truelsen T, Gronbaek M, Schnohr P, Boysen G. Intake of beer, wine, and spirits and risk of stroke: The Copenhagen City Heart Study. *Stroke* 1998;29:2467–72

43. Mortensen EK, Jensen HH, Sanders SA, Reinisch JM. Better psychological function and higher social status may largely explain the apparent health benefits of wine: A study of wine and beer drinking in young Danish adults. *Arch Intern Med* 2001;161:1844–8

44. Fletcher GF. Exercise in the prevention of stroke. *Health Rep* 1994;6:106–10

45. Sacco RL, Gan R, Boden-Albala B, *et al*. Leisure-time physical activity and ischemic stroke risk: The Northern Manhattan Stroke Study. *Stroke* 1998;29:380–7

46. Lee IM, Hennekens CH, Berger K, *et al*. Exercise and risk of stroke in male physicians. *Stroke* 1999;30:1–6

47. Lee IM, Paffenbarger RS Jr. Physical activity and stroke incidence: The Harvard Alumni Health Study. *Stroke* 1998;29:2049–54

48. Haheim LL, Holme I, Jhermann I, Leren P. Risk factors of stroke incidence and mortality. A 12-year follow-up of the Oslo Study. *Stroke* 1993;24:1484–9

49. Wannamethee G, Shaper AG. Physical activity and stroke in British middle aged men. *Br Med J* 1992;304:597–601

50. Abbott RD, Rodriguez BL, Burchfiel CM, Curb JD. Physical activity in older middle-aged men and reduced risk of stroke: The Honolulu Heart Program. *Am J Epidemiol* 1994;139: 881–93

51. Keily DK, Wolf PA, Cupples LA, *et al*. Physical activity and stroke risk: The Framingham Study. *Am J Epidemiol* 1994;140:608–20

52. Lindenstrom E, Boysen G, Nyboe J. Lifestyle factors and risk of cerebrovascular disease in women. The Copenhagen City Heart Study. *Stroke* 1993;24:1468–72

53. Blair SN, Kampert JB, Kohl HW III, *et al.* Influences of cardiorespiratory fitness and other precursors on cardiovascular disease and all-cause mortality in men and women. *J Am Med Assoc* 1996;276:205–10

54. Wannamethee SG, Shaper AG. Physical activity and the prevention of stroke. *J Cardiovasc Risk* 1999;6:213–16

55. Blumenthal JA, Sherwood A, Gullette EC, *et al.* Exercise and weight loss reduced blood pressure in men and women with mild hypertension: Effects on cardiovascular, metabolic, and hemodynamic functioning. *Arch Intern Med* 2000;160:1947–58

56. Manson JE, Rimm EB, Stampfer MJ, *et al.* Physical activity and incidence of non-insulin-dependent diabetes mellitus in women. *Lancet* 1991;338:774–8

57. From the Centers for Disease Control and Prevention. Prevalence of leisure-time physical activity among overweight adults – United States, 1998. *J Am Med Assoc* 2000;283:2650–1

58. Lakka TA, Salonen JT. Moderate to high intensity conditioning leisure time physical activity and high cardiorespiratory fitness are associated with reduced plasma fibrinogen in eastern Finnish men. *J Clin Epidemiol* 1993;46:1119–27

59. Wang JS, Jen CJ, Chen HI. Effects of exercise training and deconditioning on platelet function in men. *Arterioscler Thromb Vasc Biol* 1995;15:1668–74

60. Williams PT. High-density lipoprotein cholesterol and other risk factors for coronary heart disease in female runners. *N Engl J Med* 1996;334:1298–303

61. Physical activity and cardiovascular health: NIH Consensus Development Panel on Physical Activity and Cardiovascular Health. *J Am Med Assoc* 1996;276:241–6

62. Caicoya M, Rodriguez T, Corrales C, *et al.* Alcohol and stroke: A community case-control study in Asturias, Spain. *J Clin Epidemiol* 1999;52:677–84

63. Beghi E, Boglium G, Cosso P, *et al.* Stroke and alcohol intake in a hospital population: A case-control study. *Stroke* 1995;26:1691–6

64. Romelsjo A, Leifman A. Association between alcohol consumption and mortality, myocardial infarction, and stroke in 25 year follow up of 49 618 young Swedish men. *Br Med J* 1999;319:821–2

65. Lee TK, Huang ZS, Ng SK, *et al.* Impact of alcohol consumption and cigarette smoking on stroke among the elderly in Taiwan. *Stroke* 1995;26:790–4

66. Iso H, Kitamura A, Shimamoto T, *et al.* Alcohol intake and the risk of cardiovascular disease in middle-aged Japanese men. *Stroke* 1995;26:767–73

67. Kiyohara Y, Kato I, Iwamoto H, *et al.* The impact of alcohol and hypertension on stroke incidence in a general Japanese population: The Hisayama Study. *Stroke* 1995;26:368–72

68. Shinton R, Sagar G. Lifelong exercise and stroke. *Br Med J* 1993;307:231–4

69. Gillum RF, Mussolino ME, Ingram DD. Physical activity and stroke incidence in women and men: The NHANES I Epidemiologic Follow-up Study. *Am J Epidemiol* 1996;143:860–9

Chapter 19

I. Antiplatelet therapies for prevention of first and recurrent stroke

Stanley N. Cohen, MD

INTRODUCTION

Antithrombotic agents remain the cornerstone of a therapeutic strategy for both primary and secondary stroke prevention. Currently there are four antiplatelet agents with Food and Drug Administration approval in the USA for this purpose: aspirin, ticlopidine, clopidogrel and combination aspirin and extended release dipyridamole (ASA/ER-DP). There has been a plethora of clinical trials testing the safety and efficacy of these medications in this setting, yet, opinion remains diverse regarding the best agent or agents for stroke prevention. The clinical trials can be separated arbitrarily into those primarily evaluating primary prevention and those evaluating secondary prevention. In this chapter we shall review the mechanism of action of the antiplatelet agents and the indications for their use, and make recommendations based on the evidence.

THE ANTIPLATELET AGENTS: SECONDARY STROKE PREVENTION

The choice of a first-line antiplatelet agent for secondary stroke prevention is controversial.

Each of the four approved antiplatelet agents has been shown, in controlled clinical trials, to have advantages and disadvantages. In addition, the mechanism of action, proven risks and proven efficacy vary with each of these agents. In order to optimize therapy for the individual patient, the doctor must weigh the relative risks and benefits of each agent as it applies to each patient.

Aspirin both inhibits and promotes thrombogenesis[1]. It inhibits thrombogenesis by irreversibly inactivating platelet cyclooxygenase. This results in the inhibition of thromboxane A2, a potent stimulator of platelet activation and vasoconstriction. This inhibition lasts for the lifespan of the platelet (about seven to ten days). Aspirin impairs platelet aggregation but not adhesion. It actually promotes thrombogenesis by blocking the production of endothelial prostacyclin, which causes vasodilation and de-aggregation. The pro-thrombogenetic effect is reversible, ceasing as soon as aspirin levels fall below a certain point, which partially accounts for why the drug's antiplatelet effect is predominant. Aspirin has a rapid onset of antiplatelet activity, with maximal effect occurring within 15 to 30 minutes[2]. In the doses commonly used for stroke prevention (50 to 1300 mg/day), aspirin prolongs bleeding time for 24 to 48 hours. Restoration of normal bleeding time is probably due to the new production of unexposed platelets.

Both ticlopidine and clopidogrel are thienopyridine derivatives[3]. Each drug is metabolized in the liver and each irreversibly inhibits platelet aggregation by inhibiting the platelet adenosine diphosphate (ADP) receptor. Ticlopidine, given 250 mg twice a day, inhibits platelet function within 24 to 48 hours of administration and peaks at three to seven days. The effect lasts for the lifespan of the platelet[4]. Bleeding time is doubled and remains prolonged for four to ten days after the last dose. Clopidogrel's antiplatelet effect is dose-related, with 75 mg causing a prolongation of bleeding time roughly equivalent to 500 mg of ticlopidine[3]. After a loading dose of 300 mg, there is an 80% inhibition of platelet function at five hours[5], and peak platelet inhibition occurs between three and seven days. As with ticlopidine, bleeding time remains prolonged for four to ten days after the last dose of clopidogrel.

Dipyridamole (DP) reversibly inhibits platelet adhesion by blocking platelet phosphodiesterases and potentiating the effects of adenosine on the platelet[6]. It also acts by direct stimulation of prostacyclin synthesis and potentiation of prostacyclin-induced platelet inhibition as well as increasing platelet cyclic AMP. Dipyridamole is metabolized in the liver and is highly protein bound. For the standard release formulation, the time to peak concentration varies from 34 to 75 minutes[7]. Standard release dipyridamole falls below its therapeutic level about six to eight hours after the last dose. Because its inhibition of platelet function is reversible, four daily doses of the drug are necessary to maintain the desired effect[8]. By contrast ER-DP reportedly requires twice daily dosing, achieving a steady

therapeutic state after approximately 48 hours of treatment. Combining aspirin with ER-DP has the potential benefit of inhibiting both platelet aggregation and adhesion. Theoretically, using a combination of platelet inhibitors with different mechanisms of action can maximize effectiveness.

Clinical trials of antiplatelet agents in patients at risk for recurrent cerebral ischemia have been conducted for over 20 years. But, in spite of the abundance of data, controversy remains in almost all aspects of drug selection. There are various interpretations of the data, partly because of disparity between and weaknesses within the designs of the different trials, including sample size, choice of agents and dose, dropout rates and choice of endpoints. A critical endpoint in a secondary stroke prevention trial is the ability of the agents to prevent recurrent stroke[9]. If only the incidence of recurrent stroke is analyzed, however, a high rate of death prior to the patient's having a recurrent stroke could confound the results. In clinical trials, therefore, it is important to consider both incidence of stroke and incidence of stroke plus death as endpoints.

Stroke patients are at risk for coronary heart disease, with myocardial infarction (MI) being the most common long-term cause of death in patients with a history of stroke. Some have suggested that trials of antiplatelet agents given to prevent recurrent cerebrovascular events should also show benefit in reducing the rate of subsequent MI[10]. The rate of MI in the first two years after stroke, however, is only between 1% and 2.5%[11,12]. For this reason it is unlikely that a clinical trial with just a two-year follow-up would have the power to find clinically significant differences in the rate of MI in patients who were taking different antiplatelet agents following a cerebrovascular event. By using a combined endpoint of stroke, MI, or vascular death, the number of patients required in a trial involving secondary stroke prevention can be smaller.

Table 1 Prospective randomized trials comparing aspirin (ASA) with placebo for the prevention of secondary stroke

Study	Patients, n	Mean follow-up, months	ASA dose, mg/day	Ischemic strokes in ASA group, n (%)	Ischemic strokes in placebo group, n (%)	Strokes and deaths in ASA group, n (%)	Strokes and deaths in placebo group, n (%)
AITIA[13]	178	6	1300	5 (6)	10 (11)*	7 (8)	14 (16)
CCS[14]	283	26	1300	22 (15)	20 (14)*	26 (18)	30 (22)
Reuther and Dorndorf[18]	58	24	1500	1(3)	4 (13)*	1 (3)	4 (13)
Danish[19]	203	25	1000	17 (17)	11 (11)*	21 (21)	17 (17)
AICLA[15]	402	36	990	17 (9)	31 (15)**	27 (14)	38 (19)
Swedish[20]	505	24	1500	32 (13)	32 (13)*	65 (26)	65 (26)
Danish[21]	301	21	50–100	9 (6)	11 (7)*	21 (14)	17 (11)
UK-TIA[17]	2435	48	300 or 1200	201 (12)	238 (15)*	346 (21)	205 (25)
SALT[22]	1360	32	75	82 (12)	105 (15)*	138 (20)	171 (25)
ESPS 2[16]	6602	24	50	206 (12.2)	250 (15.2)**	330	378

*, difference in number of strokes between drug and placebo groups is not significant; **, difference in number of strokes between drug and placebo groups, $p < 0.05$

There have been ten prospective randomized trials testing the efficacy of aspirin *vs.* placebo for secondary stroke prevention (Table 1). Fields and colleagues reported the first of these trials in 1977[13]. These investigators reported on 178 patients with hemispheric transient ischemic attacks (TIAs) who were not referred for carotid endarterectomy. The selection of patients for surgical or medical treatment was not done on a randomized basis. Patients were treated with 650 mg aspirin twice daily or placebo. They found that the overall number of unfavorable outcomes (death, cerebral or retinal infarction, or failure to reduce the number of transient ischemic attacks in a three-month period) was significantly lower at six months in the aspirin group compared to the placebo group. No difference was found, however, in the individual endpoints of ischemic stroke, retinal infarction, or death.

The Canadian Cooperative Study (CCS) was another large, prospective, randomized trial to address the role of antiplatelet agents in stroke prevention[14]. In this study a total of 585 patients with TIA or stroke were randomized to receive aspirin, sulfinpyrazone, aspirin plus sulfinpyrazone, or placebo. The women who participated in this trial had relatively few endpoints, and analyses performed on participants of both genders as a whole yielded no significant differences for the various treatments. Subsequent analyses, therefore, included only men. When comparing men taking aspirin (the aspirin alone group plus the aspirin and sulfinpyrazone group) to those not taking aspirin (the sulfinpyrazone alone group plus the placebo group), the researchers found that during an average follow-up of 26 months, the men taking aspirin were significantly less likely to have continuing TIA, have a stroke, or die. There was no difference between groups when stroke was considered as the endpoint. It is important to note that the CCS was not powered to evaluate aspirin's effectiveness in decreasing the risk of stroke as an isolated endpoint, but only to identify a treatment that could reduce the combined outcome of TIA, stroke and death.

Since the CCS many other trials have set out to examine aspirin's potential benefit in preventing recurrent stroke. Unfortunately, the individual trial results have been less than definitive. Of ten trials comparing aspirin to placebo[13-22], only two – the French Accidents, Ischemiques Cerebraux Lies a l'Atherosclerose (AICLA) study and the European Stroke Prevention Study 2 (ESPS 2)[15,16] – demonstrated significant reductions in the rate of stroke with aspirin therapy. Nevertheless, many of the trials did find significantly lower incidences of other unfavorable vascular outcomes with aspirin. Most of the controversy over aspirin's efficacy in preventing stroke or vascular death comes from conflicting results of individual studies[23]. It is possible that some of these studies missed modest risk reductions owing to the relatively small numbers of study participants and endpoints. To address this possibility, several meta-analyses of pooled data have been reported.

In 1988, the Antiplatelet Trialists' Collaboration analyzed the results of 25 trials that used antiplatelet medications (aspirin, dipyridamole, sulfinpyrazone and ticlopidine) in 29 000 patients with TIA, ischemic stroke, unstable angina, or myocardial infarction[11]. They found that antiplatelet treatment in general reduced the odds of vascular mortality by 15%, non-fatal MI or stroke by 30%, and unfavorable vascular events by 25%. In the 13 cerebrovascular trials, the odds reduction for non-fatal stroke was 22%. Unfortunately, separate analyses for the various agents used were not included in this report.

Sze and colleagues performed a meta-analysis of ten randomized trials that compared antiplatelet drugs to placebo in 1928 patients with TIA or minor stroke[24]. In the five trials (involving 1118 patients) in which aspirin was compared to placebo, they found a non-significant 15% odds reduction in stroke risk. For aspirin combined with dipyridamole or sulfinpyrazone, there was a significant odds reduction of 39% in stroke risk ($p < 0.05$). On the negative side, however, the risk of serious gastrointestinal (GI) effects was 350% higher with aspirin combinations than with placebo

($p < 0.05$). Aspirin alone did not have a significantly higher risk of GI complications compared to placebo. Neither aspirin alone nor aspirin combinations carried any significant reduction in mortality.

In 1994, the Antiplatelet Trialists' Collaboration analyzed data from 145 trials comparing antiplatelet therapy to control in about 70 000 high-risk and 30 000 low-risk patients[25]. The high-risk group included 18 studies entering 11 707 patients with prior stroke or TIA. The meta-analysis found an odds reduction of about 25% in vascular events for each of the four main categories of high-risk patients (prior MI, acute MI, prior stroke/TIA and other high risk). Subgroup analyses showed that the reductions were statistically significant in middle-aged patients as well as in the elderly, in both men and women, in both hypertensive and normotensive patients, and in both diabetic and nondiabetic patients. For patients presenting with stroke or TIA, antiplatelet therapy resulted in a significant 23% odds reduction in subsequent non-fatal stroke, but there was no significant reduction in fatal stroke events. The authors concluded that in this same group of patients, prolonged antiplatelet therapy reduced both vascular mortality and all-cause mortality.

In a meta-analysis of nine trials that compared aspirin to placebo in 9256 patients with a history of TIA or minor stroke, Gelmers and Tijssen reported that aspirin therapy resulted in a small but significant 15% reduction in both the risk of all vascular events and the risk of stroke[26]. In 1999, Albers and Tijssen presented a meta-analysis that included the results of the ESPS 2 trial[27]. In the ten trials comparing aspirin to placebo, there was a 19.5% rate of vascular events in the aspirin group compared to 22.3% in the placebo group. This is a relative risk reduction of 13% ($p = 0.001$).

The results of each meta-analysis must be viewed with caution since data are pooled from heterogeneous groups of trials (focusing, for instance, on TIA, stroke, surgical procedures, MI and unstable angina), heterogeneous groups of endpoints (including non-fatal stroke, non-fatal MI, vascular death and death from all causes), heterogeneous patient populations and various antiplatelet medications at various doses. In addition, several of the meta-analyses reported their results in terms of odds ratio reduction, whereas others used relative risk reduction. While both are legitimate methods of reporting results, each will produce a different numeric outcome. Despite the varying results from the prospective trials and meta-analyses, it is generally agreed that aspirin offers a statistically significant benefit and is at least marginally clinically effective at preventing recurrent ischemic stroke. However, the optimal dose for aspirin in stroke prevention remains controversial[28,29]. Prospective trials have used doses ranging from 30 to 1500 mg per day. Of these, only the United Kingdom Transient Ischemic Attack (UK-TIA) trial compared both moderate dose (300 mg/day) and high dose (1200 mg/day) aspirin therapy with placebo[17]. No difference was found between the two aspirin doses in terms of stroke prevention, but the moderate-dose aspirin group had significantly fewer GI side-effects. Given the power of this study, though, differences of up to 25% could have been missed.

The Dutch trial compared moderate-dose (283 mg/day) and very-low-dose (30 mg/day) aspirin therapy in 3131 patients who had had a TIA or minor stroke[30]. They found no difference between the two doses in prevention of vascular death, non-fatal stroke, or MI. Again, the lower-dose group had fewer adverse effects.

In a meta-analysis, Albers and Tijssen reported that trials using high-dose (900 to 1500 mg/day) aspirin and low dose (50 to 75 mg/day) aspirin each demonstrated significant (13%) relative risk reductions in vascular outcomes[27]. In another meta-analysis, including eleven trials with a total of 9629 patients with symptomatic cerebrovascular disease assigned

to receive aspirin or placebo, Johnson and colleagues looked for a dose–response relationship with aspirin therapy[31]. They found a consistent relative risk reduction of approximately 15% across all doses, which ranged from 50 to 1500 mg/day. The authors concluded that the absence of a dose–response relationship supports the use of low-dose aspirin.

One of the few studies to find a difference between the efficacy of different aspirin doses in favor of high-dose aspirin was a post hoc, retrospective analysis, conducted by the North American Symptomatic Carotid Endarterectomy Trial (NASCET) investigators[32]. They found that patients taking high-dose (650 to 1300 mg/day) aspirin had significantly fewer postoperative strokes after carotid endarterectomy than did patients taking lower doses (81 to 350 mg/day). Based on these results, Taylor and colleagues organized the ASA and Carotid Endarterectomy (ACE) trial, a prospective, randomized trial of aspirin dosing in the 90-day period beginning just prior to carotid endarterectomy[33]. They found that patients taking low-dose aspirin had significantly fewer unfavorable outcomes than those assigned to a high dose. This is opposite to the conclusion of the initial post-hoc analysis of the NASCET data. Perhaps the most important message to take away from this trial, therefore, is that post hoc, retrospective analyses should be interpreted with caution, even when they are generated from large, carefully designed, prospective trials.

The data from the ACE trial suggest that low-dose aspirin is better than high-dose aspirin for preventing vascular events in the postoperative period[33]. Because of the short duration of follow-up and the probable differences in the pathophysiology between postoperative stroke and atherosclerotic stroke, the ACE trial cannot address the issue of the optimal aspirin dose for long-term stroke prevention. In fact, to date, there are no convincing data to show that any particular dose of aspirin is superior to another in preventing stroke over a long period of time in a population at high risk for stroke.

The GI hemorrhage rate for aspirin in a stroke population is not negligible. Roderick and colleagues performed a meta-analysis of aspirin trials, and reported a 2.48% GI hemorrhage rate, with 1.7% requiring hospitalization[34]. In a more recent meta-analysis, Derry and Loke reported virtually the same GI hemorrhage rate of 2.47% in patients taking aspirin compared with 1.68% taking placebo[35]. The number needed to harm was 106 based on 28 months of therapy. In stroke prevention trials reporting the rate of serious GI hemorrhages with aspirin dosing from 30 to 1300 mg per day, the hemorrhage rate ranged from approximately 2% to 3%[17,22,30,33]. Roderick and colleagues as well as Derry and Loke found no significant relationship between the dose of aspirin and GI hemorrhage rate[34,35].

In the VA Cooperative Asymptomatic Carotid Artery Stenosis Study, all patients were initially given 650 mg of regular (non-enteric-coated) aspirin twice a day[36,37]. Only 25% had no adverse effects and were still taking that dose of regular aspirin at the end of the study. There were 837 adverse reactions to aspirin during the 4954 follow-up visits, with 45% of patients experiencing adverse GI effects. The authors concluded that high-dose aspirin therapy is poorly tolerated, and that adverse reactions to even low-dose enteric-coated aspirin are common.

There have been two large, prospective, randomized trials of ticlopidine's effectiveness in preventing recurrent ischemic stroke. The Ticlopidine Aspirin Stroke Study (TASS) randomized 3069 patients with TIA or mild ischemic stroke within three months of the event to receive either ticlopidine 250 mg twice a day or aspirin 650 mg twice a day, and followed them for a mean of 3.4 years[38]. The authors reported that ticlopidine significantly reduced the risk of stroke (relative risk reduction,

21%; $p = 0.024$) and the risk of stroke plus death (relative risk reduction, 12%; $p = 0.048$) as compared to aspirin in the intent-to-treat analysis. In the efficacy analysis, in which only the patients remaining on the assigned treatment at the time of the endpoint or at the end of the trial were considered for analysis, ticlopidine's relative risk reduction for stroke rose to 27% ($p = 0.011$)[39]. Only about half of the patients remained on treatment at the end of the trial.

The Canadian-American Ticlopidine Study (CATS) compared ticlopidine to placebo in 1053 patients who had had an ischemic stroke in the previous month, and followed these patients for a mean of two years[40]. In the intent-to-treat analysis, ticlopidine reduced the endpoint of stroke, MI, or vascular death (relative risk reduction 23%; $p = 0.02$), but did not show a benefit for reducing the risk of stroke alone. The efficacy analysis, however, did show a significant risk reduction for stroke or stroke plus death (relative risk reduction 34%; $p = 0.008$) in favor of ticlopidine. In TASS and CATS, the ticlopidine groups had approximately a 1% incidence of severe but reversible neutropenia requiring discontinuation of the drug[38,40]. Almost all cases of severe neutropenia occurred in the first three months after the initiation of therapy and reversed with cessation of the drug. Compared to those taking aspirin, the ticlopidine patients had significantly more diarrhea and rash, but significantly less gastritis, ulcer, or GI bleeding. Although the patients assigned to ticlopidine had a mean rise in total cholesterol of 9%, this elevation did not result in an increase in fatal or non-fatal MI, and cholesterol level was not a predictor of MI.

Bennett and colleagues reported 60 cases of thrombotic thrombocytopenic purpura (TTP) associated with ticlopidine use, twelve within three weeks of starting the drug[41]. Only one developed TTP later than twelve weeks after the start of ticlopidine therapy.

In a post hoc, retrospective analysis of data from TASS, Grotta and colleagues reported ticlopidine to be significantly more effective than aspirin in preventing subsequent strokes in patients whose angiograms did not show associated high grade stenosis (stroke rates were 10% for ticlopidine versus 19% for aspirin)[42]. Other subgroup analyses from TASS have reported benefit from ticlopidine in women, Blacks, patients with minor stroke and diabetics[39,43,44]. As noted previously, however, caution must be used when interpreting post hoc subgroup analyses.

There has been only one large, prospective, randomized trial assessing the safety and efficacy of clopidogrel in stroke patients, the Clopidogrel Versus Aspirin in Patients at Risk of Ischemic Events (CAPRIE) trial[12]. This study included 19 185 patients, of whom 6431 were enrolled with ischemic stroke as their qualifying event. The remainder of the patients enrolled in the study had MI and peripheral arterial disease (PAD) as the qualifying event. Stroke patients had to have an atherosclerotic etiology, and cardioembolic strokes were excluded. Forty percent of the stroke patients had lacunar infarctions. Patients were entered up to six months after the qualifying event. In the intent-to-treat analysis of the whole cohort, clopidogrel showed a reduction in the rate of recurrent stroke, MI, or vascular death compared to aspirin (5.32% per year for clopidogrel versus 5.83% per year for aspirin). For the subgroup entering with stroke, the rate of stroke, MI, or vascular death was 7.15% with clopidogrel and 7.71% with aspirin. This represents a statistically non-significant relative risk reduction of 7.3% ($p = 0.26$). The recurrent stroke rate in these patients was 5.2% for the clopidogrel group and 5.7% for aspirin – a non-significant difference. The response differed between the three subgroups entering the study, with only the PAD subgroup showing an overall improvement with clopidogrel compared to aspirin. It is important to remember that the study was designed with the power to find a difference in total

atherosclerotic complications from all groups, but not in each of the three subgroups. Clopidogrel's adverse effect profile was roughly equivalent to that of aspirin, with no difference in neutropenia. The clopidogrel group had more rashes and diarrhea, while the aspirin group had more gastric irritation and GI hemorrhage. Major criticisms of the CAPRIE trial include the relatively small magnitude and marginal statistical significance of the absolute difference between treatments, the apparent heterogeneity of the findings between the three populations studied and the absence of corroborating data from other studies[45].

Recently, several cases of thrombotic thrombocytopenic purpura (TTP) and one case of hemolytic uremic syndrome have been reported in association with clopidogrel use[46,47]. The number of reported cases of TTP is small, making it appear to be a very infrequent occurrence. All cases reported occurred shortly after starting the drug.

There have been five prospective trials comparing dipyridamole and aspirin, alone or in combination, in the treatment of patients with a history of TIA and stroke. Although earlier placebo-controlled trials (AICLA and the Toulouse TIA trial) indicated an advantage for aspirin plus dipyridamole over placebo in decreasing stroke risk[15,48], both AICLA and the American-Canadian Cooperative Study failed to show a benefit for aspirin plus dipyridamole compared to aspirin alone in preventing stroke or death[15,49]. It is important to keep in mind, however, that in these two trials the number of endpoints studied was small and over 40% of patients taking high-dose aspirin withdrew from treatment. It is possible that these factors contributed to a lack of power to find a difference in the efficacy of the two treatments.

The European Stroke Prevention Study (ESPS) compared combination treatment with aspirin 330 mg plus dipyridamole 75 mg, taken three times a day, versus placebo in 2500 patients, with a two-year follow-up[50]. The study reported that aspirin plus dipyridamole reduced the primary endpoints of stroke plus death (from any cause) by 34% ($p < 0.001$) and stroke alone by 38% ($p < 0.001$). They reported no gender difference, with both men and women having significantly reduced endpoints ($p < 0.001$ for each). Specifically, the reduction in the rate of stroke was 40% for men ($p < 0.001$) and 38% for women ($p = 0.018$)[51]. Because this trial did not compare aspirin plus dipyridamole with aspirin alone, the results cannot be directly compared with the results of earlier trials that included an aspirin-only group.

Gelmers and Tijssen performed a meta-analysis of trials, conducted prior to ESPS 2, that compared aspirin alone and aspirin plus dipyridamole with placebo for stroke prevention[26]. They found a 39% relative risk reduction with a combination of dipyridamole and aspirin versus placebo that was statistically significant. When they analyzed only studies that compared aspirin alone to aspirin plus dipyridamole, the addition of dipyridamole had no clear benefit in reducing the risk of mortality or stroke. In their study report the authors did not favor discarding the aspirin plus dipyridamole combination from the therapeutic armamentarium on the basis of their findings, but called for further study.

In the ESPS 2, 6602 patients were randomized to aspirin alone (50 mg/day), ER dipyridamole alone (400 mg/day), a combination of aspirin plus ER dipyridamole, or placebo, with a two-year follow-up[16]. Compared with placebo, aspirin alone reduced the risk of stroke by 18% ($p = 0.013$), dipyridamole alone reduced it by 16% ($p = 0.039$), and the combination therapy reduced it by 37% ($p < 0.001$). When compared to aspirin alone, the combination therapy had a relative risk reduction for stroke of 23% ($p = 0.006$). In general, the aspirin-treated groups had an 8.5% risk of bleeding from any site, significantly higher than for placebo ($p < 0.001$). The incidence of severe or

fatal hemorrhage was 1.5%. There are several criticisms of this trial. First, the dose of aspirin was lower than that normally used in North America. The use of very-low-dose aspirin in stroke prevention is more common in Western Europe[52]. Second, the use of a placebo arm in a stroke prevention trial raises ethical questions because proven effective treatments are available. In their defense, in the late 1980s when their study was designed, the second antiplatelet trialists' meta-analysis had not yet been published, and the investigators believed the benefit of aspirin had not yet been clearly established[53]. Third, there were allegations of fraud at one of the study centers in the trial. The authors went public with this problem, however, and the data from the tainted center were excluded prior to trial unblinding. This approach by the investigators should add credibility to the trial[54].

In the updated meta-analysis that included the ESPS 2 trial results, Tijssen reported a 15% vascular event rate for the dipyridamole plus aspirin group (2473 patients) and a 17% rate for those in the aspirin-alone group (2436 patients)[55]. This is a 15% relative risk reduction for the combination therapy compared to aspirin alone ($p = 0.012$). Comparing the combination of aspirin plus dipyridamole to placebo, the combination therapy had an event rate of 14% (3239 events) versus placebo at 20% (3259 events). This is a relative risk reduction of 30% ($p < 0.00001$). Tijssen concluded that the addition of ER dipyridamole to aspirin in high-risk patients would reduce the vascular event rate by an additional 15% compared to aspirin alone.

Taking the plethora of data on antiplatelet agents in stroke prevention and applying the results to the individual patient is no easy task. The choice of whether to use aspirin or one of the newer antiplatelet agents remains controversial (as does the optimal dose of aspirin). Table 2 summarizes the characteristics of each of the approved antiplatelet agents that might

Table 2 Comparison of antiplatelet agents used in stroke prevention

Antiplatelet agent	Dose (mg)	Dose frequency	Mechanism of action	Efficacy in stroke prevention (RRR compared to aspirin)	Possible serious adverse effects	Most frequent minor adverse effects	Retail cost per month
Aspirin	50–1300	Once daily	Irreversible inhibition of platelet cyclooxygenase	N/A	GI bleeding	GI irritation	< $3
Ticlopidine	250	Twice daily	Irreversible inhibition of platelet ADP receptor	21%	Severe neutropenia, uncommon TTP	Diarrhea, rash	$118.67*
Clopidogrel	75	Once daily	Irreversible inhibition of platelet ADP receptor	7%	Rare TTP	Diarrhea, rash	$96.30†
Aspirin + ER-DP	25/200	Twice daily	Irreversible inhibition of platelet cyclooxygenase + reversible inhibition of platelet phosphodiesterase and uptake of adenosine	22%	GI bleeding	GI irritation, headache, diarrhea, vomiting	$88.50†

RRR, relative risk reduction; *, based on Roche Pharmaceuticals Wholesale Price list, 7/10/01; ticlopidine is also available as a generic; †, based on retail prices cited in: Heidebrink JL. *Arch Intern Med* 2001;161:1236; ER-DP, extended release dipyridamole; GI, gastrointestinal; TTP, thrombotic thrombocytopenic purpura. Adapted with permission from *Federal Practitioner* 2001;18:46–57 help in selecting the optimal therapy for an individual. Aspirin is the least expensive, is available without a prescription, has a once daily dosing schedule, and has an acceptable level of adverse side-effects. The major disadvantages to aspirin are that it is only a weak protector against recurrent stroke (about 15% better than placebo) and it carries a risk of causing serious GI bleeding (about 1 to 3%/year). A frequent minor adverse effect is GI irritation, as it can interfere with adherence. Aspirin dosing remains controversial. In one survey about half of the European neurologists who used aspirin in stroke prevention used a low dose (30 to 175 mg/day) and the other half used a medium dose (200 to 400 mg/day)[52]. Among North American neurologists who were surveyed, about 60% used a medium dose and about 40% used a high dose (500 to 1300 mg/day)[52]. In the absence of a clear advantage of one dose over another for secondary stroke prevention, doses from 50 to 1300 mg/day are considered acceptable[56].

Ticlopidine has a 20% advantage of preventing recurrent stroke in high-risk patients compared to aspirin, and causes less frequent GI pain, GI hemorrhage and peptic ulcers. Its disadvantages include expense, twice daily dosing, a high frequency of minor adverse effects and the need for frequent blood testing. The blood testing is mandatory because of the 1% risk of severe neutropenia. To monitor for this, complete blood counts must be taken every two weeks for the first three months after initiating therapy. Unlike the bleeding risk associated with aspirin, that persists as long as aspirin is used, the risk of severe neutropenia associated with ticlopidine is present only during the first three months of therapy. Blood monitoring, therefore, is not needed after that point. The frequency of ticlopidine-associated TTP is unknown. While the majority of reported cases with this adverse effect occurred within the first three months of therapy, cases have been reported beyond that time too.

The most frequent minor adverse effects of ticlopidine are diarrhea and rash, each of which occurs about twice as often as with aspirin. The risk of developing diarrhea can be reduced by initiating ticlopidine therapy at 250 mg/day after meals for the first week, and then increasing to the usual dose of 250 mg twice a day.

Clopidogrel's advantages include a somewhat increased effectiveness in preventing vascular endpoints in patients with atherosclerosis (9% relative risk reduction), once daily dosing and significantly less GI hemorrhage, indigestion, nausea and vomiting as compared to aspirin. Its main disadvantage is expense. Although clopidogrel's minor adverse effect profile is very low, the risk of rash and diarrhea are increased compared to aspirin.

While the relative risk reduction for combined endpoints in the CAPRIE study was significant, the absolute risk reduction for stroke recurrence was very small[12]. Considering all outcomes, there was a 0.5% per year reduction for all patients. One would need to transfer about 200 patients from aspirin to clopidogrel to prevent one stroke. The absolute risk reduction of 0.6% per year for those entering the study with stroke was neither statistically nor clinically significant.

The main advantage of the combination of aspirin plus extended release dipyridamole (ER-DP) is that it is more effective than aspirin alone in preventing stroke in high-risk patients. It has the disadvantages of twice daily dosing and an adverse effect profile that combines the effects of aspirin and ER-DP. The relative risk reduction for stroke as an endpoint was 23% ($p = 0.006$), with an absolute risk reduction of 2.1%, compared to that obtained with aspirin alone[16].

In a consensus statement for the American College of Chest Physicians (ACCP), Albers and colleagues stated that every patient who has had a non-cardioembolic stroke or TIA and has no contraindication should receive an antiplatelet agent[57]. They indicated that

Table 3 Suggested guidelines for choosing a first-line antiplatelet therapy for secondary stroke prevention

Therapeutic agent	*Indicated as first line therapy when...*
Aspirin 81 mg to 325 mg once daily	cost is the major factor in selecting a drug
Clopidogrel 75 mg once daily	the patient has true aspirin intolerance
Aspirin 325 mg/day plus clopidogrel 75 mg once daily	compliance with twice daily dosing is in question or the patient requires nasogastric tube feeding or the patient has unstable angina in addition to his cerebrovascular symptoms or the patient presents with crescendo TIAs
Aspirin 25 mg plus extended release dipyridamole 200 mg twice daily	cost, compliance with twice daily dosing, inability to swallow pills, and unstable angina are not considerations

Adapted with permission from *Federal Practitioner* 2001;18:46–57

aspirin, the combination of ER-DP and aspirin, and clopidogrel are all acceptable options for initial therapy. Guidelines for selecting one of these agents as first-line therapy for secondary stroke prevention are presented in Table 3. Aspirin has been the gold standard for many years. In view of its low cost, ease of use and accepted greater efficacy of 15% compared with placebo, it remains an appropriate initial choice in selected patients[31]. Because the efficacy is small, the use of aspirin as initial therapy may be reserved for patients for whom the cost of medications is the major consideration in the choice of drugs.

Because of the relatively high frequency of serious adverse events and the availability of other agents approved for stroke prevention, many feel that ticlopidine should no longer be considered a first-line option as an antiplatelet agent for this purpose. The subset analysis from TASS indicated that ticlopidine may be more effective and have a lower adverse effect profile in African-Americans[43]. To learn more about the potential use of ticlopidine in this group of patients, a prospective, randomized trial comparing ticlopidine to aspirin in African-Americans is under way[58]. Until the results of that study are reported, however, the use of ticlopidine as a routine first-line therapy is not recommended.

Although clopidogrel is less inconvenient and has fewer risks than ticlopidine, its small benefit

relative to aspirin, along with its expense, makes aspirin a better choice in most patients. Clopidogrel as a single agent would be appropriate for first-line therapy in patients who are unable to take aspirin. The combination of aspirin plus clopidogrel has never been tested in a large trial in secondary stroke prevention. There is a trial that is ongoing but the results are not expected for several years. The long-term safety and efficacy of this combination are unknown in this setting, though it has a theoretical advantage over either drug used alone. Because each component is a once-a-day drug, it can be used when adherence issues make drugs requiring twice-a-day administration undesirable. Because each drug can be crushed, it can be used in patients requiring nasogastric tube feedings. The Clopidogrel in Unstable Angina to Prevent Recurrent Events (CURE) trial recently reported a 20% benefit in preventing MI, stroke or vascular death using this combination compared to using aspirin alone in patients with acute coronary syndromes[59]. This reduction was statistically significant. However, the patients receiving the combination had a 38% higher rate of major bleeding complications compared to those on aspirin alone. That was also statistically significant. Based on the results of this study, patients presenting with unstable angina and TIA or stroke should be considered as candidates for clopidogrel plus aspirin. However, care must be taken in regard to the potential for bleeding complications with long-term use of this combination. Both aspirin and clopidogrel, when given in a loading dose, have a fairly rapid onset of action. Most feel that patients presenting with crescendo TIAs benefit from antithrombotic therapy started as quickly as possible. While there are no data to support its use, the combination of aspirin plus clopidogrel, given with a loading dose, is not unreasonable in the setting of crescendo TIAs.

The combination of aspirin plus ER-DP for secondary stroke prevention is verified. According to the ACCP's consensus statement, this combination 'is more effective than aspirin alone for the prevention of stroke and, based on indirect comparisons, [it]… may be more effective than clopidogrel and has a similarly favorable profile in terms of serious adverse effects'[57]. Based on the data reviewed above, we use this combination as initial therapy for secondary stroke prevention in non-cardioembolic strokes unless the patient has one of the exceptions listed in the above paragraphs.

THE ANTIPLATELET AGENTS: PRIMARY STROKE PREVENTION

While there is a wealth of clinical trial data on the role of antiplatelet agents in secondary stroke prevention, there are only a few large prospective randomized trials on antiplatelet agents in primary stroke prevention. In the Physicians' Health Study 22 071 male physicians were randomized to aspirin 325 mg every other day or placebo[60]. With a mean follow-up of 60.2 months, the aspirin group demonstrated a statistically significant 44% reduction in the rate of MI. The benefit was especially noteworthy in those aged over 50 years. However, the risk of stroke was slightly increased (mostly owing to hemorrhagic stroke). A smaller British trial randomized 5139 healthy male doctors who were given aspirin 500 mg per day or no treatment[61]. The authors reported a non-significant 10% reduction in total mortality in the aspirin arm but no reduction in incidence of or mortality from stroke, MI, or other vascular conditions. In a meta-analysis of low-risk patients in primary prevention studies, allocation to antiplatelet therapy for just over five years showed a 29% reduction in the rate of non-fatal MI that was significant[25]. However, the absolute difference was small and one would need to treat 200 patients for five years to prevent one MI. The meta-analysis showed a small but significant increase in fatal and non-fatal stroke in the aspirin-treated patients.

A prospective study of 87 678 female nurses responding to a questionnaire about aspirin use reported a statistically significant 32% reduction in the incidence of first MI in women taking one to six aspirin a week compared to those taking none[62]. For those aged over 50 years, the risk reduction was 39%. Aspirin use did not alter the risk of stroke.

Overall, there are no data to justify the use of any antiplatelet agent for primary stroke prevention in low-risk patients, independent of gender. There are data to justify the use of aspirin for primary prevention of MI, especially in patients over the age of 50.

References

1. Helgason CM, Bolin KM, Hoff JA, *et al.* Development of aspirin resistance in persons with previous ischemic stroke. *Stroke* 1994;25:2331–6
2. Schafer AI. Antiplatelet therapy. *Am J Med* 1996;101:199–209
3. Bousser MG, Roberts RS, Gent M. Ticlopidine and clopidogrel in secondary stroke prevention. *Cerebrovasc Dis* 1997;7(Suppl 6):17–23
4. Quinn MJ, Fitzgerald DJ. Ticlopidine and clopidogrel. *Circulation* 1999;100:1667–72

5. Mills DC, Puri R, Hu CJ, *et al.* Clopidogrel inhibits the binding of ADP analogues to the receptor mediating inhibition of platelet adenylate cyclase. *Arterioscl Thromb* 1992;12: 430–6

6. Fitzgerald DJ. Vascular biology of thrombosis. *Neurology* 2001;57(Suppl 2):S1–S4

7. Mahony C, Wolfram KM, Cocchetto DM, Bjornsson TD. Dipyridamole kinetics. *Clin Pharmacol Ther* 1982;31:330–8

8. Dresse A, Chevolet C, Delapierre D, *et al.* Pharmacokinetics of oral dipyridamole (Persantine) and its effect on platelet adenosine uptake in man. *Eur J Clin Pharmacol* 1982;23: 229–34

9. Albers GW. Choice of endpoints in antiplatelet trials. *Neurology* 2000;54:1022–8

10. Wilterdink JL, Easton JD. Dipyridamole plus aspirin in cerebrovascular disease. *Arch Neurol* 1999;56:1087–92

11. Antiplatelet Trialists' Collaboration. Secondary prevention of vascular disease by prolonged antiplatelet treatment. *Br Med J* 1988;296: 320–31

12. CAPRIE Steering Committee. A randomized blinded trial of clopidogrel versus aspirin in patients at risk of ischaemic events (CAPRIE). *Lancet* 1996;348:1329–39

13. Fields W, Lemak NA, Frankowski RF, Hardy RJ. Controlled trial of aspirin in cerebral ischemia. *Stroke* 1977;8:301–6

14. Canadian Cooperative Study Group. A randomized trial of aspirin and sulfinpyrazone in threatened stroke. *N Engl J Med* 1978;299: 53–9

15. Bousser MG, Eschwege E, Haguenau M, *et al.* "AICLA" controlled trial of aspirin and dipyridamole in the secondary prevention of atherothrombotic cerebral ischemia. *Stroke* 1983;14: 5–14

16. Diener HC, Cunha L, Forbes C, *et al.* European Stroke Prevention Study 2. Dipyridamole and acetylsalicylic acid in the secondary prevention of stroke. *J Neurol Sci* 1996;143(1–2):1–13

17. UK-TIA Study Group. United Kingdom transient ischaemic attack (UK-TIA) aspirin trial: interim results. *Br Med J* 1988;296:316–20

18. Reuther R, Dorndorf W. Aspirin in patients with cerebral ischemia and normal angiograms or non-surgical lesions. In: Breddin K, Dorndorf W, Loew D, Marx R, eds. *Acetylsalicylic Acid in Cerebral Ischaemia and Coronary Heart Disease.* Stuttgart, Germany: Schattauer, 1978:97–106

19. Sorensen PS, Pedersen H, Marquardsen J, *et al.* Acetylsalicylic acid in the prevention of stroke in patients with reversible cerebral ischemic attacks: a Danish cooperative study. *Stroke* 1983;14:15–22

20. Swedish Cooperative Study. High-dose acetylsalicylic acid after cerebral infarction. *Stroke* 1987;18:325–34

21. Boysen G, Sorensen PS, Juhler M, *et al.* Danish very-low-dose aspirin after carotid endarterectomy trial. *Stroke* 1988;19:1211–15

22. SALT Collaborative Group. Swedish Aspirin Low-Dose Trial (SALT) of 75 mg aspirin as secondary prophylaxis after cerebrovascular ischaemic events. *Lancet* 1991;338:1345–9

23. Millikan C, Futrell N. The strange story of aspirin and the prevention of stroke. *J Stroke Cerebrovasc Dis* 1995;5:248–54

24. Sze P, Reitman D, Pincus MM, *et al.* Antiplatelet agents in the secondary prevention of stroke: meta-analysis of the randomized control trials. *Stroke* 1988;19:436–42

25. Antiplatelet Trialists' Collaboration. Collaborative overview of randomised trials of antiplatelet therapy. I: Prevention of death, myocardial infarction, and stroke by prolonged antiplatelet therapy in various categories of patients. *Br Med J* 1994;308:81–106

26. Gelmers H, Tijssen J. Platelet antiaggregants in secondary prevention after stroke: does dipyridamole add to the effect of aspirin? *J Stroke Cerebrovasc Dis* 1993;3:115–20

27. Albers GW, Tijssen JG. Antiplatelet therapy: new foundations for optimal treatment decisions. *Neurology* 1999;53(Suppl 4):S25–S31

28. Hart RG, Harrison MJG. Aspirin wars: the optimal dose of aspirin to prevent stroke. *Stroke* 1996;27:585–7

29. Barnett HJM, Kaste M, Meldrum H, Eliasziw M. Aspirin dose in stroke prevention: Beautiful hypothesis slain by ugly facts. *Stroke* 1996;27: 588–92

30. Dutch TIA. Trial Study Group. A comparison of two doses of apirin (30 mg vs. 283 mg a day) in patients after a transient ischemic attack or minor ischemic stroke. *N Engl J Med* 1991;325:1261–6

31. Johnson ES, Lanes SF, Wentworth CE, *et al.* A metaregression analysis of the dose-response effect of aspirin on stroke. *Arch Intern Med* 1999;159:1248–53

32. Barnett HJM, Eliasziw M, Meldrum HE. Drug therapy: drugs and surgery in the prevention of ischemic stroke. *N Engl J Med* 1995;332: 238–48

33. Taylor DW, Barnett HJM, Haynes RB, *et al.* Low-dose and high-dose acetylsalicylic acid for patients undergoing carotid endarterectomy: a randomized controlled trial. ASA and Carotid Endarterectomy (ACE) Trial Collaborators. *Lancet* 1999;353:2179–84

34. Roderick J, Wilkes HC, Meade TW. The gastrointestinal toxicity of aspirin: an overview of randomized controlled trials. *J Clin Pharmacol* 1993;35:219–26

35. Derry S, Loke YK. Risk of gastrointestinal hemorrhage with long term use of aspirin: meta-analysis. *Br Med J* 2000;321:1183–7

36. Veterans Administration Cooperative Study Group. Role of carotid endarterectomy in asymptomatic carotid stenosis. *Stroke* 1986;17: 534–9

37. Krupski WC, Weiss DG, Rapp JH, *et al.* Adverse effects of aspirin in the treatment of asymptomatic carotid artery stenosis. VA Cooperative Asymptomatic Carotid Artery Stenosis Study Group. *J Vasc Surg* 1992;16:588–600

38. Hass W, Easton JD, Adams HP, *et al.* A randomized trial comparing ticlopidine hydrochloride with aspirin for the prevention of stroke in high-risk patients. Ticlopidine Aspirin Stroke Study Group. *N Engl J Med* 1989;321:501–7

39. Ticlopidine Aspirin Stroke Study Group. Ticlopidine versus aspirin for stroke prevention: on-treatment results from Ticlopidine Aspirin Stroke Study. *J Stroke Cerebrovasc Dis* 1993;3:168–76

40. Gent M, Easton JD, Hachinski VC, *et al.* The Canadian American Ticlopidine Study (CATS) in thromboembolic stroke. *Lancet* 1989;1: 1215–20

41. Bennett CL, Weinberg PD, Rozenberg-Ben-Dror K, *et al.* Thrombotic thrombocytopenic purpura associated with ticlopidine. *Ann Intern Med* 1998;128:541–4

42. Grotta JC, Norris JW, Kamm B. Prevention of stroke with ticlopidine: who benefits most? TASS Baseline and Angiographic Data Subgroup. *Neurology* 1992;42:111–15

43. Weisberg LA. The efficacy and safety of ticlopidine and aspirin in non-whites: analysis of a patient subgroup from the Ticlopidine Aspirin Stroke Study. *Neurology* 1993;43:27–31

44. Harbison JW. Ticlopidine versus aspirin for the prevention of recurrent stroke: analysis of patients with minor stroke from the Ticlopidine Aspirin Stroke Study. *Stroke* 1992;23:1723–7

45. Gorelick PB, Born GVR, D'Agostino RB, *et al.* Therapeutic benefit: aspirin revisited in light of the introduction of clopidogrel. *Stroke* 1999; 30:1716–21

46. Bennett CL, Connors JM, Carwile JM, *et al.* Thrombotic thrombocytopenic purpura associated with clopidogrel. *N Engl J Med* 2000;342: 1773–7

47. Moy B, Wang JC, Raffel GD, Marcoux JP. Hemolytic uremic syndrome associated with clopidogrel: a case report. *Arch Intern Med* 2000;160:1370–2

48. Guiraud-Chaumeil B, Rascol A, David J, *et al.* Prevention des recidives des accidents vasculaires cerebraux ischemiques par les anti-agregants plaquettaires. *Rev Neurol* 1982;138: 367–85

49. American-Canadian Co-operative Study Group. Persantine aspirin trial in cerebral ischemia part II: endpoint results. *Stroke* 1985;16:406–15

50. European Stroke Prevention Study Group. European stroke prevention study. *Stroke* 1990;21:1122–30

51. Sivenius J, Laakso M, Penttila IM, *et al.* The European stroke prevention study: results acording to sex. *Neurology* 1991;41:1189–92

52. Masuhr F, Busch M, Einhäupl KM. Differences in medical and surgical therapy for stroke prevention between leading experts in North America and Western Europe. *Stroke* 1998;29: 339–45

53. Gorelick PB. Aspirin plus extended-release dipyridamole: a new combination antiplatelet agent for secondary stroke prevention. *Stroke Clin Updates* 2000;10:1–4

54. Cohen SN. Dipyridamole plus aspirin in cerebrovascular disease. *Arch Neurol* 2000;57: 1086–7

55. Tijssen JGP. Low-dose and high-dose acetylsalicylic acid, with and without dipyridamole: a review of clinical trial results. *Neurology* 1998;51(Suppl 3):S15–S16

56. Albers GW, Easton JD, Sacco RL, Teal P. Antithrombotic and thrombolytic therapy for ischemic stroke. *Chest* 1998;114:683S–698S

57. Albers GW. Amarenco P. Easton JD, *et al.* Antithrombotic and thrombolytic therapy for ischemic stroke. *Chest* 2001;119(1 Suppl): 300S–320S

58. Gorelick PB, Leurgans S, Richardson D, *et al.* African-American Antiplatelet Stroke Prevention Study (AAASPS): clinical trial design. AAASPS investigators. *J Stroke Cerebrovasc Dis* 1998;7:426–34

59. The Clopidogrel in Unstable Angina to Prevent Recurrent Events Investigators. Effects of clopidogrel in addition to aspirin in patients with acute coronary syndromes without ST segment elevation. *N Engl J Med* 2001;345: 494–502

60. Steering Commmittee of the Physicians' Health Study Research Group. Final report on the aspirin component of the ongoing Physicians' Health Study. *N Engl J Med* 1989;321:129–35

61. Peto R, Gray R, Collins R, *et al.* Randomised trial of prophylactic daily aspirin in British male doctors. *Br Med J* 1988;296:313–16

62. Manson JE, Stampfer MJ, Colditz GA, *et al.* A prospective study of aspirin use and primary prevention of cardiovascular disease in women. *J Am Med Assoc* 1991;266:521–7

II. Anticoagulation for stroke prevention

Michael J. Schneck, MD

INTRODUCTION

The choice of antithrombotic therapy for stroke prevention is predicated on a clear understanding of the underlying mechanism that might result in a first-ever or recurrent stroke. Anticoagulants were typically the antithrombotic agents of choice until about twenty years ago, when better definitions of stroke mechanism through neuroimaging, clearer understanding of the relative risks of anticoagulation, and increasing evidence for the role of antiplatelet agents in stroke prevention led to a more restricted use of anticoagulants. The strongest evidence for oral anticoagulation is found in atrial fibrillation, where numerous studies have demonstrated a clear and convincing benefit for warfarin. There are also strong indications for the use of anticoagulants in those patients with valvular heart disease or who have intracardiac thrombus, but the indications for other conditions are less well defined.

MECHANISMS OF CLOT AND THERAPY WITH HEPARINOIDS AND DICOUMAROL DERIVATIVES

The development of a clot is a direct response to the injury of blood vessels or disruption of normal vascular flow, and is dependent on a complex interaction between circulating blood platelets that help form a plug at the immediate site of injury[1]. Subsequently, through a complex series of protein, calcium, and phospholipid interactions, the coagulation cascade is activated, resulting in development of a fibrin clot. Rudolph Virchow described this triad of thromboembolic factors in the mid-nineteenth century. Thrombosis occurs in the context of endothelial injury, coagulable states and circulatory stasis. When thrombus occurs, a platelet-rich clot is frequently seen in areas of fast flow and has been described as a 'white clot', whereas the predominantly fibrin-enriched clot ('red' clots) are seen in more sluggish swirling areas of vascular flow such as the venous system and the intracardiac chambers. However, mixed clots are not uncommon.

The conversion of factor X to factor Xa, followed by conversion of the prothrombin complex to thrombin, leads to the cleavage of peptides from fibrinogen and subsequent polymerization of fibrin with the resultant creation of a fibrin clot. The activation of this thrombin–fibrin system may occur through two parallel sequences. These are referred to as the intrinsic system, involving circulating compounds within the blood, and the extrinsic system, which is dependent on tissue-based factors. Therapeutic manipulations of the coagulation system began with the discovery of heparin by Mclean and Howell in 1916. Heparin was subsequently purified and characterized by Erik Jorpes in 1935[2,3]. Shortly thereafter, Jorpes and Craaford in Sweden and Charles Best in Toronto, Canada, applied heparin clinically to prevent post-operative thrombosis[2]. The heparinoids work through activation of antithrombin III, that then acts to inhibit the binding of thrombin and factor Xa. Whereas unfractionated heparin (UH) inactivates thrombin and factor Xa, low molecular weight heparinoids (LMWH) have a more selective anticoagulant effect that is mediated mainly through factor Xa inhibition. The presumed advantages of LMWHs are less non-specific binding to plasma proteins and reduced binding to platelets, leading to fewer hemorrhagic complications and a lower incidence of heparin-induced thrombocytopenia as compared with unfractionated heparin. Newer factor Xa and direct thrombin inhibitors – such as the pentasaccharides and hirudin derivatives – are under investigation and may provide even greater selective anti-thrombotic effects. Additional anticoagulant therapies are also being studied[4]. However unfractionated intravenous heparin still has an important role in the anticoagulant therapy of stroke patients because of its short half-life, that allows the drug to be stopped quickly in case a patient requires surgery or develops an unexpected systemic or intracerebral hemorrhage. The partial thromboplastin time (PTT) or activated partial thromboplastin time (aPTT) is used to monitor the efficacy of anticoagulation. The usual therapeutic goal is to aim for a PTT approximately 1.5 to 2 times 'normal'. Patients being treated with unfractionated heparin for prevention of recurrent cerebral ischemic events typically do not receive a bolus of heparin because of concerns of hemorrhagic conversion by an infarct with a loading dose of heparin.

There are no established indications for heparinoids in acute ischemic stroke, but these agents are often used either as a bridge to long-term therapy with an oral anticoagulant for prevention of recurrent cerebral ischemia, or in the specific circumstances of high-risk stroke patients who have an indication for anticoagulation but for whom warfarin is contraindicated because of an allergic reaction or pregnancy[5,6]. Oral anticoagulation is contraindicated during pregnancy because of fetal teratogenicity and fetal bleeding complications associated with coumarin derivatives. Pregnant patients with cerebral venous thrombosis (CVT) should be maintained, therefore, on a low molecular weight heparinoid during the pregnancy. There is no contraindication, however, to coumarin derivatives post-partum and patients may even breast-feed their children if desired[6].

Warfarin is the main oral anticoagulant in clinical use in the United States. Investigators at the University of Wisconsin, investigating a hemorrhagic disease of cattle, identified dicumoral as the etiologic agent in the 1920s[7]. Warfarin (derived from Wisconsin Agricultural Research Foundation) was initially developed as a rat poison and, in the late 1940s, was brought into clinical use. Warfarin does not have direct anticoagulant activity[7], instead it blocks vitamin K metabolism in the liver. This blocks gamma-carboxylation of glutamic acids that serve as calcium binding sites on factors II, VII, IX, and X (as well as proteins C, S and Z) necessary for the generation of activated thrombin. Monitoring of coumadin therapy uses the international normalized ratio (INR) as a calibration standard to correct for variations in different laboratory tissue thromboplastin agents for assay of the 'prothrombin time'. Adequacy of anticoagulation can vary widely in patients, depending on changes in the intake of vitamin K-rich foods and changes in absorption and/or protein-binding with other drug therapies[7].

On the basis of pooled data that tested anticoagulation therapy in various atrial fibrillation clinical trials, the optimal anticoagulation range for most patients is an INR of 2.5 ± 0.5 (a range of 2.0 to 3.0). In some circumstances, such as in patients with mechanical heart valves, an INR as high as 3.5 may be desirable. When the INR is greater than 4.0 the risk of hemorrhage dramatically increases[8]. Conversely, when the INR is 1.7 or less, the odds of an ischemic stroke double as compared with an INR of 2.0[9]. Close monitoring of warfarin is necessary because of this narrow therapeutic index and, whenever possible, substitution of warfarin preparations from different manufacturers should be avoided.

CARDIOEMBOLIC STROKE

Evidence-based justification for anticoagulation exists for atrial fibrillation, prosthetic heart valves, dilated cardiomyopathies, left ventricular thrombus and large anterior wall myocardial infarction. There is also some evidence suggesting a role for anticoagulation of patients with strokes associated with patent foramen ovale, atrial septal aneurysms and aortic arch atheroma. Justification for the use of anticoagulants in other potential cardiac sources of embolism such as mitral valve prolapse, mitral annular calcifications and valvular strands is less clear. Chronic atrial fibrillation (AF) provides the clearest indication for the use of anticoagulation to prevent cardioembolic stroke.

Atrial fibrillation

Numerous trials provide strong evidence that adjusted-dose warfarin reduces stroke risk by approximately two-thirds as compared to placebo in patients with atrial fibrillation. Aspirin, as an alternative therapy, provides a modest 20% risk reduction, but is probably a reasonable option in patients with lone atrial fibrillation and no other risk factors for stroke. Low-intensity anticoagulation with or without aspirin is no better than aspirin alone. Limited data are currently available regarding alternative antiplatelet treatments[10-13]. The risk of stroke appears to be similar for those patients with paroxysmal or persistent chronic atrial fibrillation. Therefore, unless the patient falls into the low-risk category of lone atrial fibrillation, long-term anticoagulation is also indicated for patients with paroxysmal atrial fibrillation[13-15].

A continuing challenge in clinical practice is to determine which patients with atrial fibrillation should not be anticoagulated. There are possibly more studies demonstrating under-utilization of anticoagulants in AF than studies confirming anticoagulant efficacy. In individual circumstances, when there is doubt, anticoagulation should be favored. Risk stratification analysis based on randomized trials has led to three categories of patient[10]. Low-risk patients are those with no prior history of stroke or transient ischemic attack (TIA) and no clinical or echocardiographic evidence of cardiovascular disease, and who are under 65 years old. Such patients can be treated with aspirin alone since their stroke risk is estimated to be approximately 0.5% per year[11]. Patients in an intermediate risk category have only one of the following risk factors: age 65–75 years, diabetes mellitus, or coronary artery disease without left ventricular (LV) dysfunction. In such patients the risk/benefit ratio supports the use of either warfarin or antiplatelet therapy. If any of these patients have more than one of these factors, however, they should be considered as being at high risk. Any patient with the following risk factors should be considered at high risk of cerebral ischemia and should be treated with adjusted-dose anticoagulation: history of stroke or TIA or systemic embolus, history of hypertension (treated or untreated), poor left ventricular systolic function, rheumatic mitral valve disease, prosthetic heart valves, and age over 75 years. Increased age is a particularly important predictor of increased risk. Even though older patients with atrial fibrillation on anticoagulation have a higher risk of bleeding complications, they have an even greater risk of cardioembolic ischemic stroke. Yet, many physicians tend to avoid warfarin in older patients while treating younger patients, whose risk is actually lower[11,16–20].

Patients being considered for elective cardioversion should receive anticoagulants for at least three weeks preceding and at least four weeks following DC cardioversion[10]. Transesophageal echocardiographic demonstration of the absence of intracardiac thrombus may eliminate the need for anticoagulation in some patients prior to cardioversion but, following cardioversion, even these patients should be anticoagulated for at least four weeks, with some clinicians advocating as long as three months[10]. The risk of recurrent atrial fibrillation is high even when a patient converts to sinus rhythm. Van Gelder *et al.* reported that only 42% of patients in atrial fibrillation remained in sinus rhythm one year following cardioversion; the percent in sinus rhythm was projected to fall to 36% at two years[21]. Long-term anticoagulation may be an appropriate option even for those patients who are successfully cardioverted who are otherwise in the high-risk atrial fibrillation group[13]. The benefit of long-term anticoagulation in other atrial arrhythmias has not been established but short-term anticoagulation at the time of cardioversion has been suggested for these patients as well.

Prosthetic valves

Prosthetic heart valves are associated with a definite and significant thromboembolic risk that is dependent on their type and location, the risk being higher for mitral than for aortic valves. The thromboembolic risk is upwards of 5% per year for mechanical valves, with modern caged-ball or caged-disk valves having a risk of 2.5% per year, tilting-disk valves having a risk of 0.7% per year and bi-leaflet valves having a risk of approximately 0.5% per year. The thromboembolic risk is lower for bioprosthetic valves, ranging from approximately 0.2% to 2.6% per year, although the risk is 2–3 times higher in the first three months post insertion. Because of the high thromboembolic risk, the consensus is that all patients with mechanical heart valves should be chronically anticoagulated[22]. Since the long-term risk of bioprosthetic valves is lower, anticoagulation for these valves is warranted only in the first three months following insertion of the valve unless there are other risk factors for systemic embolism. Long-term anticoagulation for these patients is not associated with a sufficient degree of stroke-risk reduction to offset the increased risk of hemorrhage. After the first three months, antiplatelet therapy is considered sufficient antithrombotic prophylaxis for bioprosthetic valves.

The intensity of anticoagulation is also different, depending on the type and location of the prosthetic valve[22]. In general, an INR of 2.5 ± 0.5 is appropriate, but an INR of 3.0 ± 0.5 is recommended for mechanical mitral valves. Combination anticoagulant and antiplatelet therapy may also be appropriate for patients with mechanical valves. Fixed low-dose warfarin plus aspirin has been shown to have less benefit than adjusted-dose warfarin in the context of atrial fibrillation. In contrast, there are good data to support combining thromboembolic prophylaxis by using adjusted-dose warfarin and low-dose aspirin (80–100 mg) daily in patients with prosthetic valves. By analogy with prosthetic valve cases, combination adjusted-dose warfarin and antiplatelet therapy may also be appropriate for patients with atrial fibrillation, but further investigation in this area is warranted.

Cardiac failure (ischemic and non-ischemic) and myocardial infarction

Cardiac failure is associated with a 2–3 times increased risk of cardioembolic stroke, and is the second most common cause of cardioembolic stroke after atrial fibrillation[23]. Although the stroke rates in various heart failure trials are relatively low, ranging from 1.3% to 3.5% per year[23], and the stroke rate is not directly related to the severity of heart failure, the rate of stroke does increase significantly as the cardiac ejection fraction declines[23]. There appears to be no difference in the risk of stroke between ischemic and non-ischemic etiologies of heart failure[23]. A prior history of stroke, however, markedly increases stroke risk[24].

Warfarin decreases the risk of stroke in patients with myocardial infarction as compared with placebo[23,25], but it is unclear whether warfarin is more efficacious than antiplatelet agents. In patients with chronic heart failure and a low ejection fraction, there are, as yet, no definitive clinical trials that demonstrate a convincing benefit for warfarin over antiplatelet therapy. The Warfarin Versus Aspirin in Reduced Cardiac Ejection Fraction (WARCEF) and the Warfarin and Antiplatelet Therapy in Chronic Heart Failure (WATCH) are two on-going trials that may clarify whether anticoagulation is better than aspirin in chronic heart failure for the prevention of stroke and death. Additionally, WATCH will include clopidogrel as a third arm and so may provide information on the relative efficacy of a newer antiplatelet agent versus warfarin. Another primary endpoint in the WATCH trial is myocardial infarction. Until data from these trials become available, current guidelines recommend early administration of heparin followed by warfarin for up to three months in patients with acute myocardial infarction at increased risk for systemic embolism because of a prior history of systemic or pulmonary embolism, anterior wall Q-wave infarction, severe left ventricular dysfunction or echocardiographic evidence of left ventricular thrombus[25]. In patients with an ejection fraction less than 30% who have had a prior TIA or stroke, anticoagulation is reasonable given the increased risk of recurrent cerebral ischemia in such patients. Whether anticoagulation is useful in the primary prevention of stroke for patients with a low cardiac ejection fraction remains to be determined. Until further clinical trial data are forthcoming, it is reasonable to anticoagulate patients with a very low ejection fraction (arbitrarily less than 10%). Either antiplatelet or anticoagulant therapy would also be reasonable for patients with an ejection fraction of 10 to 30% who have no other cardioembolic risk factors. For patients with an ejection fraction of greater than 30%, antiplatelet therapy seems more appropriate unless there are other cardioembolic risk factors for stroke, although this assertion is arbitrary and requires more data.

Patent foramen ovale and atrial septal aneurysms

As a result of improved echocardiographic techniques, inter-atrial septal abnormalities can be identified in stroke patients with increasing frequency. However, an asymptomatic patent foramen ovale (PFO) may be present in approximately one-third of the population and atrial septal aneurysms (ASA) may be present in upwards of 10% of the population[26]. Because of this high frequency, in some stroke patients the PFO may be a coincidental finding[27]. However the prevalence of PFO in patients with 'cryptogenic' stroke, particularly in those under the age of 55, is much higher than in non-stroke patients[26–28]. A recent meta-analysis of case–control studies that examined the association of stroke and atrial septal abnormalities calculated an odds ratio of 6.0 (95% CI, 3.72–9.68) for the risk of stroke in patients under the age of 55 with a PFO[28]. The risk of stroke may also be higher in patients who have a PFO and atrial septal aneurysm, a large PFO or PFO with an increased right to left shunt[26].

Because the presumed mechanism of embolization with PFO and/or ASA is from either the venous system or the atrial chambers ('red clot'), anticoagulation is a logical initial therapeutic option. However, the choice of therapy should be determined by the risk of stroke. Because PFO is much more common in the general population than stroke, especially in younger persons, prophylactic therapy against a cerebral ischemic stroke in a patient with a PFO is not warranted. Treatment to prevent recurrent cerebral ischemia would depend on the rate of recurrent events. If the stroke recurrence rate is less than one or two percent, then treatment with warfarin may not be justifiable because chronic warfarin therapy is also associated with a 1–2% risk of intracranial hemorrhage[7,8].

Enthusiasm for percutaneous endovascular closure of PFO has recently developed. However, the long-term course of closure devices remains to be defined. A decision-analysis model suggested that when the risk of recurrence was over 0.8%, closure of a PFO was better than antiplatelet therapy in reducing stroke, but the analysis model was based on limited, non-randomized data. A clinical trial of anticoagulation versus PFO closure has been proposed but is not yet underway. Until more information becomes available younger patients (less than 50–60 years old) who have no other cause of stroke, have a large PFO with significant inter-atrial shunting or who have recurrent ischemic events despite antiplatelet therapy, may benefit from anticoagulation. PFO closure is also a reasonable alternative in such patients who are opposed to life-long

anticoagulation. PFO closure is also indicated in those patients who have a recurrent stroke despite being on anticoagulation, are at high risk for bleeding complications, or who cannot take warfarin for other reasons (e.g. pregnancy)[27].

NON-CARDIOEMBOLIC STROKE

The benefit of anticoagulation in any atherothrombotic stroke or TIA has not been confirmed, but data are available from the SPIRIT trial and the Warfarin–Aspirin Recurrent Stroke Study (WARSS) trial. SPIRIT was a randomized European study comparing low-dose aspirin at 30 mg per day with high-dose anticoagulation (INR 3–4.5)[29]. This study was terminated early because of an excess of serious bleeding events in the anticoagulation arm after 1316 patients had been enrolled with mean follow-up of 14 months. The hazard ratio for an excess of complications with anticoagulation was 2.3 (95% CI, 1.6–3.5). There were 27 intracranial hemorrhages, of which 17 were fatal, in the anticoagulation arm and only three intracranial hemorrhages (with one fatality) in the antiplatelet arm. There was no significant difference in the number of recurrent ischemic events between the arms. The excess hemorrhage rate was clearly attributable to the high intensity of anticoagulation; the bleeding incidence increased by a factor of 1.43 (95% CI, 0.96–2.13) for each 0.5 unit increase of the achieved INR.

The WARSS trial is a recently completed study of warfarin with lower intensity anticoagulation (INR 1.4–2.8) versus 325 mg aspirin in 2206 patients with two-year follow-up[30]. The mean INR achieved in the anticoagulation group was 2.0–2.1 over the two-year follow-up. The study found no statistical difference between the arms for the risk of recurrent ischemic events or hemorrhagic complications. Concerns about the generalizability of these data include the possibility that the INR in the anticoagulated patients was too low to test efficacy. A higher mean INR of 2.5 might have resulted in fewer recurrent strokes for warfarin. In addition, the WARSS cohort comprised a large percentage (> 50%) of patients with lacunar strokes. Therefore, the possibility that warfarin might be more beneficial in large artery atherothrombotic stroke cannot be excluded. Further information about subgroup analyses may be forthcoming after publication of the initial WARSS report. In addition, another study, the Warfarin Aspirin Symptomatic Intracranial Disease (WASID) prospective study, may shed light on therapy for intracranial arterial stenosis[31].

Still another trial, the European/Australian Stroke Prevention in Reversible Ischemia (ESPRIT) trial, may shed light on the role of medium intensity anticoagulation as compared with antiplatelet therapy[32]. This is a trial enrolling 4500 stroke patients with a mean follow-up of three years who will be randomized to either dipyridamole (400 mg daily) plus aspirin (any dose from 30 mg to 325 mg daily) or anticoagulation with an INR between 2.0 and 3.0. The planned primary outcome is a combined endpoint of recurrent stroke, myocardial infarction, vascular death, or major bleeding complications. This study will be of particular interest because it compares anticoagulation at a range typically utilized in most stroke patients in the United States with one of the newer combination antiplatelet agents that are now being increasingly used instead of aspirin. At present, however, the use of an anticoagulant as first-line therapy for non-cardioembolic stroke is unsupported by evidence from clinical trials. However, expert opinion or non-randomized studies suggests that there may be a role for anticoagulation in cervical arterial dissection, severe extracranial carotid stenoses awaiting endarterectomy, transient anticoagulation following acute carotid occlusion, stroke as a result of certain hypercoagulable states, and perhaps in those patients who 'failed' all other antiplatelet therapy combinations and have experienced a recurrent stroke or TIA[10].

Intracranial stenosis

Studies from the 1960s through the early 1980s suggested that warfarin might reduce the risk of recurrent stroke or TIA. However, these studies were flawed by lack of defined entry criteria, the small numbers of patients enrolled and a retrospective design. In 1995 the WASID study investigators reported their own retrospective experience in 151 patients with angiographically confirmed intracranial arterial stenoses[33]. They reported a relative risk reduction of 0.46 (95% CI, 0.23–0.86) for stroke, MI or sudden death with the use of warfarin rather than aspirin. The main benefit of warfarin was in stroke prevention. The stroke rate was 10.4 per 100 patient-years on aspirin but only 3.6 per 100 patient-years on warfarin. Patients with posterior circulation strokes had a higher rate of recurrent strokes than patients with stroke in the anterior circulation. There was no obvious difference in benefit of warfarin for posterior circulation stenosis compared with anterior circulation stenosis. The WASID study provided better defined patient entry criteria and specific definitions for 50–99% angiographically confirmed stenosis. However, despite these improvements in design, the WASID study still had significant methodological problems. For example, the study only considered patients on aspirin and thus provided no data on the role of the newer antiplatelet agents. Furthermore, the aspirin dose was not uniform for all patients. Like earlier studies, this study had a selection bias in that it was a non-randomized and retrospective cohort. The WASID investigators have recently initiated a randomized, double-blind, prospective study of adjusted-dose warfarin (INR 2.0–3.0) and high-dose aspirin (1300 mg daily) for angiographically defined 50–99% symptomatic intracranial arterial stenosis[31] but results are not yet available. Until completion of that study, the choice of antiplatelet versus anticoagulant therapy may be based on an assessment of risks (for example, tendency to fall, poor compliance) and possible benefits of anticoagulation. Antiplatelet therapy, including the newer combination therapies, may be appropriate. Conventional angiography is still preferred in determining the degree of stenosis, since non-invasive modalities such as transcranial Doppler ultrasonography or magnetic resonance angiography may overestimate the degree of stenosis.

Extracranial carotid atherosclerotic disease

Anticoagulation is frequently utilized for patients with high-grade stenosis or occlusion of the carotid arteries despite the lack of evidence to definitively support this practice. Anticoagulation is more likely to be used by physicians for patients with seventy percent or greater carotid stenosis, patients with recent TIA or stroke, and patients with surgical contraindications[34]. A survey of physicians showed that, compared with surgeons, non-internist primary care physicians were 5.32 times more likely (95% CI, 3.79–7.45), internists 3.65 times more likely (95% CI, 2.63–5.06) and neurologists only 1.88 times more likely (95% CI, 1.40–2.35) to use an anticoagulant in treating patients at risk of stroke or stroke recurrence. This survey failed to distinguish between short-term intravenous or oral anticoagulation prior to endarterectomy and long-term oral anticoagulation. This limits our understanding of the physician's rationale for anticoagulation in carotid disease. Internists and neurologists also had an approximately two-thirds higher odds ratio of using antiplatelet therapies compared with surgeons, but there was no difference between surgeons and non-internist primary care physicians in the use of antiplatelet therapy in carotid artery disease. The American Heart Association guidelines recognize that there may be a role for short-term anticoagulation despite being on antiplatelet therapy following a transient ischemic attack (TIA) or crescendo TIAs while a diagnostic evaluation is urgently in progress. As yet, no adequate data are available to support or refute this practice[35].

The best available trial data on the use of anticoagulation in specific stroke types is derived from a subgroup analysis of the Trial of Org 10172 in Acute Stroke Treatment (TOAST) trial[36]. This trial failed to show an overall benefit for the low molecular weight heparinoid danaparoid following an acute ischemic stroke. However, an exploratory analysis suggested a favorable outcome at both 7 days and 3 months for patients with duplex evidence of a greater than 50% stenosis or occlusion of the carotid artery who were on danaparoid compared with those on placebo. At 7 days 53.8% of the patients on danaparoid and only 38% of the patients on placebo had a favorable outcome ($p = 0.023$). At 3 months, 69.3% of the patients on danaparoid and 53.2% of the patients on placebo had a favorable outcome ($p = 0.021$). The benefit from danaparoid may have resulted from decreased microemboli developing at the carotid artery plaque that could disseminate downstream. In fact, microemboli, as detected by transcranial Doppler studies, are frequent in patients with high-grade carotid stenoses and may actually occur more frequently with acute carotid artery disease than in patients with a potential cardioembolic source[37,38]. Therefore, short-term intravenous or even oral anticoagulation may be appropriate for patients admitted with a fairly recent stroke or TIA who are not immediate candidates for endarterectomy. Given the meager available evidence and the inherent hemorrhagic risks of anticoagulation, long-term anticoagulation may not be appropriate for patients with extracranial carotid disease.

Aortic arch atheroma

Atheromatous plaque in the aortic arch is often discussed in the context of cardioembolic stroke. The pathophysiology of stroke attributed to such lesions is most probably due to cholesterol-laden and platelet-enriched artery-to-artery emboli and, by analogy with carotid artery disease, stroke secondary to aortic arch atheroma should be classified as large-vessel disease.

With improvements in vascular ultrasound, these lesions have been more frequently identified and shown to represent an independent risk factor for stroke[39-44]. Typically, aortic arch atheroma has been visualized by transesophageal echocardiography, but new techniques allow visualization of the aortic arch through a supraclavicular approach in those patients undergoing carotid ultrasonography[41,45]. In the French Study of Aortic Plaques in Stroke Groups (FAPS), those subjects who had aortic arch plaque with a thickness of 4 mm or more had a recurrent stroke rate of 11.9 per 100 person-years[44]. By comparison, the risk of recurrent stroke with an aortic wall thickness of 1.0 to 3.9 mm was 3.5 per 100 person-years, and it was 2.8 per 100 person-years when the thickness was less than 1 mm. In that study, aortic arch plaque was found to be a significant independent predictor of recurrent stroke ($p = 0.0012$) as well as a predictor for a combined endpoint of all vascular events ($p < 0.001$). Ulcerated plaque was not associated with an increased risk but soft plaque at least 4 mm thick, without evidence of calcification, had a significant increased risk of stroke[43]. Other large series have described similar results, suggesting that large mobile aortic arch plaques had a significant increased risk of stroke. A series of case–control studies

also suggested a significantly increased risk of stroke with large aortic plaque[39,40,42], especially in patients aged 60 years or older with large mobile aortic arch atheroma and an otherwise cryptogenic stroke. Di Tullio and colleagues reported an odds ratio of 3.4 (95% CI, 1.2–11.2) in a population-based series for a population of patients from Northern Manhattan[40] and Amarenco and colleagues reported an odds ratio of 4.7 (95% CI, 2.2–10.1) in a French population[39].

Despite the increased risk of stroke associated with significant aortic arch atheromatous plaque, an optimal treatment has not yet been established, although there has been some suggestion that warfarin is the treatment of choice[46]. However, based on the mechanism of stroke with carotid artery disease, antiplatelet therapy will remain the first-line therapy for primary and secondary stroke prevention until further clinical trial data are available[44].

Cervical artery dissection

Recognition of cervical artery dissection has certainly increased with improved neuroimaging techniques. The estimated incidence of internal carotid artery (ICA) dissection is approximately 2.6–2.9 per 100 000 population and the estimated incidence of vertebral artery dissections is approximately one third that of ICA dissection[47,48]. The majority of ICA dissections occur in young adults. Such lesions may account for upwards of 20% of all strokes in adults under the age of 50[48-50]. The presumptive mechanism of infarction for patients with dissection is an embolus from the false lumen that develops when a tear occurs in the arterial media of the dissected artery. This embolus occludes arterial branches downstream from the dissection. Anticoagulation is the accepted treatment and is continued for approximately one to six months until the stenosis from the dissection improves. Even if the artery is occluded by the dissection, anticoagulation is continued for one to six months. Thereafter, patients with carotid artery dissection may be maintained on antiplatelet therapy. If the patient has little or no clinical deficits and minimal radiological evidence of infarction, antiplatelet therapy alone may be sufficient. Alternatively, intravascular placement of a vascular stent, in addition to antiplatelet therapy, is an option for those patients with intracranial extension of the dissection, particularly if they are experiencing major or recurrent clinical events[47,51]. Antiplatelet therapy is also appropriate if the dissection extends intracranially because such extension increases the risk of subarachnoid hemorrhage. Moreover there are no controlled trials showing that warfarin is superior to antiplatelet therapy for dissection of either the carotid or vertebral arteries[47].

Cerebral venous thrombosis

Cerebral venous thromboses (CVT) have remarkably diverse presentations, including focal neurological deficits, seizures or increased intracranial pressure with headache or papilledema[52,53]. Though patients of any age or either sex may have CVT, such lesions occur predominantly in woman of child-bearing age. CVT should be included in the differential diagnosis of a pregnant or post-partum patient with neurological symptoms or signs[52,54]. The role of intravenous anticoagulation in treating CVT has been studied in retrospective series and small randomized trials[53,55,56]. American College of Chest Physician (ACCP) consensus guidelines recommend heparin or low molecular weight heparinoids in the acute phase of CVT even when hemorrhagic infarcts are also present, followed by oral anticoagulation for approximately three to six months[10]. Heparinoid therapy has a relative contraindication in patients with CVT with large intracranial hematomas. In those instances, supportive therapy or local infusion of thrombolytic agents within the occluded venous sinus may be considered[10,53,57].

Hypercoagulable states

Prothrombotic states associated with disorders of coagulation may be acquired or inherited. Factor V Leiden mutations are associated with resistance to activated protein C and are present in up to 8% of the normal population, making this the most common of the inherited hypercoagulable disorders[58,59]. Other less common inherited syndromes are associated with protein S, protein C and antithrombin deficiencies. All of these syndromes are associated with venous thromboembolism but they may also be seen in hepatic disease, nephrotic syndromes, systemic malignancy, and in patients who are pregnant or on oral contraceptives. The antiphospholipid syndromes that are associated with abnormal antiphospholipid antibodies, including the anticardiolipin epitopes or an abnormal lupus anticoagulant, represent the best recognized of the acquired hypercoagulable states[60,61]. Hypercoagulable syndromes are often seen with systemic lupus erythematosus. Hypercoagulability also occurs in Sneddon's syndrome, a disorder characterized by antiphospholipid antibodies, livedo reticularis and stroke.

The routine screening of stroke patients for hypercoagulable disorders is not cost-efficient because they are relatively rare[62]. Empiric therapy of adults with hypercoagulable disorders discovered incidentally without associated thromboembolic events is of unproven benefit. Nonetheless, in those with a stroke or TIA in whom a homozygous factor V Leiden mutation, protein S, protein C or antithrombin deficiency has been identified, long-term oral anticoagulation is usually recommended. Such patients, particularly those with protein C or S deficiencies, should first receive heparin prior to oral anticoagulation because of the possible risk of increased hypercoagulability when starting warfarin[63]. A clear consensus about choosing antiplatelet agents versus anticoagulant drugs for the antiphospholipid antibody syndromes is lacking[60,64,65].

SPECIAL CONSIDERATION: RESUMPTION OF ANTICOAGULATION IN THE CONTEXT OF INTRACEREBRAL HEMORRHAGE

The absolute risk of intracerebral hemorrhage in the general population ranges from 0.3% to 1.7% per year[66]. With high-intensity anticoagulation, the risk of hemorrhage is 6–11 fold higher than this rate[67]. However, the risk of an ischemic cerebral event in patients with an intracerebral hemorrhage who otherwise have an absolute indication for anticoagulation may also be high and has been estimated at upwards of 1% per day in the first two weeks. Other estimates of early stroke recurrence are much lower[10]. Several small series and a larger retrospective series from the Mayo Clinic suggest that, when absolutely necessary, resumption of oral anticoagulation after one to two weeks is associated with a low short-term embolic risk and no major complications of recurrent hemorrhage[68–74]. Intravenous heparin or continuation of oral anticoagulation without cessation, after demonstrating a cardiac thrombus in a patient with intracerebral hemorrhage or a cerebral infarct with hemorrhagic conversion, is less clear. It is hard to ignore the danger of emboli posed by the presence of an intracardiac thrombus, visualized on echocardiography, even though the risk over the short term is low. Pessin *et al.* reported their experience with anticoagulation in 12 patients who did well despite hemorrhagic infarction[75]. Leker and Abramsky also described good outcomes in four patients who received early heparin therapy despite having had an intracerebral bleed[71]. Nevertheless, anticoagulation in such circumstances is certainly controversial[74].

CONCLUSIONS

Oral and intravenous anticoagulants provide important therapeutic options in the primary and secondary prevention of cerebral ischemic events. The indications for anticoagulation for stroke prevention are not yet well established, except for atrial fibrillation, prosthetic cardiac valves, recent anterior wall myocardial infarction and intracardiac thrombus. Because of the high risk of serious bleeding complications, anticoagulants should be reserved for the specific conditions described in this chapter. Anticoagulation with a high INR (> 4.0) is associated with more frequent hemorrhagic complications. However, inadequate anticoagulation (INR < 1.4) has its own problems, such as increased risk of recurrent stroke. The initiation of anticoagulants requires close and continued monitoring to maintain the appropriate intensity. After stabilization, the INR should be followed monthly, mindful of the possibility that diet and new drugs may substantially affect the degree of anticoagulation.

References

1. Rosenberg RD. Vascular-bed – specific hemostasis and hypercoagulable states. *N Engl J Med* 1999;340(20):1555–64
2. Davies MK. Heparin. *Heart* 1998;80(2):120
3. Shampo MA. Erik Jorpes – pioneer in the identification and clinical applications of heparin. *Mayo Clin Proc* 1997;72(11):1056
4. Weitz JI. New anticoagulant drugs. *Chest* 2001;119(Suppl 1):95S–107S
5. Kalafut MA, Kidwell CS, Saver JL. Safety and cost of low molecular weight heparin as bridging anticoagulant therapy in subacute cerebral ischemia. *Stroke* 2000;31: 2563–8

6. Ginsberg JS, Hirsch J. Use of antithrombotic agents during pregnancy. *Chest* 2001;119 (Suppl 1):122S–131S

7. Keller C, Kemkes-Matthes B. Pharmacology of warfarin and clinical implications. *Semin Thromb Hemost* 1999;25(1):13–16

8. Hylek EM. Risk factors for intracranial hemorrhage in outpatients taking warfarin. *Ann Intern Med* 1994;120(11):897–902

9. Hylek EM, Sheehan MA, Singer DE. An analysis of the lowest effective intensity of prophylactic anticoagulation for patients with nonrheumatic atrial fibrillation. *N Engl J Med* 1996;335(8):540–6

10. Albers GW, Easton JD, Sacco RL, Teal P. Antithrombotic and thrombolytic therapy for ischemic stroke. *Chest* 2001;119(Suppl 1): 300S–320S

11. Hart RG. Atrial fibrillation and stroke: concepts and controversies. *Stroke* 2001;32:803–8

12. Hart RG, McBride R, Pearce LA. Antithrombotic therapy to prevent stroke in patients with atrial fibrillation. *Ann Intern Med* 1999;131:492–501

13. Falk RH. Atrial fibrillation. *N Engl J Med* 2001;344(14):1067–78

14. Hart RG, Rothbart RM, McAnulty JH, *et al.* Stroke with intermittent atrial fibrillation: incidence and predictors during aspirin therapy. *J Am Coll Cardiol* 2000;35:183–7

15. Atrial Fibrillation Investigators. Risk factors for stroke and efficacy of antithrombotic therapy in atrial fibrillation. Analysis of pooled data from five randomized controlled trials. *Arch Intern Med* 1994;154:1449–57

16. Beyth RJ, Covinsky KE, Miller DG, *et al.* Why isn't warfarin prescribed to patients with non-rheumatic atrial fibrillation? *J Gen Intern Med* 1996;11(12):721–8

17. Antani MR, Covinsky KE, Anderson PA, *et al.* Failure to prescribe warfarin to patients with nonrheumatic atrial fibrillation. *J Gen Intern Med* 1996;11(12):713–20

18. Brass LM, Krumholz HM, Scinto JD, *et al.* Warfarin use following ischemic stroke among Medicare patients with atrial fibrillation. *Arch Intern Med* 1998;158:2093–100

19. Sudlow M, Thwaites B, Rodgers H, Kenny RA. Prevalence of atrial fibrillation and eligibility for anticoagulants in the community. *Lancet* 1998;352:1167–71

20. Smith NL, Furberg CD, White R, *et al.* Temporal trends in the use of anticoagulants among older adults with atrial fibrillation. *Arch Intern Med* 1999;159:1574–8

21. Van Gelder IC, Van Gilst WH, Verwer R, Lie KI. Prediction of uneventful cardioversion and maintenance of sinus rhythm from direct-current electrical cardioversion of chronic atrial fibrillation and flutter. *Am J Cardiol* 1991;68: 41–6

22. Stein PD, Bussey HI, Dalen JE, Turpie AGG. Antithrombotic therapy in patients with mechanical and biological prosthetic heart valves. *Chest* 2001;119:220S–227S

23. Pullicino PM, Thompson JLP. Stroke in patients with heart failure and reduced left ventricular ejection fraction. *Neurology* 2000;54:288–94

24. Sacco RL, Zamanillo MC, Kargmen ME. Predictors of mortality and recurrence after hospitalized cerebral infarction in an urban community: the Northern Manhattan Study. *Neurology* 1994;44:626–34

25. Cairns JA, Lewis HD Jr, Ezekowitz M, Meade TW. Anthithrombotic agents in coronary artery disease. Chest 2001;119(Suppl 1): 228S–252S

26. Devuyst G. Status of patent foramen ovale, atrial septal aneurysm, atrial septal defect and aortic arch atheroma as risk factors for stroke. *Neuroepidemiology* 1997;16(5):217–23

27. Chambers J. Should percutaneous devices be used to close a patent foramen ovale after cerebral infarction or TIA? *Heart* 1999;82(5):537–8

28. Overell JR, Lees KR. Interatrial septal abnormalities and stroke: a meta-analysis of case-control studies. *Neurology* 2000;55(8):1172–9

29. Anonymous. A randomized trial of anticogulants versus aspirin after cerebral ischemia of presumed arterial origin. The Stroke Prevention in Reversible Ischemia Trial (SPIRIT) Study Group. *Ann Neurol* 1997;42:857–65

30. Mohr JP, Thompson JL, Lazar RM. Warfarin–Aspirin Recurrent Stroke Study Group. A comparison of warfarin and aspirin for the prevention of recurrent ischemic stroke. *N Engl J Med* 2001;345:1444–51

31. Benesch CG. Best treatment for intracranial arterial stenosis? 50 years of uncertainty. The WASID Investigators. [letter; comment]. *Neurology* 2000;55(4):465–6

32. De Schryver EL. Design of ESPRIT: an international randomized trial for secondary prevention after non-disabling cerebral ischaemia of arterial origin. European/Australian Stroke Prevention in Reversible Ischaemia Trial

(ESPRIT) group. *Cerebrovasc Dis* 2000;10(2): 147–50

33. Chimowitz MI, Strong J, Brown MB, *et al.*, for the Warfarin-Aspirin Symptomatic Intracranial Disease Study Group. The Warfarin-Aspirin Symptomatic Intracranial Disease Study. *Neurology* 1995;45(1):1488–93

34. Goldstein LB, Matchar DB, Duncan PW, Samsa GP. US national survey of physician practices for the secondary and tertiary prevention of ischemic stroke: medical therapy in patients with carotid artery stenosis. *Stroke* 1996;27(9):1473–8

35. Albers GW, Lutsep HL, Newell DW, Sacco RL. AHA Scientific Statement. Supplement to the guidelines for the management of transient ischemic attacks: a statement from the ad hoc committee on guidelines for the management of transient ischemic attacks, stroke council, American Heart Association. *Stroke* 1999; 30(11):2502–11

36. Adams HP Jr, Leira E, Chang KC, *et al.* Antithrombotic treatment of ischemic stroke among patients with occlusion or severe stenosis of the internal carotid artery: a report of the Trial of Org 10172 in Acute Stroke Treatment (TOAST). *Neurology* 1999;53(1):122–5

37. Valton L, Arrue P, Geraud G, Bes A. Asymptomatic cerebral embolic signals in patients with carotid stenosis. *Stroke* 1995;26:813–15

38. Sliwka U, Stohlmann WD, Schmidt P, *et al.* Prevalence and time course of microembolic signals in patients with acute stroke. *Stroke* 1997;28(2):358–63

39. Amarenco P, Tzourio C, Bertrand B, *et al.* Atherosclerotic disease of the aortic arch and the risk of ischemic stroke. *N Engl J Med* 1994; 331:1474–9

40. Di Tullio MR, Gersony D, Nayak H, *et al.* Aortic atheromas and acute ischemic stroke: a transesophageal echocardiographic study in an ethnically mixed population. *Neurology* 1996; 46:1560–6

41. Geraci A. Natural history of aortic arch atherosclerotic plaque. *Neurology* 2000;54(3): 749–51

42. Jones EF, Tonkin AM, Donnan GA. Proximal aortic atheroma. An independent risk factor for cerebral ischemia. *Stroke* 1995;26(2):218–24

43. Cohen A, Bertrand B, Chauvel C, *et al.* Aortic plaque morphology and vascular events: a follow-up study in patients with ischemic stroke. FAPS Investigators. French Study of Aortic Plaques in Stroke. *Circulation* 1997; 96(11):3838–41

44. The French Study of Aortic Plaques in Stroke Group. Atherosclerotic disease of the aortic arch as a risk factor for recurrent ischemic stroke. *N Engl J Med* 1996;334:1216–21

45. Weinberger J, Newfield A, Godbold J, Goldman M. Plaque morphology correlates with cerebrovascular symptoms in patients with complex aortic arch plaque. *Arch Neurol* 2000;57(1):81–4

46. Wein TH. Stroke prevention. Cardiac and carotid-related stroke. *Neurol Clin* 2000;19(2): 321–41

47. Schievink W. Spontaneous dissection of the carotid and vertebral arteries. *N Engl J Med* 2001;344(12):898–906

48. Mokri B. Spontaneous dissections of cervicocephalic arteries. In Welch K, Caplan LR, Reis DJ, *et al.*, eds. *Primer on Cerebrovascular Diseases.* San Diego, CA: Academic Press, 1997:390–6

49. Chimowitz M. Ischemic stroke in the young. In Welch K, Caplan LR, Reis DJ, *et al.*, eds. *Primer on Cerebrovascular Diseases.* San Diego, CA: Academic Press, 1997:330–2

50. Llinas R. Evidence-based treatment of patients with ischemic cerebrovascular disease. *Neurol Clin* 2001;19(1):79–105

51. Liu AY, Marcellus ML, Steinberg GK, Marks MP. Long-term outcomes after carotid stent placement treatment of carotid artery dissection. *Neurosurgery* 1999;45(6):1368–73

52. Ameri A. Cerebral venous thrombosis. *Neurol Clin* 1992;10:87–111

53. Bousser MG. Cerebral venous thrombosis: nothing, heparin, or local thrombolysis? *Stroke* 1999;30(3):481–3

54. Cantu C. Cerebral venous thrombosis associated with pregnancy and puerperium. *Stroke* 1993;24:1880–4

55. Einhaupl KM, Meister W, Meharacin S, *et al.* Heparin treatment in sinus thrombosis. *Lancet* 1992;338:597–600

56. de Bruijn SF, Stam J. Randomized placebo-controlled trial of anticoagulant treatment with low molecular weight heparin for cerebral sinus thrombosis. *Stroke* 1999;30:484–8

57. Frey JL, McDougall CG, Dean BL, Jahnke HK. Cerebral venous thrombosis: combined intra-thrombus rtPA and intravenous heparin. *Stroke* 1999;30:489–94

58. Ridker PM, Hennekens CH, Buring JE. Ethnic distribution of factor V Leiden in 4047 men and women. Implications for venous

thromboembolism screening. *J Am Med Assoc* 1997;16:23–30

59. Ridker PM, Lindpaintner K, Stampfer MJ, *et al.* Mutation in the gene coding for coagulation factor V and the risk of myocardial infarction, stroke, and venous thrombosis in apparently healthy men. *N Engl J Med* 1995; 332(14):912–17

60. Feldmann E. Cerebrovascular disease with antiphospholipid antibodies: immune mechanism, significance, and therapeutic options. *Ann Neurol* 1995;37(S1):S114–S130

61. D'Olhaberriague L, Salowich-Palm L, Tanne D, *et al.* Specificity, isotype, and titer distribution of anticardiolipin antibodies in CNS diseases. *Neurology* 1998;51(5):1376–80

62. Bushnell CD. Diagnostic testing for coagulopathies in patients with ischemic stroke. *Stroke* 2000;31(12):3067–78

63. Sallah S, Gagnon GA. Recurrent warfarin induced skin necrosis in kindreds with protein S deficiency. *Haemostasis* 1998;28: 25–30

64. Anonymous. Anticardiolipin antibodies and the risk of recurrent thrombo-occlusive events and death. The Antiphospholipid Antibodies and Stroke Study Group (APASS). *Neurology* 1997;48(1):91–4

65. McCrae KR. Antiphospholipid antibody associated thrombosis: a consensus for treatment? [Review]. *Lupus* 1996;5(6):560–70

66. Hart RG, Anderson DC. Oral anticoagulants and intracranial hemorrhage: facts and hypotheses. *Stroke* 1995;26:1471–7

67. Gebel JM. Intracerebral hemorrhage. *Neurol Clin* 2000;19(2):419–38

68. Crawley F, Wren D. Management of intracranial bleeding associated with anticoagulation: balancing the risk of further bleeding against thromboembolism from prosthetic heart valves. *J Neurol Neurosurg Psychiatry* 2000; 69(3):396–8

69. Bertram M, Hacke W, Schwab S. Managing the therapeutic dilemma: patients with spontaneous intracerebral hemorrhage and urgent need for anticoagulation. *J Neurol* 2000;247: 209–14

70. Hacke W. The dilemma of reinstituting anticoagulation for patients with cardioembolic sources and intracranial hemorrhage: how wide is the strait between Scylla and Charybdis. *Arch Neurol* 2000;57(12):1682–4

71. Leker RR, Abramsky O. Early anticoagulation in patients with prosthetic heart valves and intracerebral hematoma. *Neurology* 1998;50:1489–91

72. Phan TG, Widjicks EFM. Safety of discontinuation of anticoagulation in patients with intracranial hemorrhage at high thromboembolic risk. *Arch Neurol* 2000;57(12):1710–13

73. Widjicks EF, Brown RD, Mullany CJ. The dilemma of discontinuation of anticoagulation therapy for patients with intracranial hemorrhage and mechanical heart valves. *Neurosurgery* 1998;42:769–73

74. Widjicks EF, Brown RD, Mullany CJ, *et al.* Early anticoagulation in patients with prosthetic heart valves and intracerebral hematoma (comment and response). *Neurology* 1999; 52(3):676–7

75. Pessin MS, Lafranchise F, Caplan LR. Safety of anticoagulation after hemorrhagic infarction. *Neurology* 1993;43(7):1289–303

Chapter 20

Carotid endarterectomy for symptomatic and asymptomatic carotid stenosis

James D. Fleck, MD, and José Biller, MD

INTRODUCTION

The importance of stroke, its risk factors, and its medical management are all expertly discussed in other chapters within this book. The goal of this chapter is to define the appropriate use of carotid endarterectomy (CEA) for symptomatic and asymptomatic patients with extracranial internal carotid artery stenosis. In this chapter the term stroke will imply an ischemic stroke and not a hemorrhagic stroke. Chiari is credited as being the first to propose that occlusive disease of the extracranial blood vessels could be responsible for neurological symptoms. In 1905 he reported that four out of seven patients in a series of 400 autopsies with thrombus superimposed on atherosclerosis near the carotid bifurcation had suffered a cerebral embolism[1]. However, the landmark publication describing the relationship between carotid artery disease and transient ischemic attacks (TIA) and stroke was written by Dr C. Miller Fisher in 1951[2]. He initially described the clinical history and premortem studies and available postmortem examinations of the carotid arteries of eight patients with stroke. He later published the clinicopathologic

results of 45 more patients with occlusion or near-occlusion of the carotid arteries[3]. In 1954 Eastcott and colleagues were the first to publish a description of a surgical intervention on the carotid artery in a patient with neurological symptoms[4]. Over the ensuing years, and especially in the early 1980s, the number of carotid endarterectomies increased rather dramatically to a peak of over 100 000 operations in the United States in 1985[5]. In the 1970s platelet antiaggregating agents such as aspirin were found to be helpful in preventing ischemic strokes. The number of operations then declined in the late 1980s and early 1990s because of reports of high complication rates and uncertainty as to which patients were most appropriate for the treatment[6]. A number of large, randomized and controlled clinical trials were then conducted to address the questions regarding the efficacy of CEA combined with best medical treatment, typically in comparison to best medical therapy alone. We plan to clarify the usefulness of CEA for extracranial internal carotid artery (ICA) stenosis based on the outcomes of these trials.

Table 1 Results from the North American Carotid Endarterectomy Trial; any stroke

Stenosis	Any ipsilateral stroke				Any stroke				Any stroke or death			
	M, %	S, %	RR, %	p	M, %	S, %	RR, %	p	M, %	S, %	RR, %	p
70–99%	26.0	9.0	65	< 0.001	27.6	12.6	54	< 0.001	32.3	15.8	51	< 0.001
50–69%	22.2	15.7	29	0.045	32.3	23.7	26	0.026	43.3	33.2	23	0.005
< 50%	18.7	14.9	20	0.16	26.2	25.7	2	0.88	37.0	36.2	2	0.97

M, medical management; S, medical management plus endarterectomy; RR, relative risk reduction; *p*, *p*-value

EXTRACRANIAL INTERNAL CAROTID ARTERY STENOSIS

Patients with extracranial ICA disease usually come to a physician's attention in one of three ways: (1) an asymptomatic lesion is found on some type of screening test, most often a carotid ultrasound, (2) a carotid bruit is auscultated on physical examination, or (3) a stenosis is found during the evaluation of a patient with a previous stroke or TIA symptoms. Those with symptoms referrable to the carotid artery would have cerebral hemisphere difficulties or symptoms of retinal ischemia. Our discussion begins with those patients who have symptomatic extracranial ICA disease.

Carotid endarterectomy for symptomatic internal carotid artery stenosis

The most influential study in the USA regarding symptomatic ICA stenosis was the North American Symptomatic Carotid Endarterectomy Trial (NASCET)[7,8]. A total of 2885 patients with a TIA or non-disabling ischemic stroke ipsilateral to an extracranial ICA stenosis were randomized to receive either optimal medical therapy or optimal medical therapy plus carotid endarterectomy. Notable exclusion criteria included: (1) no angiographic visualization of both carotid arteries and their intracranial branches, (2) intracranial stenosis/lesion more severe than the surgically accessible lesion, (3) kidney, liver or lung failure or cancer judged likely to cause death within five years, (4) a cerebral infarction on either side that deprived the patient of all useful function in the affected territory, (5) symptoms attributable to non-atherosclerotic disease, (6) obvious cardiac source of embolus, and (7) previous ipsilateral CEA. The patients were eventually stratified by the degree of stenosis into three groups: less than 50% stenosis (1368 patients), 50–69% stenosis (858 patients) and 70–99% stenosis (659 patients). The results clearly showed that those patients with severe (70–99%) stenosis who had CEAs had significantly fewer subsequent strokes (Tables 1 and 2). These patients were followed for approximately two years and the study was stopped early in the severe stenosis group because of the robustly positive results in favor of CEA. In a secondary analysis of these patients, there appeared to be a stenosis-dependent trend related to the degree of risk reduction, with absolute risk reduction being higher in the 90–99% stenosis group, intermediate in the 80–89% stenosis group and lower in the 70–79% stenosis group. The results from the other two stratums of patients were published in 1998. The average follow-up of these patients was five years. In those patients with a 50–69% stenosis, CEA reduced the number of subsequent strokes over optimal medical therapy alone (Tables 1 and 2). However, the benefit was not as great as in the 70–99% stenosis group. Observations from this cohort of patients suggested that the long-term benefit of surgery is greater for men than for women, for patients who have had a stroke

Table 2   Results from the North American Carotid Endarterectomy Trial; major stroke

Stenosis	Major ipsilateral stroke				Any major stroke				Any major stroke or death			
	M, %	S, %	RR, %	p	M, %	S, %	RR, %	p	M, %	S, %	RR, %	p
70–99%	13.1	2.5	81	< 0.001	13.1	3.7	72	< 0.001	18.1	8.0	56	< 0.01
50–69%	7.2	2.8	61	0.054	10.3	5.3	49	0.070	25.2	18.3	27	0.03
< 50%	4.7	4.6	3	0.95	8.0	8.7	–	0.56	21.9	21.7	1	0.70

M, medical management; S, medical management plus endarterectomy; RR, relative risk reduction; *p*, *p*-value

Table 3   Approximate equivalent degrees of internal carotid artery stenosis in two clinical trials, the North American Symptomatic Carotid Endarterectomy Trial (NASCET) and the European Carotid Surgery Trial (ECST)

NASCET (% stenosis)	ECST (% stenosis)
30	65
40	70
50	75
60	80
70	85
80	91
90	97

than for those with TIAs, for patients with hemispheric rather than retinal symptoms and for those taking 650 mg or more of aspirin per day[8]. Carotid endarterectomy added no additional benefit over medical therapy in those patients with less than 50% stenosis.

Other studies have confirmed the benefit of CEA in patients with certain degrees of symptomatic extracranial carotid artery stenosis. The European Carotid Surgery Trial (ECST) also randomized patients with varying degrees of symptomatic carotid stenosis to medical management alone or medical management plus CEA. The technique for measuring the degree of stenosis differed between NASCET and ECST, so the results are not exactly comparable. However, approximate equivalent degrees of carotid stenosis are listed in Table 3[9]. Initial results from the ECST were published in

1991. Those patients with a mild (0–29%) stenosis had no benefit from CEA. Those with a 'severe' stenosis (70–99%) had a risk of ipsilateral stroke or perioperative death of 10.3% versus 16.8% for patients treated medically[10]. The final results of the ECST were published in 1998 and failed to prove an outstanding benefit from CEA in patients with moderate stenosis. For the combined outcome of surgical events, ipsilateral major ischemic stroke and other major stroke, there was no overall benefit below about 70–80% stenosis. There was a clear decreasing trend in the benefit of surgery from the 90–99% category to the 80–89% category of stenosis. It was suggested that the value of stenosis above which CEA is beneficial, on average, would lie somewhere in the range of 70 to 79%[11]. A Veterans' Affairs study on CEA was terminated early because of the initial results of NASCET and ECST. The results were published in 1991[12]. In this study, 189 men with carotid artery stenosis greater than 50% ipsilateral to the presenting symptoms were randomized to best medical therapy or CEA plus best medical therapy and followed for a mean of 11.9 months. There was a statistically significant reduction in stroke or crescendo TIAs in those undergoing CEA (7.7%) compared with non-surgical patients (11.7%). The benefit of surgery was greater in those with greater than 70% stenosis.

The surgical risk must be carefully weighed in every patient being considered for CEA. The surgeons in the NASCET study had to prove their experience and low complication rate in performing CEA before being allowed to participate in the study. In the patients who underwent CEA, the perioperative stroke and death rate was 5.8% in those with a 70–99% stenosis and 6.7% in those with less than 70% stenosis. In a patient with a high-grade stenosis the benefit of surgery would vanish if the rate of major surgical complications approached 10%[7]. The margin of benefit is even narrower for patients with moderate stenosis (50–69%). It is estimated that for every increase of 2 percentage points in the surgical complication rate above the level of 6–7%, the five-year benefit would be reduced by 20%[5]. In the 1415 patients who underwent CEA in NASCET, several baseline variables emerged that appeared to increase the perioperative stroke and death rate: (1) hemispheric versus retinal TIAs as the qualifying event, (2) left-sided CEA, (3) contralateral carotid occlusion, (4) ipsilateral ischemic lesion on CT scan, (5) irregular or ulcerated ipsilateral plaque, and (6) lack of collateral circulation in the hemisphere with a severe carotid stenosis[13,14]. Some clinicians are concerned about performing CEA in elderly patients. While surgical risk may be greater among the elderly, much of this risk is attributable to comorbidities. In generally healthy older individuals, age *per se* may not be a potent risk for surgical morbidity or mortality. Because the risk of stroke unrelated to any surgical procedure does increase as a patient gets older, age alone should not be considered a contraindication to CEA[15]. Certainly, not every person with a symptomatic carotid artery stenosis should automatically undergo CEA. Careful contemplation of their surgical risk is as important as determining their degree of carotid stenosis.

Several other interesting pieces of information have been learned from the symptomatic CEA trials, mostly from NASCET. While these data largely come from post-hoc analysis they are worth noting. Some surgeons consider it dangerous to operate on symptomatic carotid arteries that are nearly occluded, while others consider it an emergency. In those patients with severe (70–99%) stenosis in NASCET, only 1 of 58 (1.7%) with near occlusion treated medically had a stroke within one month, suggesting that the procedure is not emergent[16]. In medically treated patients with 90–94% stenosis, the one-year stroke risk was 35%, but fell to 11.1% in those with near occlusion and a 'string sign'. In those patients who underwent CEA for near occlusion, the perioperative stroke risk was 6.3%, and the risk of stroke at one year was reduced by nearly half. However, this reduction was not statistically significant because of the relatively small number of patients analyzed.

Is surgery appropriate in patients with a symptomatic ICA stenosis who also have a contralateral ICA occlusion? Again, patients in the severe stenosis (70–99%) arm of the NASCET study were analyzed regarding outcomes if they had a contralateral stenosis or occlusion[17]. A total of 659 patients were grouped into 3 categories based on the degree of contralateral carotid artery stenosis: mild-to-moderate (< 70%, 559 patients), severe (70–99%, 57 patients), occlusion (43 patients). At two years, medically treated patients were more than twice as likely to have an ipsilateral stroke if they had a contralateral occlusion (69.4%) than if they had either a severe (29.3%) or mild-to-moderate (26.2%) contralateral stenosis. Despite a relatively high perioperative risk of stroke or death (14%) if an occluded contralateral artery was present, the two-year risk of an ipsilateral stroke was decreased to 22% in those patients who had a CEA. In patients with a contralateral occlusion the rates of any stroke or any stroke or death were also lower in the surgically treated group, but the analysis involved relatively small numbers. The presence of angiographically defined ulcerations also appears to increase the risk of subsequent ipsilateral stroke. In medically treated patients with a severe (70–99%) carotid stenosis, the risk of ipsilateral stroke at two years increased incrementally from 26.3% to 73.2% as the degree of stenosis associated with an ulceration increased from 75% to 95%. Overall, CEA reduced the risk of ipsilateral stroke at two years by at least 50%[18].

Patients experiencing a lacunar stroke as their qualifying event were not excluded from NASCET despite the theoretical mechanism for their stroke being more probably a small vessel event than a large-artery event secondary to the carotid stenosis. In patients presenting with a non-lacunar stroke and a 50–99% ipsilateral stenosis, there was a relative risk reduction of 61% for ipsilateral stroke at three years with CEA (9.7%) versus those treated only medically (24.9%). For patients presenting with a possible or probable lacunar stroke, the relative risk reduction in favor of CEA was 53% and 35%, respectively. Neither of these reductions was statistically significant. In general, there was a trend towards a beneficial effect of CEA in patients presenting with a lacunar stroke and an ipsilateral carotid stenosis, but the results were not as convincing as in those patients presenting with non-lacunar strokes[19]. Again, the number of patients analyzed was too small to make a definitive statement.

The question of when to perform a carotid endarterectomy on an appropriate patient with a stroke has been a bit controversial. Because of concerns over a higher complication rate (either hemorrhagic transformation of the infarct or recurrent ischemic events) in patients operated on immediately after a stroke compared with those who are asymptomatic or had TIAs, CEA may be delayed for 4 to 6 weeks. This risk must be weighed against the possibility of an early spontaneous recurrent ischemic event. Patients with a stable neurologic deficit, a CT scan showing no infarct or a small infarct without significant shift, whose level of consciousness is normal, can undergo CEA shortly after their stroke[20–22].

Carotid endarterectomy for asymptomatic internal carotid artery stenosis

Carotid endarterectomy for patients with asymptomatic carotid artery stenosis has been studied in four prospective randomized controlled clinical trials (Table 4)[23–26]. The Veterans' Affairs Cooperative Study included transient hemispheric and retinal symptoms as endpoints. When all strokes and death were analyzed, there was virtually no difference between the surgically treated and medically treated groups. Mortality, including the post-operative deaths, was primarily due to coronary events[24]. The Mayo Asymptomatic Carotid Endarterectomy Study (MACE) was terminated early because of a significantly higher number of myocardial infarctions and TIAs in the surgical group than in the medical group. The use of aspirin was discouraged in the surgical group, emphasizing the importance of continuing such medical care in all patients. Too few cerebral ischemic events occurred before termination of the study to judge the comparative effectiveness of CEA versus low-dose aspirin in patients with asymptomatic carotid stenosis[25]. The Carotid Artery Stenosis with Asymptomatic Narrowing: Operation Versus Aspirin (CASANOVA) study enrolled 410 patients at multiple centers. Interpretation of the results was difficult because the study design was complicated. Overall, CEA was not more beneficial than medical treatment for carotid stenosis less than 90%. Furthermore, patients with 90–99% asymptomatic stenosis were excluded from the study on the recommendation from the ethics committee that patients with this degree of stenosis should undergo CEA[26]. The largest and most influential of these trials was the Asymptomatic Carotid Atherosclerosis study (ACAS)[23]. In this study

Table 4 Randomized trials of carotid endarterectomy for patients with asymptomatic carotid artery stenosis

Trial	Patients, n	Men, %	Follow-up period (yr)	Stenosis	Outcome	Results, %		RRR, %	p value	Perioperative stroke/death
						M	S			
ACAS	1662	66	2.7	60–99%	Ipsilateral stroke or any perioperative stroke or death	11.0	5.1	53	< 0.004	2.3%
					Any stroke or death	31.9	25.6	20	0.08	
					Any major stroke or death	25.5	20.7	19	0.16	
VA	444	100	4	50–99%	Ipsilateral TIA/TMB/stroke	20.6	8.0	38	< 0.001	4.3%
					Total TIA/TMB/stroke	24.5	12.8	51	< 0.002	
					All stroke, stroke death, any death	44.2	41.2			
MACE	71	58		50–99%	Terminated early because of excessive myocardial infarction rate in surgical group which was encouraged to not use aspirin. Too few cerebral events to compare effectiveness of CEA vs. 81 mg aspirin					
CASANOVA	410	73	3	50–90%	Study design complicated, making interpretation of results difficult. CEA not more beneficial than medical treatment					

ACAS, Asymptomatic Carotid Atherosclerosis Study; VA, Veterans' Affairs Cooperative Study; MACE, Mayo Asymptomatic Carotid Endarterectomy Study; CASANOVA, Carotid Artery Stenosis with Asymptomatic Narrowing: Operation Versus Aspirin; M, medically treated arm of study; S, surgically treated arm of study; RRR, relative risk reduction; TIA, transient ischemic attack; TMB, transient monocular blindness; CEA, carotid endarterectomy

medical therapy with 325 mg of aspirin and vascular risk factor modification was compared to medical therapy plus CEA in patients with a 60–99% stenosis (Table 4). While the relative risk reduction due to surgery over medical therapy alone was 53%, the absolute difference in the estimated rate for ipsilateral stroke or any perioperative stroke or death was only 5.9%. This reduction translates into an annual absolute difference of 1.2%. When the outcome of any stroke or death was used, there was no statistical difference between the surgical and medically treated arms. The perioperative stroke and death rate was extremely low (2.3%). Included in this is a stroke complication rate of 1.2% from the cerebral angiogram performed on all patients prior to surgery. It is estimated that increasing the perioperative complication rate by 2% would reduce the benefit by more than 30%,

which essentially negates the benefit of CEA[5]. Diabetes mellitus, contralateral siphon stenosis and never drinking alcohol were associated with a higher perioperative stroke rate. A history of a previous stroke, contralateral stenosis greater than 60% and never drinking alcohol were associated with a higher risk of all perioperative complications[27]. It also appeared that CEA was not notably beneficial in women with asymptomatic 60–99% stenosis, probably because the perioperative complication rate was higher in women (3.6%) than in men (1.7%)[23]. Comparing patients with 60–69%, 70–79%, and 80–99% stenosis, there was no statistically significant gradation in reduction of the risk of ipsilateral stroke and any perioperative stroke or death. However, the sample size in each category of stenosis was, perhaps, too small. This is a bit counter-intuitive, and other studies have indicated that the risk of stroke ipsilateral to an asymptomatic artery increases as the degree of stenosis increases[28]. In the ECST study, the three-year risk of stroke in the distribution of the asymptomatic carotid artery increased when the stenosis reached 70–79%. The risks were 1.8%, 2.1% and 5.7% for degrees of stenosis of 0–29%, 30–69% and 70–99%, respectively[29]. In the NASCET trial the five-year risk of ipsilateral stroke on the asymptomatic side also increased as the degree of stenosis increased. The risks were 7.8%, 12.6%, 14.8% and 18.5% for initially asymptomatic stenosis of less than 50%, 50–59%, 60–74% and 75–94%, respectively. All of these risks were less than the risk of stroke in the territory of an artery with symptomatic stenosis[30]. One should also keep in mind the possibility that causes of stroke other than ICA stenosis may be present in any given individual. In looking at the NASCET outcome strokes, the data suggest that approximately 20% of strokes in the territory of symptomatic carotid arteries, and approximately 45% of strokes in the territory of asymptomatic carotid arteries were unrelated to carotid stenosis[31]. The other common causes of stroke were cardioembolic and lacunar strokes, as would be expected.

While one should not discount the primary outcome of ACAS, we do not feel that the evidence is compelling enough to advocate performing a CEA on every patient with an asymptomatic carotid stenosis of 60–99%. Because of much of the information stated above, we often prefer to treat patients medically unless the asymptomatic carotid stenosis reaches approximately 80%. Certainly, the available information should be discussed with the patient so that an informed decision can be made on an individual basis. More data would be helpful and, it is hoped, an ongoing European trial, the Asymptomatic Carotid Surgery Trial (ACST), will shed more light on the best use of CEA in asymptomatic patients[32].

GENERAL STATEMENTS

Some general statements regarding the care of patients with vascular risk factors and ICA stenosis need to be emphasized. All patients must have their modifiable vascular risk factors well managed. These include hypertension, diabetes mellitus, cigarette smoking, hyperlipidemia and excessive alcohol consumption. These, as well as other vascular risk factors, are discussed in other chapters. Patients undergoing CEA should receive aspirin therapy, beginning before surgery unless there are contraindications[33].

Controversy still exists as to the appropriate imaging methods necessary before CEA[34,35]. Techniques include conventional angiography, carotid ultrasonography, and magnetic resonance angiography (MRA). Conventional cerebral angiography was performed in all patients undergoing CEA in all of the major trials discussed in this chapter; it remains the gold standard to which other imaging studies are compared in the measurement of carotid stenosis. The aortic arch, the entirety of the common carotid, internal carotid and external carotid arteries as well as the intracranial circulation can be adequately viewed with a conventional angiogram. This test does carry with it some risk – generally small – especially of stroke. We do not feel, at this time, that carotid ultrasound should be used as the only imaging method before CEA. It does not adequately image the aortic arch, proximal common carotid artery or intracranial internal carotid artery or its branches. It may miss internal carotid near-occlusions. MRA technology is evolving quickly but the quality of the images and the accuracy of stenosis measurement still varies among institutions. MRA has a tendency to overestimate the degree of stenosis. On the other hand, it non-invasively images all of the necessary vessels. The relatively new technique of CT angiography (CTA) appears to detect carotid occlusion, but it may be unable to reliably distinguish between moderate and severe ICA stenosis[36]. We are comfortable enough with the carotid ultrasonography and MRA images at our institution to bypass conventional angiography in a few clinical scenarios. In a symptomatic patient with a severe (70–99%) stenosis, we feel there is enough margin of efficacy in these patients to avoid the small risk of angiography. If, however, doubt remains regarding the percent stenosis in marginal cases, we feel conventional angiography should be used.

SUMMARY RECOMMENDATIONS

Listed below are the guidelines we typically use in selecting patients for CEA. The percentage stenosis is based on NASCET criteria.

(1) CEA is beneficial for symptomatic patients with a recent carotid territory TIA or non-disabling ischemic stroke and an ipsilateral 70–99% internal carotid artery stenosis.

(2) CEA should be considered in patients with a recent carotid territory TIA or non-disabling stroke and an ipsilateral 50–69% internal carotid artery stenosis. The patient's surgical risk should be less than 7%.

(3) CEA has not been proven to be of benefit over medical therapy for symptomatic patients with a less than 50% ipsilateral internal carotid artery stenosis.

(4) CEA may be considered for asymptomatic patients with a 60–99% internal carotid artery stenosis. However, their procedure-related risk for stroke or death must be less than 3%. Because it appears that the risk for stroke increases as the degree of carotid artery stenosis increases and the margin of benefit was narrow in the ACAS study, we prefer to operate on selected asymptomatic patients if there is an 80–99% internal carotid artery stenosis. Further studies may help clarify the usefulness of CEA in asymptomatic patients.

References

1. Fields WS, Lemak NA. *A History of Stroke: its Recognition and Treatment*. New York: Oxford University Press, 1989
2. Fisher CM. Occlusion of the internal carotid artery. *Arch Neurol Psychiatry* 1951;65:346–77
3. Fisher CM. Occlusion of the carotid arteries: further experiences. *Arch Neurol Psychiatry* 1954;72:187–204
4. Eastcott HHG, Pickering GW, Rob CG. Reconstruction of internal carotid artery in a patient with intermittent attacks of hemiplegia. *Lancet* 1954;2:994–6
5. Chassin MR. Appropriate use of carotid endarterectomy. *N Engl J Med* 1998;339(20): 1468–71
6. Tu JV, Hannan EL, Anderson GM, *et al*. The fall and rise of carotid endarterectomy in the United States and Canada. *N Engl J Med* 1998;339(20): 1441–7
7. North American Symptomatic Carotid Endarterectomy Trial Collaborators. Beneficial effect of carotid endarterectomy in symptomatic patients with high-grade carotid stenosis. *N Engl J Med* 1991;325(7):445–53
8. Barnett HJ, Taylor DW, Eliasziw M, *et al*. Benefit of carotid endarterectomy in patients with symptomatic moderate or severe stenosis. North American Symptomatic Carotid Endarterectomy Trial Collaborators. *N Engl J Med* 1998;339(20):1415–25
9. Donnan GA, Davis SM, Chambers BR, *et al*. Surgery for prevention of stroke. *Lancet* 1998; 351:1372–3
10. European Carotid Surgery Trialists' Collaborative Group. MRC European Carotid Surgery Trial: interim results for symptomatic patients with severe (70–99%) or with mild (0–29%) carotid stenosis. *Lancet* 1991;337(8752): 1235–43
11. European Carotid Surgery Trialists' Collaborative Group. Randomised trial of endarterectomy for recently symptomatic carotid

stenosis: final results of the MRC European Carotid Surgery Trial (ECST). *Lancet* 1998;351(9113):1379–87

12. Mayberg MR, Wilson SE, Yatsu F, *et al.* Carotid endarterectomy and prevention of cerebral ischemia in symptomatic carotid stenosis. Veterans Affairs Cooperative Studies Program 309 Trialist Group. *J Am Med Assoc* 1991;266(23):3289–94

13. Ferguson GG, Eliasziw M, Barr HW, *et al.* The North American Symptomatic Carotid Endarterectomy Trial: surgical results in 1415 patients. *Stroke* 1999;30(9):1751–8

14. Henderson RD, Eliasziw M, Fox AJ, *et al.* Angiographically defined collateral circulation and risk of stroke in patients with severe carotid artery stenosis. North American Symptomatic Carotid Endarterectomy Trial (NASCET) Group. *Stroke* 2000;31(1):128–32

15. Cheitlin MD, Gerstenblith G, Hazzard WR, *et al.* AHA Conference Proceedings: Do existing databases hold the answers to clinical questions in geriatric cardiovascular disease and stroke? Executive Summary. Database Conference, January 27–30, 2000. Washington, DC, USA. *Circulation* 2001;104(7):E39

16. Morgenstern LB, Fox AJ, Sharpe BL, *et al.* The risks and benefits of carotid endarterectomy in patients with near occlusion of the carotid artery. North American Symptomatic Carotid Endarterectomy Trial (NASCET) Group. *Neurology* 1997;48(4):911–15

17. Gasecki AP, Eliasziw M, Ferguson GG, *et al.* Long-term prognosis and effect of endarterectomy in patients with symptomatic severe carotid stenosis and contralateral carotid stenosis or occlusion: results from NASCET. *J Neurosurg* 1995;83(5):778–82

18. Eliasziw M, Streifler JY, Fox AJ, *et al.* Significance of plaque ulceration in symptomatic patients with high-grade carotid stenosis. North American Symptomatic Carotid Endarterectomy Trial. *Stroke* 1994;25(2):304–8

19. Inzitari D, Eliasziw M, Sharpe BL, *et al.* Risk factors and outcome of patients with carotid artery stenosis presenting with lacunar stroke. North American Symptomatic Carotid Endarterectomy Trial Group. *Neurology* 2000;54(3):660–6

20. Whittemore AD, Ruby ST, Couch NP, *et al.* Early carotid endarterectomy in patients with small, fixed neurologic deficits. *J Vasc Surg* 1984;1(6):795–9

21. Pritz MB. Timing of carotid endarterectomy after stroke. *Stroke* 1997;28(12):2563–7

22. Gasecki AP, Ferguson GG, Eliasziw M, *et al.* Early endarterectomy for severe carotid artery stenosis after a nondisabling stroke: results from the North American Symptomatic Carotid Endarterectomy Trial. *J Vasc Surg* 1994;20(2):288–95

23. Executive Committee for the Asymptomatic Carotid Atherosclerosis Study. Endarterectomy for asymptomatic carotid artery stenosis. *J Am Med Assoc* 1995;273(18):1421–8

24. Hobson RWII, Weiss DG, Fields WS, *et al.* Efficacy of carotid endarterectomy for asymptomatic carotid stenosis. The Veterans Affairs Cooperative Study Group. *N Engl J Med* 1993;328(4):221–7

25. Mayo Asymptomatic Carotid Endarterectomy Study Group. Results of a randomized controlled trial of carotid endarterectomy for asymptomatic carotid stenosis. *Mayo Clin Proc* 1992;67(6):513–18

26. The CASANOVA Study Group. Carotid surgery versus medical therapy in asymptomatic carotid stenosis. *Stroke* 1991;22(10):1229–35

27. Young B, Moore WS, Robertson JT, *et al.* An analysis of perioperative surgical mortality and morbidity in the asymptomatic carotid atherosclerosis study. ACAS Investigators. *Stroke* 1996;27(12):2216–24

28. Norris JW, Zhu CZ, Bornstein NM, *et al.* Vascular risks of asymptomatic carotid stenosis. *Stroke* 1991;22(12):1485–90

29. The European Carotid Surgery Trialists Collaborative Group. Risk of stroke in the distribution of an asymptomatic carotid artery. *Lancet* 1995;345(8944):209–12

30. Inzitari D, Eliasziw M, Gates P, *et al.* The causes and risk of stroke in patients with asymptomatic internal carotid artery stenosis. North American Symptomatic Carotid Endarterectomy Trial Collaborators. *N Engl J Med* 2000;342(23):1693–700

31. Barnett HJ, Gunton RW, Eliasziw M, *et al.* Causes and severity of ischemic stroke in patients with internal carotid artery stenosis. *J Am Med Assoc* 2000;283(11):1429–36

32. Halliday AW, Thomas D, Mansfield A. The Asymptomatic Carotid Surgery Trial (ACST). Rationale and design. Steering Committee. *Eur J Vasc Surg* 1994;8(6):703–10

33. Biller J, Feinberg WM, Castaldo JE, *et al.* Guidelines for carotid endarterectomy: a

statement for healthcare professionals from a Special Writing Group of the Stroke Council, American Heart Association. *Circulation* 1998; 97(5):501–9

34. Barnett HJ, Eliasziw M, Meldrum HE. The identification by imaging methods of patients who might benefit from carotid endarterectomy. *Arch Neurol* 1995;52(8):827–31

35. Strandness DE Jr. Angiography before carotid endarterectomy – no. *Arch Neurol* 1995;52(8): 832–3

36. Anderson GB, Ashforth R, Steinke DE, *et al.* CT angiography for the detection and characterization of carotid artery bifurcation disease. *Stroke* 2000;31(9):2168–74

Endovascular approaches to stroke prevention: thrombolysis, angioplasty/ stenting, aneurysm coiling, and treatment of intracerebral vasospasm

Glen Geremia, MD, Bradley Strimling, MD, and Nilay Patel, MD

INTRODUCTION

Endovascular therapies have evolved over the past twenty years to a level where they are currently effective in the treatment of many intracerebral vascular problems. Technical advances in digital (computer-based) subtraction angiography, catheter polymer science, metallurgy, device engineering and contrast and pharmaceutical development have all contributed to their success. Early endovascular techniques were considered, at best, ineffective and often dangerous. They have since proved to be safe, effective and necessary as an integral component of treatment at major medical centers. This chapter concentrates on the application of endovascular therapies in the treatment of intracerebral vascular and related diseases.

THROMBOLYSIS IN STROKE

Stroke is the third most common cause of death in the United States, following heart disease and cancer[1]. Each year there are more than 500 000 new strokes, with over 150 000 deaths. Stroke causes an estimated 30 billion dollars in medical expenses, rehabilitation and loss of employment. The majority of ischemic strokes are caused by thromboembolic arterial occlusions, with 75% in the territory of the carotid artery[2,3]. Interest in cerebral fibrinolysis has been prompted by the success of thrombolysis in patients suffering from acute myocardial infarction. The FDA has approved intravenous recombinant tissue plasminogen activator (rtPA) for the treatment of acute ischemic stroke within three hours of the onset of symptoms.

Conservative medical management of non-hemorrhagic stroke results in severe neurologic deficit or death in many patients[4]. The 30-day and 5-year mortality rates for stroke in the carotid distribution are 17% and 40% respectively[5]. Saito *et al.*, in a study of clinical outcomes in 33 patients with M-1 occlusions, reported that 26 (79%) died or were severely disabled, and only three (9%) had a good outcome[6]. Clinical outcome in patients with vertebrobasilar occlusion is even less favorable, with death in the majority of patients and severe deficit in most survivors[7]. Because of the very poor outcome in patients with vertebrobasilar occlusions, in 1983 Zeumer *et al.* treated five patients with local intra-arterial fibrinolysis, achieving successful recanalization in three, all of whom experienced subsequent neurologic improvement[8]. One year later Zeumer *et al.* reported treating two patients who had occlusion of the distal internal carotid artery with urokinase, both of whom improved clinically[9]. Since then other series have been published. Neurologic improvement was variable in these studies, with minimal or no neurologic deficit reported in 15–75% of patients. This wide variation in outcome is most probably due to several factors, including (1) the grading system used for assessing outcome, (2) the dose of thrombolytic agent used, (3) differences in baseline patient demographics (age, baseline neurologic status), and (4) the site of arterial occlusion.

Published studies of patients with carotid distribution stroke reported a mortality rate of 5 to 45%[6]. The results of Jahan and colleagues are within this range (38%) and do not exceed the mortality rates in other published reports of intra-arterial thrombolytic treatment for stroke[4].

Intravenous (iv) thrombolytic therapy

The results from the National Institute of Neurological Disorders and Stroke recombinant Tissue Plasminogen Activator stroke study (the NINDS, rtPA stroke study) prompted the FDA to approve rtPA therapy. In this trial the majority of patients were treated within three hours of the onset of symptoms, with many receiving treatment within 90 minutes. At three months, 31–50% of patients treated with rtPA had a near complete recovery versus 20–38% of patients receiving placebo. Cerebral hemorrhage occurred in 6.4% of patients receiving rtPA, compared to 0.6% of those receiving placebo. The mortality rate in the two groups, however, was similar. In the European Cooperative Acute Stroke Study (ECASS I, II), rtPA was of no greater benefit than placebo in improving neurological outcome at three months. Patients who received rtPA had a 19.8% incidence of intracerebral hematoma versus 6.5% in the placebo group. In patients demonstrating findings consistent with edema or infarction involving greater than one-third of the territory of the middle cerebral artery, those patients receiving rtPA were less likely to have a good outcome than those receiving placebo[10]. In the ECASS, a total of 511 patients were studied. The patients all presented with acute ischemic stroke within six hours of the onset of symptoms and with moderate to severe neurologic deficit. They were randomly assigned to two groups; one received placebo, and the other received intravenous rtPA (1.1 mg/kg, of which 10% was given as a bolus and the rest given over 60 minutes; the maximum dose was 100 mg). The investigators concluded that, although rtPA administration improved some functional measures in properly selected patients, the degree of improvement did not outweigh the risks of increased mortality or parenchymal hemorrhage. Retrospective evaluation of the results of the ECASS trial reveals that there was a wide range in the results and in the risks of fibrinolytic therapy. If a stroke involved more than one-third of the middle cerebral artery territory, the mortality rate for treatment was 24%, compared with a rate of only 4% if the stroke involved less than one-third of the middle cerebral territory. If there was CT evidence of edema, the mortality rate was 17%, compared with only 2% if there was no evidence of edema[11].

Intra-arterial (ia) thrombolysis

The two largest randomized trials conducted to examine the safety and effectiveness of intra-arterial thrombolysis were the Prolyse in Acute Cerebral Thromboembolism I (PROACT I) trial and the PROACT II trial[10]. The first phase of this trial, which was organized by Abbott laboratories, demonstrated the safety of prourokinase infusion in thromboembolic occlusion of the M-1 segment of the middle cerebral artery and successful angiographic recanalization when compared with placebo. However, clinical efficacy was not proved. Patients were entered into the double-blind trial only if angiographically demonstrated occlusion could be identified and local intra-arterial therapy could be done within six hours after the acute clinical event[11].

The PROACT II trial was the first randomized trial in which intra-arterial thrombolysis unequivocally demonstrated benefit to patients who had had a stroke caused by occlusion of the middle cerebral artery. A total of 121 patients received local intra-arterial infusion of prourokinase along with low-dose intravenous heparin six hours after the onset of symptoms. These were compared with 59 patients who received only low-dose intravenous heparin during this period. The patients in these two groups were selected from a total of 12 323 patients screened, of whom 474 underwent arteriography to identify middle cerebral artery occlusion. Angiographically, there was partial or complete lysis in 67% of the 121 patients who received prourokinase infusion directly into the thrombus, compared to 18% of the 59 who received only intravenous heparin. In this

trial patients who received the combination of prourokinase and heparin fared better than those who received only intravenous heparin. The primary endpoint of the PROACT II trial was the patient's ability to live independently at three months following the stroke. This was achieved in 40% of patients treated with the combination of prourokinase and heparin, versus 25% of those treated with heparin alone. However, intracerebral hemorrhage with associated neurological deficit was found in 10% of the patients in the group receiving the combination intra-arterial prourokinase and heparin, versus 2% of those receiving intravenous heparin only. The PROACT II study results were positive. However they did not meet the FDA regulatory requirement for drug approval: a single overwhelmingly positive study or two studies sufficiently positive to prove efficacy[12]. However, it did establish 'proof of principle' that intra-arterial thrombolysis is an effective therapy, even when given in the late ischemic phase (PROACT median time to treatment was equal to 5.3 hours). Most major stroke centers today recommend intravenous thrombolysis with tPA in patients presenting within three hours after the onset of stroke symptoms. Intra-arterial thrombolysis is recommended in patients presenting 3–6 hours after the onset of symptoms[10].

Compared with the systemic infusion of intravenous rtPA, localized intra-arterial thrombolysis has the advantage of achieving faster, more complete recanalization with less fibrinolysis. A major disadvantage with intra-arterial infusion is the complexity involved in organizing an efficient neuro-interventional team that can respond and treat in a timely fashion[13].

Cerebral thrombolysis

There is no recommended established protocol for cerebral intra-arterial thrombolysis. Various combinations of catheters, wires,

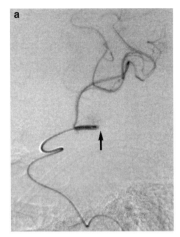

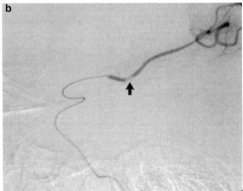

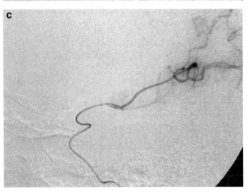

Figure 1 Angiogram of a 47-year-old woman who presents with aphasia. (a) Selective catheterization and angiography of a branch of the middle cerebral artery occluded from thrombus (arrow). (b) Partial recanalization of the vessel is seen after selective infusion of 4 mg of tissue plasminogen activator (tPA) into the clot. Notice the filling defect, thrombus (arrow) within the vessel. (c) Complete lysis of the clot with restoration of flow is seen following the infusion of 8 mg of tPA

thrombolytics, anticoagulants and antiplatelet agents have been used. We are not endorsing any single method as the best technique; rather we will describe, in general terms, some guidelines and materials that have been successful in selective intra-arterial thrombolysis.

Technique

The patient is placed on the angiography suite table in the supine position and the groin is prepped and draped in the usual sterile manner. A 6 French (F) sheath is percutaneously placed within the right femoral artery. A 5F diagnostic catheter is used to selectively cannulate the internal carotid artery. Angiography is performed and the occluded vessel is identified. The diagnostic catheter is exchanged for a 6F 90 cm guide catheter over an extended length exchange wire (260–300 cm). Through the guide catheter and in a coaxial fashion, a micro-catheter is placed (Soft-Stream or Tracker catheter, Boston Scientific, Fremont, CA; Prowler Plus, Cordis Endovascular, Miami Lakes, FL). A single-end hole catheter (Tracker or Prowler) or multi-side hole catheter (Soft Stream) is advanced until the tip lies within the clot. The thrombolytic agent selected (urokinase, rtPA, or reteplase) should be infused directly into the clot. One method is slow infusion through an intravenous pump over one to two hours. A manual infusion (pulse-spray) is also effective. When using a standard intravenous pump the thrombolytic agent is diluted into 100 ml of normal saline. In the manual pulse-spray technique, the agent is diluted into 10 ml of normal saline. Two milliliters of agent are injected with a tuberculin syringe every 30 seconds. Total dosage administered: Urokinase, 250 000–750 000 units; rtPA, from 10–15 mg up to 30 mg; reteplase, from 1–2 mg up to 4 mg. See Figure 1. A problem may arise when infusing too large a volume of thrombolytic into a middle cerebral artery thrombus. The solution may reflux into the anterior cerebral artery territory, which would prevent fresh blood and plasminogen from reaching the proximal thrombus[11].

An intravenous 2000 to 4000 unit bolus dose of heparin is usually given prior to the coaxial placement of the microcatheter within the thrombus. An activated clotting time (ACT) of approximately 200 seconds is desired. A dose of 1000 to 2000 units of heparin per hour can be administered during the fibrinolytic infusion. This relatively small amount of heparin may help prevent recurrence of a new thrombus during the fibrinolytic therapy. However, the administration of intravenous heparin may also increase the incidence of intracranial hemorrhage. Again, as with the thrombolytics, there is no definite established optimal dosage. Following the procedure the arterial sheath is left in place and the heparin is not reversed. The patient's blood pressure is monitored actively and the systolic pressure kept below 160 mmHg.

If the thrombolytic infusion does not lyse the clot and re-establish antegrade flow, a mechanical means of removing or displacing the clot should be attempted. These include (1) a snare device to remove or macerate the clot, (2) angioplasty balloon to displace the clot and re-establish distal flow, (3) wire manipulation to fragment the clot, and (4) coil embolus grabber (under development). The microsnare is currently popular.

There have been no reported randomized trials of thrombolytic treatment for vertebrobasilar stroke. A recent report on a small series of patients suggested a possible benefit of iv tPA if administered within three hours after the appearance of symptoms[14]. There have been many documented small series where intra-arterial thrombolytics have been used to successfully lyse clots within the vertebrobasilar system[10]. Cross *et al.* have recently published their results on the thrombolysis of 20 patients with basilar artery thrombosis; CT scans of the brain, neurologic examinations,

symptom duration, clot location and degree of recanalization were analyzed retrospectively[15]. Complete recanalization was obtained in 50% of patients, 60% of whom survived and 30% of whom had good neurologic outcomes. Less than complete recanalization resulted in only 10% survival. Overall survival was 35% at three months. Patients whose clot was within the distal basilar artery had a survival rate of 71% compared with only 15% survival if the clot was located in the mid-basilar or proximal regions. Outcome would not be predicted by pretreatment CT scan findings, duration of symptoms prior to treatment, age, or neurologic symptoms. The single best predictor of survival with basilar clot followed by local intra-arterial thrombolysis was clot location. Patients with a clot in the distal basilar artery fared better than those whose thrombus was more proximal. These authors concluded that since factors such as age, pretreatment neurologic status, presence of infarction on CT scan and delayed diagnosis did not predict poor outcome, they should not be considered absolute contra-indications for intra-arterial thrombolysis in patients with basilar artery thrombosis.

ANGIOPLASTY/STENTING

Background

Carotid angioplasty and stenting have recently been employed in patients who are poor candidates for carotid endarterectomy. So far, carotid stenting has not yielded results that could justify its replacing conventional surgical carotid endarterectomy[16]. Large, prospective, randomized controlled trials have demonstrated that carotid endarterectomy is an effective therapy in symptomatic patients with stenosis greater than 70% in diameter. In the North American Symptomatic Carotid Endarterectomy Trial (NASCET) study there was a 5.8% risk of perioperative stroke and death. In a subsequent NASCET study, a moderate reduction of stroke risk was found in patients with 50 to 69% stenosis. The Asymptomatic Carotid Atherosclerosis Study (ACAS) trial reported a modest benefit for asymptomatic patients with a 60–99% stenosis and a complication rate less than 3%. Recent published series of carotid angioplasty and stenting report stroke and death rates ranging from 2 to 8%[16]. However, rapidly evolving device technology should further reduce this rate and yield more favorable and competitive results.

Vitek *et al*. reported on the results of carotid artery stenting in 451 vessels (390 patients)[17]. Sixty-one patients underwent treatment for bilateral disease. Indications for stenting included symptomatic patients with at least 50% stenosis and asymptomatic patients with at least 70% stenosis. Prior carotid endarterectomy with restenosis occurred in 70 (15.5%) of the arteries that were treated. Nineteen (4%) had undergone previous radiation therapy. Technical success was achieved in 98% of all cases. Extreme vessel tortuosity precluded treatment in seven patients. There was one stent thrombosis. Self-expanding stents (Wallstent, Boston Scientific, Maple Grove, MN) were used in 70% of cases and balloon expandable stents were used in the remainder. The carotid stenosis was reduced from 74 ± 15% to 5 ± 10%. The stroke and death rate combined at 30 days was 7.9%. One patient had a non Q-wave myocardial infarction. No cranial nerve palsies were present. Death occurred in 7 (1.8%); 2 (0.5%) were neurologic and 5 (1.3%) were systemic. One death was the result of carotid artery rupture caused by over dilation. A ruptured internal carotid artery aneurysm caused death in another patient. There was a total of 4 (1.0%) major strokes. Minor disabling strokes were present in 25 (6.4%) patients. Fourteen (3.6%) had an increase in the NIHSS score of 1 and completely reversed within seven days.

Refinements in equipment, advanced levels of skill and better patient selection have resulted in an overall reduction in neurologic complications. In the opinion of Vitek's group, advanced age was the most important predictor of procedural complications, especially in patients over 80 years old. Patients with brain atrophy/dementia and Alzheimer's disease did not tolerate the procedure well. Lesion severity (greater than 90% stenosis) and length and multiplexity of stenosis were associated with more embolic complications. Emphasis has been placed on the use of antiplatelet therapy prior to and after stenting in order to prevent related embolic stroke[17].

Balloon expandable stents were used initially, but most investigators currently prefer self-expanding stents. The stent should be at least 1–2 mm larger than the largest vessel segment within which the stent will be deposited. Oversizing the stent within the internal carotid artery does not cause any acute or late problems[17]. The stent length chosen is dependent upon the lesion length. Recently, non-shortening, self-expanding stents have come into use[18]. They are less rigid, have a lower profile tip, and can be placed more precisely using the distal and proximal markers. These stents have a tendency to 'jump' distally if released too quickly. In order to avoid this, 3 mm to 5 mm of the distal stent is slowly deployed and fully expanded before the remainder of the stent is released.

Self-expanding stents have a tendency for late, progressive expansion[19]. Ulcerations may continue to fill following the acute release of a stent, and these lesions tend to heal with time[20]. Bradycardia and hypotension commonly occur during predilation and stent postdilation, especially when the lesion is located at the origin of the internal carotid artery. These usually resolve within seconds to minutes following balloon deflation. Hypotension usually resolves with a 300–500 ml iv bolus of normal saline. Bradycardia can be reversed with 0.5–1.0 mg of iv atropine.

Technique

Pre-procedure

The patient is placed on antiplatelet therapy for at least three days prior to the procedure (aspirin 325 mg daily and clopidogrel 75 mg once daily). Pre-procedural laboratory tests include a complete blood and platelet count, blood urea nitrogen and creatinine, prothrombin time and partial thromboplastin time.

Procedure

A sheath (7–9F) is placed percutaneously within the femoral artery. Another 5F sheath is placed in the ipsilateral femoral vein through which a transvenous cardiac pacemaker wire is inserted, and the tip is placed within or near the right ventricle. An arteriogram, including injection of both the common carotid arteries, a single vertebral artery and an arch aortogram are required prior to the stent/angioplasty procedure. The diseased common carotid artery is selectively catheterized with a 5F or 6F diagnostic catheter. An exchange guidewire (0.035 in super-stiff Terumo wire or 0.035 in Amplatz stiff wire) is placed within the external carotid artery. The diagnostic catheter is exchanged for an 8F or 7F guide catheter (Envoy, Cordis Endovascular, Miami Lakes, FL) and placed within the carotid artery. After placement of the guide catheter, the patient is given an intravenous bolus of approximately 5000 units of heparin (activated clotting time greater than or equal to 250 seconds). Bradycardia and/or hypotension may be experienced during balloon dilation, especially if the stenosis lies at the origin of the internal carotid artery. Usually, 0.5–1.0 mg of atropine and a 300–500 ml bolus of normal saline will reverse these signs. If necessary, temporary cardiac

pacing can be performed through the previously placed transvenous pacemaker.

Prior to placement of the stent, predilation with a small coronary balloon is recommended. Ohki *et al.* have shown that embolic debris is potentially released in 'primary stenting' without pre-dilation[21]. Predilation with a 4 mm diameter balloon is sufficient for passage of the stent delivery system. The coronary balloon catheter, mounted on a 0.014 in exchange wire, is placed coaxially within the guide catheter. The tip of the wire traverses the stenotic lesion and is positioned at the base of the skull. The coronary balloon (4 mm × 40 mm) is advanced across the stenosis and dilated to the nominal pressure; one dilation is usually sufficient. The balloon catheter is removed and the stent (Wallstent, Boston Scientific, or Smart-Stent, Cordis Endovascular, Miami Lakes, FL) is advanced across the stenosis and deployed. Stents are usually 8 mm × 20 mm or 10 mm × 20 mm. If the stenosis is at the origin of the internal carotid artery, then the stent is positioned across the stenosis and extends from the proximal internal carotid artery into the distal common carotid artery. The stent should measure 1–2 mm greater than the largest diameter vessel within which it will be positioned (internal carotid artery or common carotid artery). If a significant residual stenosis remains (approximately 50%), then a post-dilation angioplasty balloon (5 or 6 mm × 20 mm) can be used to post-dilate the residual stenosis. Recently, it has been observed that gradual progressive dilation of a residual stenosis may be seen over time (3–6 months) following deployment of a self-expanding stent. Thus, it is unnecessary to establish complete or near complete dilation of the stenotic segment. The guide catheter is removed. Hemostasis at the groin may be achieved with a closure device or with direct manual compression over the femoral artery after the activated clotting time measures less than 200 seconds. See Figures 2 and 3.

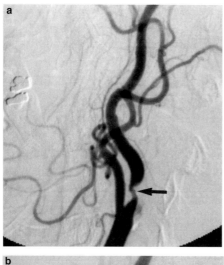

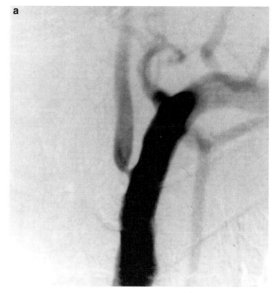

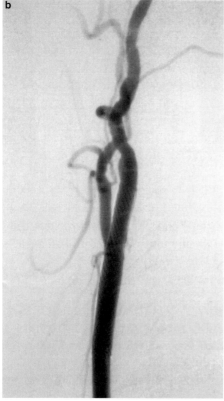

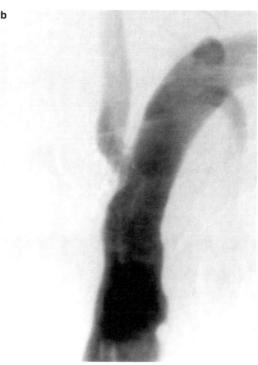

Figure 2 Angiogram of a 57-year-old man with a history of old left carotid territory stroke and crescendo TIAs. (a) Carotid angiogram reveals severe stenosis (arrow) at the origin of the left interval carotid artery. (b) The vessel is widely patent following placement of a self-expanding Wallstent (10 mm × 20 mm)

Figure 3 Angiogram of a 59-year-old man with a history of multiple posterior circulation infarcts. (a) Severe stenosis at origin of the left vertebral artery. (b) Dilation of this segment with a balloon-mounted 4 mm × 12 mm stent

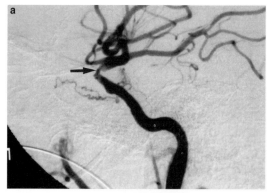

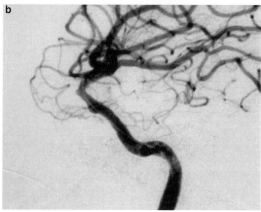

Figure 4 (a) Angiogram of a 66-year-old man with ischemic symptoms who was found to have symptomatic, severe focal stenosis of the supraclinoid internal carotid artery (arrow). (b) The vessel was dilated with a small (3.0 mm × 15.0 mm angioplasty balloon)

Post-procedure

The patient is placed on aspirin, 325 mg daily for life, and clopidogrel 75 mg once daily for four weeks following insertion of the stent.

Intracranial angioplasty and stenting

Angioplasty and stenting of intracranial carotid and vertebrobasilar arteries have shown favorable results in patients who fail conventional medical management[22,23]. Sundt *et al.* performed the first intracranial basilar artery angioplasty in 1980[24]. Many investigators have

reported good results with cerebral angioplasty, while others have reported high rates of morbidity and mortality[25-27]. Complications include vessel rupture and occlusion. Advances in coronary balloon and stent technology have reduced the occurrences of procedure-related morbidity. See Figures 4 and 5.

ENDOVASCULAR TREATMENT OF ANEURYSMS

Conventional surgical clipping of cerebral aneurysms continues to be the current mainstay for the treatment of intracranial aneurysms. Attempts have been made to augment or replace this conventional therapy by a less invasive endovascular approach. Previously-used devices used to pack the lumen of aneurysms endovascularly include balloons and pushable coils, which have been used with varying degrees of success, but the inability to accurately control the position of these devices limited their safety and effectiveness. Since then, electrically detachable coils – Guglielmi detachable coils (GDC) – have been developed, which provide the control necessary to safely and effectively pack an aneurysmal sac. The GDC is a soft platinum alloy coil bonded to a stainless steel delivery wire. Twenty to thirty percent of all aneurysms in the USA are treated with GDC.

In aneurysms with favorable geometry (sac to neck ratio ≥ 1.5; size, 0.3–1.5 cm), the GDC has provided a minimally invasive means to occlude aneurysms. As with other minimally invasive surgical procedures, the postoperative recuperative period is significantly shorter than with conventional surgery. There has been a recent trend to treat aneurysms soon after the initial acute subarachnoid hemorrhage. This philosophy decreases the risk of re-bleed and allows aggressive management of posthemorrhage vasospasm. Early surgery may not always be possible and is dependent upon the patient's clinical examination.

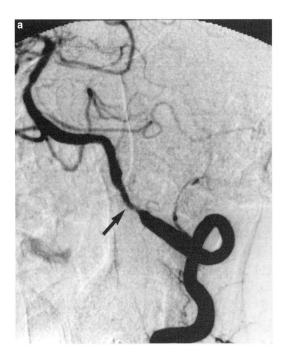 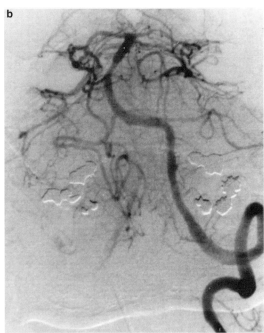

Figure 5   (a) Angiogram of a 66-year-old man with multiple posterior circulation ischemic strokes who is found to have severe stenosis of the distal left vertebral artery (arrow). (b) The segment was dilated with a balloon-mounted 3 mm × 12 mm stent

Endovascular therapy can be employed in this acute stage despite the patient's clinical condition and, at a minimum, may decrease the risk of re-rupture. GDC coiling may stabilize the patient and allow a more definitive procedure to be performed once the patient's clinical condition is more stable.

Debrun *et al.* recently published their experience with GDC endovascular treatment of aneurysms[28]. All procedures were performed with patients under general anesthesia and systemic heparinization. Follow-up angiography was performed six months, one year and two years after treatment. Aneurysms that were considered favorable for coiling included those that had a dome to neck ratio of at least 2 and an absolute neck diameter less than 5 mm. In 119 patients with 123 aneurysms considered favorable for coiling based on their geometry, there was no mortality directly related to the coiling procedure, and the permanent morbidity was limited to 1%. The degree of permanent aneurysm occlusion was associated with the geometry of the aneurysm. Complete occlusion was achieved in 72% of patients with acute ruptured aneurysms and in 80% of patients with non-acute aneurysms. These were patients whose aneurysms had a dome to neck ratio that was at least 2. The total occlusion rate dropped to 53% when the geometry was unfavorable for GDC treatment and the dome to neck ratio was less than 2. The authors concluded that these preliminary results suggest that using GDCs is a safe technique, resulting in low morbidity and mortality rates for the treatment of aneurysms in appropriately selected patients. The percentage of complete aneurysm occlusion is related to the density of coil packing, which is strongly dependent upon the geometry of the aneurysm.

Vinuela *et al.* reported the experience of eight interventional neuroradiology centers in the United States that participated in a prospective clinical study to evaluate the safety of the Guglielmi detachable coil system[29]. Reasons for exclusion from surgical treatment were anticipated surgical difficulty (69.2%), attempted and failed surgery (12.7%), poor neurological (12.2%) or medical (12.7%) status and refusal of surgery (1.2%). After excluding patients who did not qualify, there were 403 patients who presented with subarachnoid hemorrhage from a ruptured aneurysm and were entered into the GDC study. Complete aneurysm occlusion was documented in 70.8% of small aneurysms with a small neck, 35% of large aneurysms, and 50% of giant aneurysms. A small neck remnant was present in 21.4% of small aneurysms with a small neck, 57.1% of large aneurysms, and 50% of giant aneurysms. Technical complications included aneurysm perforation (2.7%), unintentional parent artery occlusion (3%), and cerebral embolization (2.5%). There was an 8.9% immediate morbidity rate related to the GDC technique. Seven deaths were related to technical complications (1.7%) and 18 (4.5%) to the severity of the primary hemorrhage.

Lot *et al.* reported on a series in which both techniques, conventional surgical clipping and coiling, were applied[30]. There were 395 consecutive patients with small or large aneurysms treated either by surgery or endovascular coiling. Coiling was chosen when the shape of the aneurysm was appropriate for treatment. Unsatisfactory results were seen in seven cases following surgery and 25 cases following coil embolization. In the overall series, surgery and embolization, good and excellent clinical outcome was noted in 90% of small aneurysms and 86.5% of large ones; mortality was 4.8%. They concluded that with appropriate selection, endovascular treatment is a good alternative for treatment of the majority of saccular aneurysms. A combination of coiling and clipping may occasionally be used when the initial procedure has resulted in an aneurysm remnant. In a poorly positioned clip, coils may help pack the residual aneurysm, or in an incompletely coiled aneurysm a clip may be necessary for definitive therapy[11].

Limitations to endovascular therapy include (1) inaccessibility to the aneurysm because of atherosclerotic disease or vessel tortuosity or stenosis, (2) broad-based aneurysms in which the sac to neck ratio is less than 2, and (3) coil compaction leading to recanalization and regrowth of the aneurysm[31]. This is especially noted in large para-ophthalmic and basilar apex aneurysms. Contraindications include severe adverse reaction to contrast material and severe vasospasm.

Aneurysm coil embolizations

Technique

The patient is endotracheally intubated and placed under general anesthesia and the groin is prepped and draped in the usual sterile manner. A 6F sheath is percutaneously placed within the femoral artery. The target vessel, that which harbors the aneurysm, is catheterized with a 5F diagnostic catheter. A diagnostic arteriogram with multiple projections is performed to define the anatomic features of the aneurysm to be treated. Precise measurements of the aneurysm are needed to determine coil selection. The working projection is one that includes the aneurysm neck and its relation to the native vessel. During coil placement it is necessary to deposit the entire coil within the aneurysm lumen without allowing it to displace into the adjacent vessel lumen. The diagnostic catheter is replaced with a 6F guide catheter, and the patient is systemically heparinized. Through the guide catheter, a micro-catheter designed for coil placement is advanced (Prowler, Cordis Endovascular, Miami Lakes, FL; Excel, Boston Scientific,

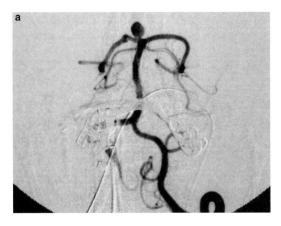
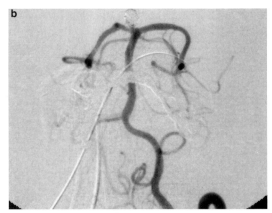

Figure 6   (a) Angiogram of a 52-year-old woman who presented with a Hunt and Hess Grade I subarachnoid hemorrhage and was found to have a distal basilar artery aneurysm. (b) The aneurysm was packed with Gugliemli detachable coils (GDCs)

Fremont, CA). The tip of the micro-catheter is slowly and carefully positioned within the aneurysm. Coils are advanced through the catheter into the aneurysm lumen.

The ideal initial coil should be the largest diameter coil that can be safely deposited within the aneurysm lumen. Also, it should take on a 3-dimensional form when unconstrained so that it can act as a basket into which other coils can be deposited. The endpoint is reached when no additional coils can be deployed safely within the aneurysm without causing displacement of the catheter tip. Excessive resistance to coil advancement within the aneurysm is also an endpoint, and indicates that coil advancement should cease. Following coil placement the micro-catheter is completely withdrawn from the guide catheter. Angiography is performed to assess the degree of coil packing. A mental inventory of all major filling arterial branches should be performed to determine vessel occlusion from thromboembolism.

The heparinized state is allowed to reverse on its own, and hemostasis at the groin should be achieved when the activated clotting time is less than 200 seconds. A follow-up arteriogram is recommended at six months to assess the long-term effects of the coils, such as coil displacement or compaction, aneurysm regrowth, native vessel occlusion, or complete aneurysm ablation. See Figure 6.

COMPLICATIONS

The most commonly reported complications are stroke related to cerebral emboli. Thromboemboli are more likely to occur in large aneurysms with broad-based necks, and they may be caused by the larger surface area of coils exposed to the intraluminal surface of the native vessel. Many centers recommend systemic heparinization for 24 hours post-coiling in these large aneurysms. No large series has been reported to determine the effectiveness of heparinization as prophylaxis against thromboembolism following coil embolization of aneurysms. In the report by Pelz *et al.* (presented at the American Society of Interventional and Therapeutic Neuroradiology, New York, New York; September 1997) the rate of acute stroke caused by thromboembolism for aneurysm coiling was 15.5%, with a 3.4% incidence of permanent deficits[11].

Rupture of an aneurysm during endovascular therapy may occur as a complication. This

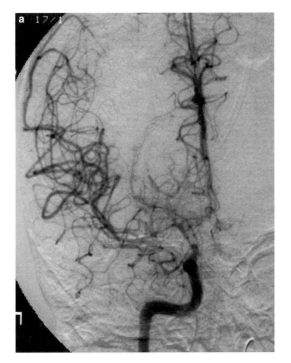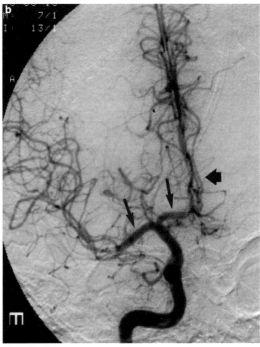

Figure 7 (a) Angiogram of a severe vasospasm of the carotid, middle and anterior cerebral arteries following subarachnoid hemorrhage. (b) The carotid, proximal middle and anterior cerebral arteries are dilated by balloon angioplasty (arrows). The more distal vessels are dilated with a 300 mg papaverine infusion (arrowhead)

may be related to poor technique, microcatheter instability, or inappropriate coil selection. Intracerebral bleeding causes a sudden increase of pressure within the subarachnoid space, which may result in clinical consequences such as instant death from herniation, vasospasm or ischemia. An arterial line during treatment is mandatory in order to discern any acute change in the patient's clinical status. Any abrupt increase in the patient's blood pressure with simultaneous decrease in pulse rate (Cushing effect) should raise the suspicion that an acute rupture has occurred. At this time reversal of the anticoagulant state is necessary. The endovascular procedure should continue so that packing of the aneurysm will reduce or stop the rate of blood flow into the intracranial fossa. Endovascular obliteration of the aneurysm sac at this time is necessary

and should be performed as expeditiously as possible. Every patient who has had an aneurysm treated by endovascular means should undergo a repeat angiogram after six months to assess the durability of the initial treatment.

TREATMENT OF VASOSPASM CAUSED BY SUBARACHNOID HEMORRHAGE

Infusion of papaverine

Papaverine is a smooth-muscle relaxant that can dilate intracranial arteries in spasm caused by subarachnoid blood. There has been no large series verifying the efficacy of intra-arterial papaverine infusion for the treatment of post subarachnoid hemorrhage vasospasm[11].

Benefit has been shown in some small series of patients[32]. Papaverine can be infused through a 5F diagnostic catheter with the tip lying within the internal carotid artery or vertebral artery. Some authors recommend intracranial catheterization with a microcatheter above the ophthalmic artery to prevent retinal infarction. We have never experienced this problem. Extracranial infusion proximal to the ophthalmic artery can cause ipsilateral mydriasis.

Papaverine infusion may be indicated when there is angiographically visible vasospasm. It can be infused directly through the diagnostic catheter. Three hundred milligrams of papaverine are mixed with 100 ml of normal saline and infused through an intravenous pump at a rate of 2 ml/minute. Thus, the entire volume is injected over 50 minutes. If necessary, this can be repeated within the same vascular territory. In up to 30–50% of patients the effects may be transient. Physiologic monitoring is necessary since there are occasionally cardiovascular side-effects including tachycardia (usually supraventricular) and hypotension. If these occur, the infusion should be discontinued. Care should be taken not to mix this solution with heparin. The papaverine may precipitate out of solution causing a stroke from microemboli. It has been suggested that a concentration greater than 0.3%

(300 mg/100 ml normal saline) could also increase the possibility of precipitate formation.

BALLOON ANGIOPLASTY

Balloon angioplasty is recommended when there is angiographically visible vasospasm within the intracranial carotid and vertebrobasilar arteries, proximal M-1 segment of the middle cerebral artery and A-1 segment of the anterior cerebral artery. Unlike papaverine infusion, dilation of a vessel with a balloon is permanent. Soft silicone balloons (Endeavor, Boston Scientific, Fremont, CA) tend to elongate longitudinally at the distal tip. The Endeavor balloon is flow directed.

The balloon system is advanced through a 6F, 90 cm guide catheter. A wire 0.014 inches in diameter can be used with the balloon catheter system to ease advancement and provide steerability. A 50% contrast solution allows easier inflation and deflation since it is not as viscous as full-strength contrast. The balloon is advanced into the narrowed segment and slowly inflated. Since the balloon elongates longitudinally along its distal end, the dilation procedure begins proximally and is slowly advanced distally. Only short inflation times of 1–2 seconds are necessary. See Figure 7.

References

1. Wolf P, Kannel W, McGee D. Epidemiology of strokes in North America. In Barnett HJM, Stein BM, Mohr J, *et al.*, eds. *Stroke: Pathophysiology, Diagnosis and Management*. New York: Churchill Livingstone, 1986:19–29
2. Zeumer H, Freitag H, Knospe V. Instravascular thrombolysis in the central nervous system cerebrovascular disease. *Neurol Clin North Am* 1992;2:359–69
3. Feussner J, Matchar DB. When and how to study the carotids. *Ann Intern Med* 1988;109:805–18
4. Jahan R, Duckwiler GR, Kidwell CS, *et al*. Intra-arterial thrombolysis for treatment of acute stroke: experience in 26 patients with long-term follow-up. *Am J Neuroradiol* 1999;20:1291–9
5. Chambers B, Norris J, Shurvell B, *et al*. Prognosis of acute stroke. *Neurology* 1987;37: 221–5
6. Saito I, Segawa H, Shiokawa Y, *et al*. Middle cerebral artery occlusion: correlation of computed tomography and angiography with clinical outcome. *Stroke* 1987;18:863–8
7. Hacke W, Zeumer H, Ferbert A, *et al*. Intra-arterial therapy improves outcomes in patients with acute vertebrobasilar disease. *Stroke* 1988;19:1216–22

8. Zeumer H, Hacke W, Ringelstein EF, *et al.* Local intra-arterial thrombolysis in vertebrobasilar thromboembolic disease. *Am J Neuroradiol* 1983;4:401–4

9. Zeumer H, Hundgen R, Ferbert A, *et al.* Local intra-arterial fibrinolytic therapy in inaccessible internal carotid occlusion. *Neuroradiology* 1984;26:315–17

10. Brott T, Bogousslavsky J. Treatment of acute ischemic stroke. *N Engl J Med* 2000;343: 710–22

11. Connors JJ, Wojak JC. Current directions in emergency stroke therapy. In Connors JJ, Wojack JC, eds. *Interventional Neuroradiology.* Philadelphia: W.B. Saunders, 1999:629–44

12. Executive Committee of the ASITN. Intra-arterial thrombolysis: ready for prime time? *Am J Neuroradiol* 2001;22:55–8

13. Strother CM. Intra-arterial thrombolysis for the treatment of patients with acute ischemic stroke. *Am J Neuroradiol* 1999;20:1580

14. Grond M, Rudolf J, Schmulling S, *et al.* Early intravenous thrombolysis with recombinant tissue-type plasminogen activator in vertebrobasilar ischemic stroke. *Arch Neurol* 1998; 55:466–9

15. Cross DT, Moran CJ, Akins PT, *et al.* Relationship between clot location and outcome after basilar artery thrombolysis. *Am J Neuroradiol* 1997;18:1221–8

16. Cloft HJ. Angioplasty and stenting of the carotid artery. *Appl Radiol* 2001;July:23–7

17. Vitek JJ, Roubin GS, Al-Mubarek N, *et al.* Carotid artery stenting: technical considerations. *Am J Neuroradiol* 2000;21:1736–43

18. Phatouros CC, Higashida RT, Malek AM, *et al.* Endovascular stenting for carotid artery stenosis: preliminary experience using the shape-memory-alloy-recoverable-technology (SMART) stent. *Am J Neuroradiol* 2000;21:732–8

19. Piamsomboon C, Roubin GS, Liu MW, *et al.* Relationship between oversizing of self-expanding stents and late loss index in carotid stenting. *Cath Cardiovasc Diagn* 1998;45: 139–43

20. Vitek JJ, Iyer SS, Roubin G. Carotid stenting in 350 vessels: problems faced and solved. *J Invasive Cardiol* 1998;10:311–14

21. Ohki T, Marin ML, Lyon RT, *et al.* Ex vivo human carotid artery bifurcation stenting; correlation of lesion characteristics with embolic potential. *J Vasc Surg* 1998;27:463–71

22. Mori T, Kazita K, Chokyu K, *et al.* Short-term arteriographic and clinical outcome after cerebral angioplasty and stenting for intracranial vertebrobasilar and carotid atherosclerotic occlusive disease. *Am J Neuroradiol* 2000; 21:249–54

23. Gomez CR, Misra VK, Liu MW, *et al.* Elective stenting of symptomatic basilar artery stenosis. *Stroke* 2000;31:95

24. Sundt TM, Smith HC, Campbell J, *et al.* Transluminal angioplasty for basilar artery stenosis. *Mayo Clin Proc* 1980;55:673–80

25. Gomez CR, Misra VK, Campbell MS, *et al.* Elective stenting of symptomatic middle cerebral artery stenosis. *Am J Neuroradiol* 2000; 21:971–3

26. Al-Muborak N, Gomez CR, Vitek JJ, *et al.* Stenting of symptomatic stenosis of the intracranial internal carotid artery. *Am J Neuroradiol* 1998;19:1949–51

27. Morris PP, Martin EM, Regan J, *et al.* Intracranial deployment of coronary stents for symptomatic atherosclerotic disease. *Am J Neuroradiol* 1999;20:1688–94

28. Debrun GM, Aletich VA, Kehrli P, *et al.* Selection of cerebral aneurysms for treatment using Guglielmi detachable coils: the preliminary University of Illinois at Chicago experience. *Neurosurgery* 1998;43:1281–95

29. Vinuela F, Duckwiler G, Mawad M. Guglielmi detachable coil embolization of acute intracranial aneurysm: perioperative anatomical and clinical outcome in 403 patients. *J Neurosurg* 1997;86(3):475–82

30. Lot G, Houdart E, Cophignon J, *et al.* Combined management of intracranial aneurysms by surgical and endovascular treatment. Modalities and results from a series of 395 cases. *Acta Neurochiraurgica* 1999;141(6): 557–62

31. Hope JK, Byrne JV, Molyneux AJ. Factors influencing successful angiographic occlusion of aneurysms treated by coil embolization. *Am J Neuroradiol* 1999;20:391–9

32. Kassell NF, Helm G, Simmons N, *et al.* Treatment of cerebral vasospasm with intra-arterial papaverine. *J Neurosurg* 1992;77: 848–52

Chapter 22

Pros and cons of screening for and ablating asymptomatic intracranial aneurysms

Sean Ruland, DO, and Dan Heffez, MD, FRCS

INTRODUCTION

Aneurysmal subarachnoid hemorrhage (SAH) has a 30-day mortality rate reported to approach 50%[1-4], and an additional 20% of patients are left dependent following SAH[2]. SAH accounts for nearly half of all mortality due to cerebrovascular disease in persons less than 35 years old[5]. The potential impact for the general population of cerebral aneurysm is difficult to measure because only limited data exist regarding the incidence of and prevalence of intracranial aneurysm (IA). Autopsy studies have suggested a mean prevalence of IA in the general population of 5%[6]. In Olmsted County, Minnesota, from 1965 to 1995, the incidence and prevalence of IA were 9.0/100 000 person-years and 83.4/100 000 person-years, respectively[7]. Whether IA should be sought in asymptomatic individuals and treated if identified are hotly debated issues. To resolve the issue, the natural history of an unruptured IA, risk of harboring an IA, risk of the treatment and the long-term cost-effectiveness of screening need to be determined.

NATURAL HISTORY

The International Study of Unruptured Intracranial Aneurysms (ISUIA) retrospectively reviewed records on 1449 patients with 1937 aneurysms and 12 023 patient-years of follow-up. Multiple aneurysms were found in 364 of the patients. Seventy-five percent of all patients were women. One-half of patients had previously suffered a SAH from a separate IA, but the other half had no previous history of SAH. In the group without previous SAH, the risk of aneurysm rupture was estimated to be 0.05%/year for IAs less than 10 mm in diameter and 1%/year for larger IAs (10–24 mm). Six percent of giant IAs ($\geq$ 25 mm) ruptured within the first year following diagnosis[6]. In the group that had suffered a previous IA rupture, the average annual rupture rate was 0.5%/year for small IAs and 1%/year for large IAs. It is important to note that, in the latter group, most of the index SAHs were due to IAs less than 10 mm in diameter[6]. In a Finnish observational study of 181 unruptured IAs followed for 40 years, the annual rate of rupture was calculated to be 1%. IAs bigger than 7 mm were 2.3 times more likely to rupture than smaller IAs[1]. The risk of IA rupture appears to vary with anatomical location. While IAs occur more commonly in the anterior circulation[7], aneurysms of the basilar, vertebral and posterior cerebral arteries may have a higher risk of rupture[6,8]. The risk within 7.5 years has been reported to be 2%, 15%, and 45% for small, large, and giant IAs of the posterior circulation, respectively[6].

An increased risk of SAH has also been reported for first degree relatives of patients who have had a SAH[8,9]. There is a four-fold increased risk of SAH at an early age for those persons having familial intracranial aneurysm (FIA) syndrome (at least two first- or second-degree relatives with intracranial aneurysms)[8]. Other factors associated with IA rupture, each with an independent effect, include younger age, smoking[1,3,9], history of hypertension[9], alcohol consumption[3,9], autosomal dominant polycystic kidney disease (ADPKD)[9] and use of oral contraceptives pills[5]. In Western Europe and the Netherlands, the attributable risk of aneurysmal SAH in the general population was 11% if there was a positive family history, 20% for smoking, 17% for hypertension, 11% for 100–299 g/week of alcohol, 21% for more than 300 g/week of alcohol, and 0.3% for ADPKD[9]. A meta-analysis of oral contraceptive use has shown a relative risk of 1.49 for SAH after controlling for hypertension and smoking[5].

RISK OF HARBORING AN INTRACRANIAL ANEURYSM

A positive family history of IA constitutes a substantial risk[3,8]. A Finnish study showed that the relative risk with one affected first-degree family member was 1.8[8]. Another study using magnetic resonance angiography in

626 first-degree relatives of patients with a SAH found aneurysms present in 25 (4%). Siblings with IA accounted for 88% of screened family members, and IAs were multiple in nearly 25%[8]. In Finland, the familial IA syndrome conferred a relative risk for IA of 4.2[3]. Another study from the Netherlands showed that the prevalence of IAs among family members was 8%[8]. The risk was highest for sibling and mother–daughter pairs. A 1–2%/year rate of subsequent new IA formation has also been reported in these families[3].

Other genetic syndromes such as ADPKD and type IV Ehler–Danlos syndrome also appear to increase the risk of IA formation. ADPKD has been associated with a relative risk for IA of 4.4 compared with matched controls. Atherosclerosis has been shown to confer an increased relative risk of 2.3 for IA[8]. Other suggested risk factors for harboring an IA include hypertension, female sex, advanced age and smoking. IA was more often detected in women and at a younger age than in men in the Olmsted County, Minnesota cohort[7].

It is estimated that 20–34% of affected individuals have more than one aneurysm[4]. Multiple IAs were found in 21% of the Olmsted County cohort[7]. Juvela performed a multivariate analysis on 266 patients with 382 IAs and found that smoking and possibly female sex and advanced age were independent risk factors for multiple aneurysms[4].

RISK OF TREATMENT

Currently, the two treatment options for IA are surgical clipping and endovascular coil embolization. The ISUIA found that the combined surgical 30-day morbidity and mortality rates were 17.5% for patients with no previous history of aneurysmal SAH and 13.6% for those with a previous history of aneurysmal SAH. The risk was related to age, ranging from 6.5% for those less than 45 years old to 14.4% for those 45–65 years old, and to 32% for those more than 65 years old[6]. Surgical risk increases with increasing size of the aneurysm, ranging from less than 3% 30-day combined morbidity and mortality for small aneurysms ($\leq$ 5 mm) to 20–50% for giant aneurysms (> 25 mm) depending, in part, on their location[3]. A meta-analysis of 61 studies and 2460 surgically treated patients showed an overall mortality rate of 2.6% and morbidity rate of 10.9%. Size correlated directly with risk of treatment. The highest risk was found for giant aneurysms that were clipped in the posterior circulation, with a mortality of 9.6% and morbidity of 37.9%[2].

There may be a relationship between the number of aneurysms operated on at a given institution and favorable outcome. According to one study in New York State, there was a 53% reduction in mortality in hospitals that performed more than ten aneurysm surgeries per year compared with hospitals with fewer such operations[10]. A Dutch study based on 18 patients concluded that there was no difference 12 months after surgical treatment of asymptomatic IA in baseline quality of life compared to the period before surgery[11]. The investigators used two quality-of-life scales (sickness impact profile and short-form 36).

Predictors of increased surgical risk include location in the posterior circulation and cavernous segment of the internal carotid artery, fusiform aneurysmal neck, association of the IA with atherosclerotic or ectatic vessels, or presence at a major arterial bifurcation[3].

Coil embolization is an alternative treatment to surgery for aneurysm obliteration[12,13]. However, there are inherent limitations and complications to coiling. The technical feasibility is largely dependent on the configuration of the aneurysm. Complete aneurysm obliteration rates have been reported to be as high as 70–80%. Aneurysms between 4 and 10 mm have the highest rate of successful occlusion. Aneurysms with wide necks are more difficult

to occlude and those with a large dome and a narrow neck may increase the success of treatment. A dome-to-neck ratio greater than 2 has been associated with an 80% complete occlusion rate versus 58% for those aneurysms with a ratio less than 2[13]. The angulation between the aneurysm and the parent vessel may limit the ability to insert the catheter and its coil into the aneurysm lumen. Proximal vascular tortuosity and atheroma may also present challenges. Risks associated with coil embolization include aneurysmal rupture (2.1–8%), inadvertent occlusion of a nutrient artery and thromboembolism (3.2–5%) and coil migration into the parent artery (1.1–1.3%)[13].

Whether coil embolization permanently occludes an IA has not been well established. In one study of ruptured IA occluded by coil embolization, no aneurysm that had been completely occluded subsequently bled again. IAs that were nearly completely (90–99%) occluded re-bled at a rate of 1.4%/year and those incompletely occluded (< 90%) re-bled at a rate of 7.3%/year; the mean follow-up in that study was 1.9 years[13]. The applicability of these data to the treatment of unruptured IAs is unclear. An aneurysm may recur after incomplete surgical clipping as well. A Japanese study of 140 ruptured and unruptured IAs which had been surgically clipped found a recurrence rate of 2.9% over a mean follow-up of 9.3 years. The rate of *de novo* aneurysm formation in those patients was 8%[14].

A retrospective review of 2069 unruptured IAs treated statewide in California between 1990 and 1998 compared 1699 (82%) treated surgically to 370 (18%) treated with endovascular therapy. Adverse events – defined as in-hospital death or discharge to a nursing home or rehabilitation – occurred in 25.4% of the surgical group and 9.7% of the endovascular treatment group. In addition, the surgical group had a 7-fold higher in-hospital mortality rate, 4.7 day longer mean length-of-stay, and an average of $27 000 more in hospital charges. The adverse event rate declined significantly from 26% to 4% over the time period from 1991 to 1998 for endovascular treatment without a significant change in percent treated surgically (26% to 21%). Centers treating higher numbers of patients with endovascular therapy had significantly less morbidity and mortality[15]. The likelihood of incomplete treatment following endovascular therapy must be weighed against the lower morbidity and mortality rates reported with this technique. However, most series of IAs treated by coil embolization included patients selected on the basis of vascular anatomy. Most were posterior circulation aneurysms with poor Hunt and Hess grades. This selection may well introduce a bias in outcomes, thus accurate comparison of endovascular therapy and surgical clipping is not straightforward.

WHO SHOULD BE CONSIDERED FOR SCREENING AND TREATMENT?

Advances in non-invasive neurovascular imaging have expanded the possibility of screening for IA by limiting the risk of catheter angiography. CT angiography and magnetic resonance angiography have the potential to detect aneurysms as small as 3 mm in diameter with variable sensitivity (69–87%) and specificity (93–100%)[3]. Each has its own technical limitations. However, the 'gold standard' of neurovascular imaging is catheter angiography, which is associated with a neurological morbidity rate of 0.5–1.0%[3]. The decision regarding the screening and treatment of unruptured IA should first consider patient age and co-morbidity. A patient with a shorter life-expectancy will derive less benefit from preventive treatment and will probably have greater procedure-related risks. In a risk analysis for treatment of unruptured IA using data derived from ISUIA,

a treatment benefit for unruptured IA was noted in patients less than 50 years old and only for those unruptured IA greater than 10 mm[16]. This analysis used the overall rupture and surgical complication rates and did not account for the variable hemorrhage and operative risks associated with aneurysms in different locations and of different morphologies. Another theoretical model of screening in 1000 patients with FIA assumed a prevalence of 9.8%, rupture risk of 0.8% and surgical morbidity including death and dependency of 8.0%. That model did not support reduced overall morbidity and mortality from screening beyond 30 years of age. Even though the assumed one-time risk of cerebral angiography was low (0.1%), if performed three times (every ten years), there were as many complications from angiography as there were from aneurysm rupture[17]. However, this analysis did not describe the difference in severity of angiography-related complications and aneurysmal SAH. A hypothetical cohort of 50-year-old women was used to perform a cost–benefit analysis that failed to show a benefit for treatment of unruptured IAs less than 10 mm in patients without a previous history of SAH. A benefit was seen for those with larger aneurysms, prior history of SAH, or local symptoms related to the volume of the aneurysm[18]. However, until outcome data are obtained prospectively in randomized homogeneous patient groups, models will have limited value in predicting outcome.

The Stroke Council of the American Heart Association (AHA) recommends that initial screening be considered in those families with the FIA syndrome. Moreover, the AHA recommends late screening in those patients with previous aneurysmal rupture because new IA formation is reported in 1–2% of such patients. Screening was not recommended for the general population, first-degree relatives of patients with aneurysm, or other genetic syndromes such as ADPKD and Ehler–Danlos syndrome. Treatment should be considered for IAs larger than 10 mm in diameter, symptomatic unruptured IA, in patients with a history of prior SAH, younger patients, patients with a positive family history, and in IA with unusual morphologic characteristics such as daughter sac formation[3]. However, the smaller anticipated benefit of prophylactic treatment in older patients must also be weighed against previous published reports of increasing incidence of aneurysmal SAH with each decade of life[19,20].

CONCLUSIONS

The long-standing dilemma regarding which patients to screen for IA, whom to treat, and how to treat has yet to be resolved. Despite the lack of prospective, randomized data to help clarify this controversy, several points seem clear: (1) small IAs are more common than larger IAs and, therefore, account for a higher absolute number of SAH; (2) small IAs are easier and safer to treat by either surgical clipping or coil embolization than larger IAs; (3) small IAs (< 10 mm) appear to have a relatively low risk of rupture (0.05%/year); (4) under the best circumstances, both surgical clipping and coil embolization may carry morbidity and mortality rates greater than the natural history of rupture of small IAs; and (5) SAH from a ruptured IA has an extremely high morbidity and mortality and remains an unpredictable occurence.

Since there appears to be a different natural history and different treatment risks associated with IAs of varying morphologies and locations, applying uniform assumptions to a heterogeneous population will have inherent limitations. For example, ISUIA, which is the largest study of unruptured IAs to date, is non-randomized, largely retrospective, and does not take morphology into account in the analysis. Therefore, ISUIA data cannot be generalized to all IAs based on size alone. Any consideration of screening for and treatment of unruptured IA must take each individual risk profile into account. It is hoped that additional research will define rupture rates better for aneurysmal subtypes, and as refinements in interventional techniques having lower complication rates evolve, an answer to the questions of whom to screen and whom to treat will be more easily answered.

References

1. Juvelo S, Porras M, Poussa K. Natural history of unruptured intracranial aneurysms: probablility of and risk factors for aneurysm rupture. *J Neurosurg* 2000;93:379–87
2. Raaymakers TW, Rinkel GJ, Limburg M, Algra A. Mortality and morbidity of surgery for unruptured intracranial aneurysms. *Stroke* 1998;29:1531–8
3. Bederson JB, Awad IA, Wiebers DO. Recommendations for the management of patients with unruptured intracranial aneurysms. *Circulation* 2000;102:2300–8
4. Juvela S. Risk factors for multiple intracranial aneuryms. *Stroke* 2000;31:392–7
5. Johnston SC, Colford JM Jr, Gress DG. Oral contraceptives and the risk of subarachnoid hemorrhage: A meta-analysis. *Neurology* 1998;51:411–18
6. ISUIA Investigators. Unruptured intracranial aneurysms: risks of rupture and risks of surgical intervention. *N Engl J Med* 1998;339:1725–33
7. Menghini VV, Brown RD Jr, Sicks MS, *et al.* Incidence and prevalence of intracranial aneurysm and hemorrhage in Olmsted County, Minnesota, 1965–1995. *Neurology* 1998;51:405–11
8. Gorelick PB. Should we be screening relatives of patients with aneurysmal subarachnoid hemorrhage for asymptomatic intracranial aneurysm? *Curr Atheroscl Rep* 2000;2:89–91
9. Ruigrok YM, Buskens E, Rinkel GJ. Attributable risk of common and rare determinants of subarachnoid hemorrhage. *Stroke* 2001;32:1173

10. Solomon RA, Mayer SA, Tarmey JJ. Relationship between the volume of craniotomies for cerebral aneurysm performed at New York state hospitals and in-hospital mortality. *Stroke* 1996;27:13–17

11. Raaymakers TW and the MARS Study Group. Functional outcome and quality of life after angiography and operation for unruptured intracranial aneurysms. *J Neurol Neurosurg Psychiatry* 2000;68:571–6

12. Kassell NF, Lanzino G. Unruptured intracranial aneurysms: In search of the best management strategy, editorial comment. *Stroke* 2001;32:603–5

13. Dovey Z, Misra M, Thornton J, *et al.* Guglielmi detachable coiling for intracranial aneurysms: The story so far. *Arch Neurol* 2001; 58:559–64

14. Keisuke KT, Ueki D, Morita A, *et al.* Risk of aneurysm recurrence in patients with clipped cerebral aneurysms: Results of long-term follow-up angiography. *Stroke* 2001;32:1191–4

15. Johnston SC, Zhao S, Dudley RA, *et al.* Treatment of unruptured cerebral aneurysms in California. *Stroke* 2001;32:597–605

16. Jakubowski PM. Risk analysis of treatment of unruptured aneurysms. *J Neurol Neurosurg Psychiatry* 2000;68:577–80

17. Crawley F, Clifton A, Brown M. Should we screen for familial intracranial aneurysm? *Stroke* 1999;30:312–16

18. Johnston SC, Gress DR, Kahn JG. Which unruptured cerebral aneurysms should be treated? A cost-utility analysis. *Neurology* 1999; 52:1806–15

19. Christie D. Some aspects of the natural history of subarachnoid haemorrhage. *Aust NZ J Med* 1981;11:22–7

20. Fogelholm R. Subarachnoid hemorrhage in Middle-Finland: Incidence, early prognosis and indications for neurosurgical treatment. *Stroke* 1981;12:296–301

Closing remarks: on stroke prevention guidelines, organization of care and future perspectives

Edward H. Wong, MBChB, FRACP, and
Vladimir Hachinski, MD, FRCPC, DSc

INTRODUCTION

Just as acute stroke care has been revolutionized by the introduction of rtPA, stroke prevention also needs a paradigm shift. Stroke prevention now goes beyond prescribing aspirin and (in selected cases) carotid endarterectomy. Randomized trials have shown the effectiveness of angiotensin-converting enzyme inhibitors and anticoagulation, and a role for statin agents in stroke prevention.

Stroke prevention needs to take a higher priority among clinicians, health administrators and health policy makers. Stroke physicians must become as adept at stroke prevention as they are at acute stroke care, because prevention remains substantially more effective than treatment.

STROKE PREVENTION GUIDELINES

Guidelines for stroke prevention have been produced by the American Heart Association[1,2] and the National Stroke Association[3]. In addition guidelines, systematic reviews and meta-analyses on the management of hypertension, atrial fibrillation, smoking, dyslipidemia and other factors have been produced by many organizations. Although these statements are developed to assist physician and patient decisions and to improve the quality of care by reducing variation, there is little evidence that guidelines have a significant effect on changing physician behavior[4].

Several potential barriers to adherence to clinical guidelines have been identified, lack of awareness, lack of familiarity and lack of agreement being the most common[5]. Therefore, clinical guidelines, must whenever possible be based on large clinical trials or systematic reviews, and furthermore need to be updated regularly. They have to be presented in a form that is accessible to their end-users, and possibly in more than one form, if there are multiple target groups.

ORGANIZATION OF CARE

Most of the known risk factors for stroke were identified decades ago from large longitudinal studies, such as the Framingham Study cohort. Subsequently, stroke risk profiles were developed with the intention that they would 'facilitate multifactorial risk factor modification'[6]. However, despite the identification of these modifiable risk factors and the development of guidelines and consensus statements, the implementation of stroke prevention strategies has been inadequate[7]. While it has been known for 20 years that treatment of hypertension could significantly reduce the risk of stroke[8], over two-thirds of hypertensive patients are untreated or inadequately treated[9]. Similarly, randomized controlled trials have clearly demonstrated that oral anticoagulation is highly effective at preventing stroke in patients with atrial fibrillation (both primary and secondary prevention). However this treatment remains under-utilized, with only 15–44% of patients without a contra-indication to anticoagulation receiving it[10]. In a survey of physicians, the perceived benefits of anticoagulation were underestimated, while the respondents overestimated the risk of hemorrhage[11].

The answer to this discrepancy between knowledge and execution/implementation lies in better organization of health services, perhaps in atherosclerosis or vascular clinics. In our practice we have recently established an Urgent TIA Clinic for rapid triage, assessment, investigation and treatment of patients with symptoms of TIA and minor stroke. It is hoped that the timely assessment and initiation of appropriate treatment will prevent a second vascular event in the first few weeks after a TIA, the time of greatest risk.

While neurologists and other specialists see only a minority of patients with stroke risk factors, they must systematically identify these people and aggressively manage these factors, especially in those that have already suffered a vascular event, as they are at greatest risk. They must also convey to primary care physicians the importance of aggressive management of the modifiable stroke risk factors both by example and by education. Traditional continuing medical education has been ineffective in changing physicians' practice. A multifaceted approach utilizing health prevention facilitators has been shown to be effective in changing family physician practice, although the improvement in performance of 11.5% is still relatively modest[12].

Population-based strategies aimed at identification and treatment of disease by altering lifestyle and behavior have had mixed results. But on a global scale they have much greater potential, especially in the developing world, where non-communicable diseases have become more prevalent, and these nations will not be able to afford many of the drugs that are effective in preventing stroke.

Although much of the risk of stroke remains unexplained (despite the identification of new stroke risk factors) and there is a lack of evidence from clinical trials that some treatment strategies are effective (for example smoking cessation, diabetic control), stroke prevention still has much greater potential for benefit than any acute intervention.

FUTURE PERSPECTIVES

Future stroke prevention initiatives will need to improve the implementation of known effective treatments through such innovations as TIA/stroke prevention clinics, as well as population-based treatments. We need to develop new drugs, or combinations of existing drugs, to treat known stroke risk factors. For example, it is only recently that a clinical trial has clearly shown that blood pressure-lowering after a stroke or TIA reduces the risk of a second event[13]. Similarly, we need to identify novel stroke risk factors, and in turn develop effective treatments for them. Perhaps most promising will be the identification of the genetic factors that predispose the individual to atherosclerosis and stroke – ideally identification of the 'at risk' individual at a pre-disease stage. Aggressive treatment of all risk factors and, in the future, manipulation of the gene(s) could result in prevention of atherosclerosis or at least its clinical manifestations.

Just as stroke physicians have eagerly learned to care for the hyperacute stroke patient, we must just as enthusiastically embrace stroke prevention, both primary and secondary. The potential benefits of prevention are far greater than any known treatment.

References

1. Wolf PA, Clagett GP, Easton JD, *et al.* Preventing ischemic stroke in patients with prior stroke and transient ischemic attack. A statement for healthcare professionals from the Stroke Council of the American Heart Association. *Stroke* 1999;30:1991–4
2. Goldstein LB, Adams R, Becker K, *et al.* Primary prevention of ischemic stroke. A statement for healthcare professionals from the Stroke Council of the American Heart Association. *Circulation* 2001;103:163–82
3. Gorelick PB, Sacco RL, Smith DB, *et al.* Prevention of a first stroke. A review of guidelines and a multidisciplinary consensus statement from the National Stroke Association. *J Am Med Assoc* 1999;281:1112–20
4. Hayward RSA. Clinical practice guidelines on trial. *CMAJ* 1997;156:1725–7
5. Cabana MD, Rand CS, Powe NR, *et al.* Why don't physicians follow clinical practice guidelines? A framework for improvement. *J Am Med Assoc* 1999;282:1458–65
6. Wolf PA, D'Agostino RB, Belanger AJ, *et al.* Probability of stroke: a risk profile from the Framingham Study. *Stroke* 1991;22:312–18
7. Gorelick PB. Stroke prevention: windows of opportunity and failed expectations? *Neuroepidemiology* 1997;16:163–73
8. Hypertension Detection and Follow-Up Program Cooperative Group. Five-year findings of the Hypertension Detection and Follow-up Program. III. Reduction in stroke incidence among persons with high blood pressure. *J Am Med Assoc* 1982;247:633–8
9. The Joint National Committee on Prevention, Detection, Evaluation and Treatment of High Blood Pressure. The sixth report of the Joint National Committee on Prevention, Detection, Evaluation and Treatment of High Blood Pressure. *Arch Intern Med* 1997;157:2413–46
10. Bungard TJ, Ghali WA, Teo KK, *et al.* Why do patients with atrial fibrillation not receive Warfarin? *Arch Intern Med* 2000;160:41–6
11. Bungard TJ, Ghali WA, McAlister FA, *et al.* Physicians' perception of the benefits and risks of Warfarin for patients with nonvalvular atrial fibrillation. *Can Med Assoc J* 2001;165:301–2
12. Lemelin J, Hogg W, Baskerville N. Evidence to action: a tailored multifaceted approach to changing family physician practice patterns and improving prevention care. *Can Med Assoc J* 2001;164:757–63
13. PROGRESS Collaborative Group. Randomised trial of a perindopril-based blood-pressure-lowering regimen among 6105 individuals with previous stroke or transient ischaemic attack. *Lancet* 2001;358:1033–41

Index